DESCRIPTION AND ANALYSIS OF THE VA National Formulary

David Blumenthal and Roger Herdman, Editors

VA Pharmacy Formulary Analysis Committee
Division of Health Care Services
INSTITUTE OF MEDICINE

NATIONAL ACADEMY PRESS
Washington, D.C.

NATIONAL ACADEMY PRESS 2101 Constitution Avenue, N.W. Washington, D.C. 20418

NOTICE: The project that is the subject of this report was approved by the Governing Board of the National Research Council, whose members are drawn from the councils of the National Academy of Sciences, the National Academy of Engineering, and the Institute of Medicine. The members of the committee responsible for the report were chosen for their special competences and with regard for appropriate balance.

Support for this study was provided by the Department of Veterans Affairs (Contract No. V-101-(93)P-1637, Task Order 10). The views presented are those of the Institute of Medicine VA Pharmacy Formulary Analysis Committee and are not necessarily those of the funding organization.

Description and Analysis of the VA National Formulary is available for sale from the National Academy Press, 2101 Constitution Avenue, N.W., Box 285, Washington, DC 20055; call (800) 624-6242 or (202) 334-3313 (in the Washington metropolitan area), or visit the NAP's on-line bookstore at **www.nap.edu.**

The full text of this report is available on line at **www.nap.edu.**

Copyright 2000 by the National Academy of Sciences. All rights reserved.

Printed in the United States of America.

The serpent has been a symbol of long life, healing, and knowledge among almost all cultures and religions since the beginning of recorded history. The image adopted as a logotype by the Institute of Medicine is based on a relief carving from ancient Greece, now held by the Staatliche Musseen in Berlin.

*"Knowing is not enough; we must apply.
Willing is not enough; we must do."*

—Goethe

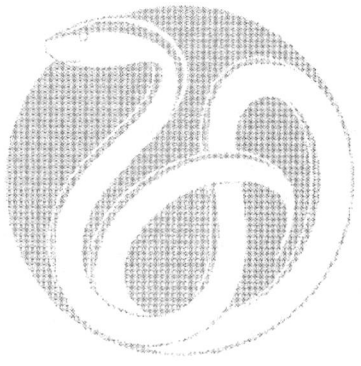

INSTITUTE OF MEDICINE
Shaping the Future for Health

THE NATIONAL ACADEMIES

National Academy of Sciences
National Academy of Engineering
Institute of Medicine
National Research Council

The **National Academy of Sciences** is a private, nonprofit, self-perpetuating society of distinguished scholars engaged in scientific and engineering research, dedicated to the furtherance of science and technology and to their use for the general welfare. Upon the authority of the charter granted to it by the Congress in 1863, the Academy has a mandate that requires it to advise the federal government on scientific and technical matters. Dr. Bruce M. Alberts is president of the National Academy of Sciences.

The **National Academy of Engineering** was established in 1964, under the charter of the National Academy of Sciences, as a parallel organization of outstanding engineers. It is autonomous in its administration and in the selection of its members, sharing with the National Academy of Sciences the responsibility for advising the federal government. The National Academy of Engineering also sponsors engineering programs aimed at meeting national needs, encourages education and research, and recognizes the superior achievements of engineers. Dr. William. A. Wulf is president of the National Academy of Engineering.

The **Institute of Medicine** was established in 1970 by the National Academy of Sciences to secure the services of eminent members of appropriate professions in the examination of policy matters pertaining to the health of the public. The Institute acts under the responsibility given to the National Academy of Sciences by its congressional charter to be an adviser to the federal government and, upon its own initiative, to identify issues of medical care, research, and education. Dr. Kenneth I. Shine is president of the Institute of Medicine.

The **National Research Council** was organized by the National Academy of Sciences in 1916 to associate the broad community of science and technology with the Academy's purposes of furthering knowledge and advising the federal government. Functioning in accordance with general policies determined by the Academy, the Council has become the principal operating agency of both the National Academy of Sciences and the National Academy of Engineering in providing services to the government, the public, and the scientific and engineering communities. The Council is administered jointly by both Academies and the Institute of Medicine. Dr. Bruce M. Alberts and Dr. William. A. Wulf are chairman and vice chairman, respectively, of the National Research Council.

www.national-academies.org

VA PHARMACY FORMULARY ANALYSIS COMMITTEE

DAVID BLUMENTHAL (*Chair*), Director, Institute for Health Policy, Professor of Medicine and Health Care Policy, Harvard Medical School

REINHARDT HENRY BODENBENDER, Director of Medical Services, Paralyzed Veterans of America, Washington, D.C.

J. LYLE BOOTMAN, Professor and Dean, Executive Director, Center for Health Outcomes and PharmacoEconomic Research, University of Arizona College of Pharmacy

JOHN P. BURKE, Professor of Medicine, Chief, Department of Clinical Epidemiology, Latter Day Saints Hospital, Salt Lake City, Utah

ELIZABETH DICHTER, Executive Vice President, PCS Health Systems, Scottsdale, Arizona

THOMAS R. FULDA, Program Director, Drug Utilization Review, U.S. Pharmacopoeia, Rockville, Maryland

MARTHA N. HILL, Professor, Director of the Center for Nursing Research, Johns Hopkins University School of Nursing

JOHN D. JONES, Director of Pharmacy Networks and Legal Affairs, Prescription Solutions, Costa Mesa, California

JAMES JONATHAN LIPSKY, Director of Clinical Pharmacology, Professor of Medicine and Pharmacology, Mayo Clinic and Foundation, Rochester, Minnesota

ALBERT SIU, Professor and Chief of General Internal Medicine, Mount Sinai School of Medicine

FRANK A. SLOAN, Professor of Health Policy and Management, Professor of Economics and Director, Center for Health Policy, Law, and Management, Duke University

RICHARD A. WANNEMACHER, JR., Associate National Legislative Director, Disabled American Veterans (DAV), Washington, D.C.

OTTO F. WOLKE, President of Schellen & Partners USA, Inc., Danville, Pennsylvania

ALLAN ZIMMERMAN, Senior Executive Vice President and General Manager, National Prescription Administrators, East Hanover, New Jersey

Consultants

JEFFREY S. BROWN, Schneider Institute for Health Policy, The Heller School, Brandeis University

ARNOLD M. EPSTEIN, Harvard School of Public Health, Department of Health Policy and Management

RICHARD FRANK, Harvard Medical School, Department of Health Care Policy

HAIDEN A. HUSKAMP, Harvard Medical School, Department of Health Care Policy

IOM Staff

ROGER HERDMAN, Study Director
CHRISTINE COUSSENS, Research Associate
RITA GASKINS, Senior Project Assistant

Preface

Medications have captured the imagination of the American people and the attention of policy makers. New scientific findings have demonstrated the extraordinary power and promise of drugs to prevent and cure disease, relieve suffering, and improve the quality of life for many Americans. Media reports, the World Wide Web, and aggressive advertising by the pharmaceutical industry have kept consumers informed of every advance, large or small, in the development of new medications. Pharmaceuticals have become as vital to good health care as hospital and physician services. Propelled by new, expensive products and consumer demand, national spending on medications is increasing at double-digit rates and may soon rival physician and even inpatient hospital expenditures.

This latter prospect has naturally attracted the interest of policy makers responsible for the publicly funded programs that have become so important to so many Americans. Most Medicaid programs have adopted measures, including formularies, to control the costs of pharmaceuticals. The Medicare program does not cover outpatient drugs, but debate rages over whether it should. If, as seems likely, Medicare does provide pharmaceutical benefits for its 39 million beneficiaries, then programs to control expenditures will be part and parcel of this reform.

As the steward of the nation's largest and most comprehensive publicly owned and managed health care program, the U.S. Department of Veterans Affairs (VA) and its Veterans Health Administration (VHA) are also confronting the opportunities and challenges associated with the national surge in the use and costs of medications. The VHA is the largest single purchaser of pharmaceuticals in the United States. It cares for a population that is disproportionately elderly and ill, including many veterans with service-related disabilities. With pharmaceutical expenditures rising at more than 10% a year, the VHA in 1997 implemented a new National Formulary intended to help control costs and improve the quality of prescribing in the VHA's 172 hospitals, more than 600 ambulatory facilities, 132 nursing homes, and other health care facilities.

The VA National Formulary generated controversy, which motivated congressional scrutiny and a directive to the VA to commission this report reviewing the experience with the National Formulary and formulary system. This Institute of Medicine committee was pleased to assist the Congress with this review, in part because the committee saw in the VHA example an opportunity to understand and anticipate problems that all publicly funded programs are likely to encounter in this new age of pharmaceuticals.

The Congress asked the committee to review the restrictiveness of the National Formulary, its impact on the costs and quality of care in the VHA, and how it compared to formularies and drug management practices in the private sector and in other public programs, especially Medicaid. Detailed in the pages that follow, the committee's findings and conclusions on these questions are, the committee believes, highly instructive, though not always in the ways that we anticipated.

The committee found that formularies and formulary systems (the many policies and procedures necessary to manage implementation of formularies) are an essential part of modern health care systems and that the VHA therefore was justified in creating its National Formulary. Further, we found that the VA National Formulary is not overly restrictive, and the limited available evidence suggests that it has probably meaningfully reduced drug expenditures without demonstrable adverse effects on quality.

This is the good news. The committee also concluded that there are manifold opportunities to improve the management of the formulary system used by the VHA. The National Formulary lacks essential systems to assure that new drugs are expeditiously reviewed for inclusion, that a responsive process for assuring access to medically necessary exceptions to the formulary is consistently in place system-wide, that therapeutic interchange is accomplished in a flexible and consistent way, sensitive to patient risks, across the far-flung VHA system, and that views of critical constituencies of both providers and patients are represented in the management of the National Formulary.

Perhaps most troubling, the committee found a dearth of information to evaluate the full impact of the National Formulary on veterans—their health and satisfaction—and on the VHA. Although the VHA has made efforts to improve quality monitoring generally, no data exist that allow an assessment of the effect of the VA National Formulary on the structure, processes, and outcomes of care received by VHA patients. Committee consultants made valiant efforts to assess quality effects using data on rates of hospitalization for conditions associated with drugs most closely regulated by the National Formulary—those in closed and preferred classes. The committee considers such analyses helpful, but insufficient to reach a satisfactory conclusion on quality effects. Available cost data do not allow a full evaluation of the indirect effects of the VA National Formulary on the use of other health care resources such as other drugs and services. Such effects have been significant in the Medicaid experience and could greatly reduce net savings on drugs themselves. There are also few data on the administrative costs of the National Formulary, including its important but subtle effects on the time health professionals must spend with and for patients in managing changes in medications.

Gaps in the information available for policy making concerning the VA National Formulary are not unique to this system. The committee found a comparable paucity of data on the quality effects of formularies in Medicaid and the private sector. Reliable information on the policies of the fast-changing private companies that manage formularies for private health care plans—so-called pharmacy benefits management companies or PBMs—were also lacking when the committee initiated its review. The committee is indebted to representatives of several PBMs who organized a survey of their companies and supplied valuable new data on their policies and procedures.

Given the rapid pace of policy development with respect to Medicare and other public and private programs, the lack of data to support decision making is disturbing. It is difficult to imagine a modern health care system that does not employ a formulary. It is also difficult to imagine how such formularies can now be effectively designed and managed given our limited understanding of their effects on cost and quality of care and patient and provider satisfaction. The VHA, because of its central control and comprehensive benefits, has a unique opportunity to study its own experience with formularies and formulary systems. The committee strongly urges the Congress and the VHA to take advantage of this opportunity.

The committee's work benefited enormously from the contributions of a dedicated and talented staff. Roger Herdman, its study director, and Christine Coussens, his assistant, accomplished an extraordinary amount of work in a very modest period of time—reviewing the copious literature on the history and current status of formularies, conducting field work to understand the National Formulary and its functioning, designing and supervising the collection of primary data on PBMs, and supervising able contractors. Drs. Herdman and Coussens were invariably rigorous in their review of data and diplomatic in their management of the committee. The committee is also indebted to Haiden Huskamp and Richard Frank, who conducted an excellent analysis of the cost effects of the National Formulary, and to Jeffrey Brown, who expertly reviewed and summarized the Medicaid experience with drug management.

The importance and salience of drug benefits in modern health care systems is more clear than ever from the committee's work. The central role of formularies in providing high-quality and affordable drug coverage is also clear. It will be hard to resolve the inevitable controversies over optimal approaches to manage drug benefits without an urgent national program of research and development on the design of formularies and formulary systems themselves.

David Blumenthal, M.D., M.P.P.
Chair

REVIEWERS

The report was reviewed by individuals chosen for their diverse perspectives and technical expertise in accordance with procedures approved by the National Research Council's Report Review Committee. The purpose of this independent review is to provide candid and critical comments to assist the authors and the Institute of Medicine in making the published report as sound as possible and to ensure that the report meets institutional standards for objectivity, evidence, and responsiveness to the study charge. The contents of the review comments and the draft manuscript remain confidential to protect the integrity of the deliberative process. The committee wishes to thank the following individuals for their participation in the report review process:

Jerome Avorn, Brigham and Women's Hospital, Boston
Enriqueta C. Bond, Burroughs Wellcome Fund, Durham, North Carolina
Christine K. Cassel, Mount Sinai Medical Center, New York City
David H. Kreling, School of Pharmacy, University of Wisconsin
Joseph P. Newhouse, Harvard University
Judith Wagner, Congressional Budget Office, Washington, D.C.
Albert L. Wertheimer, Merck and Co., West Point, Pennsylvania
Mel Worth, Senior Scholar in Residence, Institute of Medicine, Washington, D.C.

While the individuals listed above provided many constructive comments and suggestions, responsibility for the final content of the report rests solely with the authoring committee and the Institute of Medicine.

Contents

EXECUTIVE SUMMARY	1
1 INTRODUCTION	11
Legislative and Executive Branch History	11
History of the IOM Study	12
The IOM Committee	14
Formularies and Formulary Systems: History and Definitions	15
Modern Formularies and Formulary Systems	18
Economic Focus of Formularies	19
Types of Formularies and Their Restrictiveness	19
Formulary Control	21
Generic Substitution	22
Therapeutic Interchange	24
Local VA Facility and VISN Formularies and the National Formulary	27
History of VA Formulary Management Prior to the National Formulary	27
Reorganization of the VA	28
Impact of the VA Fixed Budget	29
Establishing the VA National Formulary	30
Evolution of the National Formulary	31
Medical Staff Input	33

	National Formulary Classes	34
	Formulary Relationship to Pharmaceutical Companies	35
	Report Outline	36
2	**IS THE VA NATIONAL FORMULARY OVERLY RESTRICTIVE AND DOES IT PREVENT PHYSICIANS FROM MEETING THE HEALTH CARE NEEDS OF VETERANS?**	**37**
	Background	37
	Elements of Restrictiveness	38
	Size and Coverage of the National Formulary	40
	Adequacy of the VA National Formulary	42
	Closed and Preferred Drug Classes in the VA	44
	Restrictiveness of Class Closure	46
	Excluded Drugs and Other Limits	48
	National Formulary Effects on Drug Use	49
	Addition of New Drugs and Formulary Reappraisal	50
	National Policy Regarding New Drugs	50
	VISN Addition of New FDA Approvals	51
	Evaluation of the VA Process for Adding New FDA-Approved Priority Drugs	52
	Addition of Existing Drugs by the VA	54
	Additions of Newly Approved or Existing Drugs in Other Health Care Systems	56
	The Nonformulary Process	57
	Therapeutic Interchange	61
	OTC Drug Coverage, Generic Substitution, and Physician Satisfaction	65
	Generic Substitution	66
	Veterans' Complaints	67
	VA Physician Satisfaction	68
	Summary	70
3	**WHAT ARE THE POTENTIAL COSTS TO VA HEALTH CARE ASSOCIATED WITH THE NATIONAL FORMULARY FOR DRUGS?**	**72**
	Introduction	72
	The VHA National Formulary as It Affects Costs	74
	Background	74
	Basic Economics of the VA National Formulary	76
	Features of the National Formulary	77
	VISN Implementation Issues	78
	Other Influences on VHA Pharmaceutical Spending	78
	Analytical Framework	79
	Data	79

Empirical Methods	81
Results of the IOM Committee Analysis of Cost Effects	81
How Have the VHA and the Veteran User Population Changed During the Study Period?	81
How Has the National Formulary Affected Prices for Closed and Preferred Classes?	81
How Has the National Formulary Affected Prescribing Patterns Within the Closed and Preferred Classes?	82
How Has the National Formulary Affected Pharmaceutical Spending Per Veteran User for Closed and Preferred Classes?	100
Is There Evidence That Changes in Formulary Policy Have Resulted in Increased Utilization Elsewhere in the VHA System?	109
Exploration of Changes in Hospital Discharges Per VHA User	109
Costs Associated with Implementing and Managing the National Formulary	113
Estimated National Formulary Savings	114
Conclusions	118

4 WHAT ARE THE EFFECTS OF THE NATIONAL FORMULARY AND RELATED POLICIES ON QUALITY OF CARE?   **120**

Background Information	120
Sources of Quality Data	121
Quality of Care in the VHA and Effects of the National Formulary	122
Pharmacy, Clinical, and Formulary Program Elements Relevant to Quality of Care	123
Clinical Pharmacy	123
P&T Committees	124
The VA PBM Complex	127
Additions to, and Quality of, the National Formulary	130
Policies and Procedures	131
Drug Class Reviews	131
Clinical Guidelines and Drug Utilization Reviews	133
The Nonformulary Process	134
Therapeutic Interchange, Policy, and Results	138
Effects of the National Formulary on Use of Drugs by the VHA	139
Adverse Drug Events	143
Changes in Inpatient Hospital Discharge Associated with the National Formulary	144
Patient Complaints—Advocate, Veterans of Foreign Wars, and Survey Data	145
Physician Complaints and Survey Data	146
Summary Statement	147

5	**HOW DOES THE VA NATIONAL FORMULARY COMPARE WITH PRIVATE INSURANCE FORMULARIES FOR DRUGS AND DEVICES AND WITH OTHER GOVERNMENT FORMULARIES?**	149
	Introduction	149
	Implementation of Drug Management Strategies in Managed Care	151
	Impact of State Legislation on MCO Practice	153
	Public-Sector Programs	155
	Medicaid	155
	Medicaid Fee for Service	155
	Department of Defense	178
	General Comments on Comparisons	182
6	**THE VA NATIONAL FORMULARY AND VETERANS HEALTH CARE**	183
	Introduction	183
	Background and Context	184
	The Veterans Health Administration	185
	Restrictiveness	186
	Costs	189
	Quality	193
	Comparisons	196
	REFERENCES	201
	ACRONYMS	217
	APPENDIXES	
A	Interim Report of the Committee on VA Pharmacy Formulary Analysis to the Department of Veterans Affairs and the Congress of the United States	221
B	Academy of Managed Care Pharmacy's Managed Care Formulary and Pharmacy Benefit Design Survey	227
C	Additional Cost Information	231
D	Glossary	250
E	Drug Classes and Drug Index	254
F	Committee Biographies	259

DESCRIPTION AND ANALYSIS OF THE VA National Formulary

Executive Summary

SUMMARY AND CONCLUSIONS

In 1998, the Congress (House Report 105-610) formally expressed concerns about the Department of Veteran's Affairs (VA) National Formulary. They are as follows:

> Serious concerns have been raised about the impact of the VA's new National Formulary. The Committee has learned that the formulary prevents physicians from meeting the unique health care needs of individual veterans and is overly restrictive. To address these concerns, the Committee directs the VA to contract with the Institute of Medicine to conduct an independent analysis of the effects of the National Formulary on the quality of care.
>
> Specifically, the study should be completed within 6 months and should provide the Committee with an estimate of potential costs to VA health care associated with the National Formulary for drugs, biologic products, devices, prosthetics and pharmaceutical treatment guidelines. The study should also include a comparison of the new VA formulary to private insurance formularies for drugs and devices and other government formularies, such as Medicaid.

This report was prepared by a committee appointed by the Institute of Medicine (IOM) in response to those concerns. The committee consisted of representatives from two veterans service organizations, the Disabled American Veterans and the Paralyzed Veterans of America; health professionals, including physicians and a nurse, experienced in clinical pharmacology or pharmacy and therapeutics activities; and pharmacists and others knowledgeable and experienced in the management and economics of pharmacy benefits. The committee met three times in Washington, D.C., for 5 days in all, and spent considerable additional time reviewing relevant literature, evaluating information from the

VA, and assembling new data to prepare this report. Financial support for this work was provided by the Department of Veterans Affairs.

The VA National Formulary, implemented in 1997, is a list of generic, brand name, and over-the-counter (OTC) drugs, devices, and supplies, that provides the basis for a uniform national entitlement to listed agents for all regions and facilities of the Veterans Health Administration (VHA). It also supports the prudent purchasing of drugs and drug products whose costs to the VHA escalated by almost 20% between FY 1998 and FY 1999. The National Formulary includes 22 separate regional (VISN, Veterans Integrated Service Network) and many local (VA medical center) formularies, which usually have more and different drug and supply listings than the mandatory national list. For the purposes of this report, the term "National Formulary" refers to the national drug list, the regional and local lists, and the "formulary system." Formularies are routine (92.9% or more) in other health care systems, including hospitals, medical centers, managed care organizations, and Medicaid, among others.

The formulary system consists of all the measures that the VHA employs to manage the use of agents on its lists. For example, in the case of the VA, a central directive required the establishment of a nonformulary exceptions process. Such a process entails regional and local procedures for access to drugs and supplies not on the national or other VA formularies. Systemwide drug class reviews are also performed in managing the National Formulary. Drug treatment guidelines are part of the National Formulary as well.

The VA National Formulary is partially closed, that is, some drug classes are closed or subject to restrictions, limiting choice to certain preferred or committed-use agents as a way of supporting VA negotiations for lower drug prices and meeting VHA market share objectives. Generic prescribing, generic substitution, and therapeutic interchange (that is, substitution of a formulary for a non-formulary drug within a drug class) are also employed in managing the formulary system.

In this report, the IOM committee considered pharmaceuticals the primary issue and focused on them, not on devices or supplies. This report and its summary first respond to the congressional questions and resulting VA contract, and then lay out specific and important recommendations for improvement of the National Formulary.

Restrictiveness

Elements of restrictiveness examined in this report include formulary size and quality, coverage of drugs in different classes, timeliness of new drug additions, fairness and responsiveness of the nonformulary exceptions process, and sensitivity of therapeutic interchange policies and procedures, among others. These are central elements in the implementation and management of the National Formulary, and revision of policies and procedures governing them will represent significant changes. VA controls are compared to controls more commonly used in other systems including prior authorization, specific exclusions of drugs or drug classes, and volume or quantity limits. Basic formulary and formulary system limitations of drugs in health care systems are identified. New data on restrictions in private health care formularies and formulary systems were collected for the IOM by the Academy of Managed Care Pharmacy. The VA National Formulary is not as inclusive as many Medicaid formularies, but it rarely designates drugs or drug classes as absolutely excluded or requires prior authorization of drugs as Medicaid and managed care formulary systems frequently do, nor does it impose absolute limits on numbers of prescriptions as some Medicaid formularies have done, or tiered copayments as is often the practice in managed care. *The IOM committee concluded that the VA National Formulary is not overly restrictive. In some respects it is more, but in many respects less, restrictive than other public or private formularies. The committee has identified deficiencies in the implementation and management of the National Formulary and recommended changes.*

Cost

The IOM examined VA aggregate outpatient drug use data by VISN by month for FY 1994 through FY 1999 for six drug classes that had been closed or preferred at some point by the National Formulary (omitting the luteinizing hormone-releasing hormone [LHRH] class for which data were lacking) and for eight other classes that had remained open. Person-level data were not available to support comparisons of spending for inpatients, outpatients, and pharmacy, or analyses of cost shifting and spending in various budgets associated with implementation of the National Formulary. With some gaps, average VA drug purchase price data were available by VISN by month. To arrive at expenditures for each drug, these prices were multiplied by units used. Using other data on total system users, age and other demographic factors, as well as various statistical and analytical techniques, attempts were made, within the limits of the data provided, to control for variables that might distort estimates of VHA pharmacy expenditures. For 2 years before and after implementation of the National Formulary, VA inpatient discharges for diagnoses of conditions likely to be affected by changes in treatment with drugs in closed or preferred classes were examined. The IOM assessment of cost savings associated with the VA National Formulary was limited to six drug classes and was very conservative. A recent, higher VA estimate was based on a longer time and inclusion of a wider scope and number of activities and policies. *The IOM committee found that the VA National Formulary was associated with substantial changes in utilization, prices, and market share of drugs in closed and preferred classes compared to drugs in open classes. Savings in pharmacy expenditures approaching $100 million over the approximately 2-year time span since formulary implementation have probably been realized. This figure is about 15% of the six analyzed drug class expenditures over those 2 years. An exploratory analysis of the distribution of inpatient discharges for illnesses treatable by two closed drug classes did not* reveal an association with National Formulary changes in the status of members of those classes.

Quality

Quality of health care can be assessed by examining the structure, process, and outcomes of delivery of care. The committee reviewed a number of structural elements of the VA National Formulary that might affect quality of care, such as pharmacist programs, VA regional and local pharmacy and therapeutics (P&T) committees, the VA pharmacy benefits management (PBM) group, drug class reviews, and treatment guidelines, among others. The quality of these elements was generally reassuring. Because of inconsistencies across the VA and lack of information, judgments of the quality of other structural elements were not so reassuring. For example, problems, including national inconsistency, inaccurate reporting, and variable implementation, among others, were identified in the nonformulary exceptions and therapeutic interchange programs and in other areas that could affect quality of care.

The IOM committee found almost no data relating the implementation and management of the National Formulary to the quality of the process and outcomes of veterans' care. The National Formulary affects the utilization of drugs in the treatment of veterans, but provides no evidence that would allow an assessment of how utilization changes affect quality. Such data are also scarce in the private sector. The VA has initiated programs to identify quality of outcomes, such as adverse drug events. Electronic prescribing or bar coding systems that contribute to adverse drug event control have also been initiated. These programs are not elements of the National Formulary. As noted in Chapter 3 of this report, the committee did not find changes in the distribution of hospital discharges for illnesses treatable by two of the closed drug classes comparing the 2 years before and after National Formulary implementation. The lack of any increase in hospitalizations for such conditions was somewhat reassuring, although these are crude analyses. The VA does not systematically collect other outcomes data, such as patient satisfaction. The committee found that veterans' complaints about the National Formulary comprised 0.4% of all complaints to the formal patient advocate reporting system, although one independent survey also identified complaints regarding inadequacy of information provided during therapeutic interchanges. *The committee found, based on the scarce quality data available, that there was no reason to abandon the National Formulary. As a national system, the VA also has a responsibility to provide better data on quality issues in drug treatment and formulary operations with carefully designed and implemented health services research.*

Comparisons

Using data from a variety of sources, including a survey of managed care organizations (MCOs) and PBMs carried out by the Academy of Managed Care

Pharmacy, this report compares, somewhat favorably, the VA National Formulary with private-sector and Medicaid formularies and formulary systems. These comparisons are used primarily to assess the restrictiveness and quality of the National Formulary. The task is complicated because there are multiple and highly variable private-sector and Medicaid formularies and because there is variability among VISNs in VA formularies and formulary systems. In Chapter 5, the committee collected and discussed private-sector formularies, formulary systems, and specific formulary lists, although such lists are constantly changing and evolving. In that chapter, data on every state's Medicaid formulary are also discussed. With the understanding that recent legislation will cause changes, the committee briefly compared the Department of Defense (DOD) Basic Core Formulary and formulary systems as well. VA, public-sector, and private-sector formularies variably select from an array of different controls or restrictions. *These comparisons supported the committee's conclusion that the National Formulary is not overly restrictive and that its effects on quality are likely comparable to those of formularies in private and other public-sector programs.*

Recommendations

A. **With respect to VA use of a National Formulary, the IOM committee finds:**

1. **The VA National Formulary and formulary system that enable the VHA to make quality choices among drugs and negotiate favorable prices should be maintained. The National Formulary should continue to close classes prudently and to practice generic substitution and therapeutic interchange of branded drugs to meet its particular quality and price objectives.**

Formularies (scientifically constructed lists of drugs and drug products) and formulary systems (how these lists are managed) are essential and traditional components of the cost and quality management of the pharmacy benefits of modern public and private health care systems. In many ways, the VHA is similar to those health care systems, and the need to prudently manage its pharmacy benefit may be even more urgent than in other systems given the VA's fixed overall budget. Thoughtful use of controls on drug use defines careful management of a formulary. The committee assessed how these controls were employed in the VA and in Medicaid and managed care.

Compared to Medicaid, the VA National Formulary lists fewer drugs in some classes, limits the addition of new drugs, and requires therapeutic interchange. However, the VA does not designate some drugs or drug classes as excluded, require prior approvals, or impose limits on numbers of prescriptions. The restrictions or controls in Medicaid are aimed at limiting the use of expensive drugs or limiting or excluding drugs or classes of drugs that are subject to abuse or prescribed for cosmetic, life-style, or other than significant disease-related indications. Price discounts or rebates are already determined for Medicaid by federal law.

Compared to managed care, the VA National Formulary also often lists fewer drugs in some classes or one drug choice in closed classes and imposes a fixed waiting period for adding new drugs, but it does not require prior approval, charge relatively costly copayments, or exclude categories of drugs or individual drugs. The objectives of restrictions or controls in managed care are similar to those of the VA National Formulary. They are designed to direct prescribing to ward lower-cost or preferred drugs and to drive market share in support of favorable price negotiations. Although the Federal Supply Schedule sets ceiling prices for most brand name drugs for the VA, these prices and the prices for generic and OTC drugs can still be negotiated downward. In settings without the Federal Supply Schedule, and where members make copayments, controls will differ.

Below, the IOM committee recommends improvements in the ways the VA National Formulary is managed.

B. **With respect to managing the VA National Formulary, the IOM committee finds that improvements are necessary:**

1. **The VA National Formulary should examine drugs newly approved by the Food and Drug Administration (FDA) in a timely manner and abandon the blanket policy of a fixed waiting period. Drugs that provide significant improvement in treatment options should be given priority review and serious consideration for the National Formulary based on assessments of merit by physician staffs and review committees.**

   With rare exceptions, VA National Formulary policy requires a wait of 1 year before addition of new FDA-approved drugs. This policy is inconsistent with FDA descriptions of these drugs, especially 1P priority drugs, as significant new therapies. Evidence is lacking that conclusive data will be gathered and published to significantly improve assessment of new drugs within the first year after market entry. The committee could find no clear justification for one federal agency adding a year to the approval process of another federal agency statutorily charged with assessing the safety and efficacy of new drugs. The policies on drug additions in public and private-sector formularies examined by the committee are less restrictive than those of the VA National Formulary.

2. **The balance between standardization and systemwide uniformity and deference to local autonomy and preferences in the VA National Formulary should be recalibrated towards a more uniform national approach before divergence or inconsistencies in the formularies (which sometimes exceed 100 drugs) and formulary systems increase further.**

Formulary differences among VISNs and local facilities and the National Formulary are slowly increasing. VISN and local formulary systems are not obliged to wait before evaluating and adding new FDA-approved drugs to their formularies, and many do not. If many VISNs add a new entry, it makes sense for the national system to give that drug serious consideration. In one case, more than 80% of VISNs added a new FDA-approved drug, which was then rejected for the National Formulary. Additions of drugs already on the market to VISN and local formularies outstrip additions to the National Formulary in diversity and number as well. There are also differences in therapeutic interchange and nonformulary exceptions policies and procedures. Differences among VISNs have implications for equal access to medications by veterans. Provision of equal access and consistent systemwide management must be balanced against local and regional freedom to innovate and responsiveness to local differences in standards of care.

a. **Therapeutic interchange is a necessary element of formulary management and price negotiation, but veterans and their physicians should expect consistency in important practices of interchange among therapeutic alternates and in policies of notification and control. The VA should develop and implement a policy on the frequency and number of interchanges in long-term drug therapy that can result from formulary or contract changes.**

The VHA has no policy on therapeutic interchange, except that it is a local responsibility. Scientific evaluation of the medical appropriateness, implementation, and monitoring of therapeutic interchanges should be an explicit element of drug class reviews. National standards are needed on educating and informing physicians and veterans, and protecting at-risk patients—for example, those who are stable on an existing prescription, are on multiple drugs, have significant comorbidities, or have problems with potentially compromised physiological handling of drugs. System-wide compliance with these standards should be assured. The National Formulary restrictions on a drug may change as may committed-use contracts or blanket purchase agreements that have led to interchanges. Since the VA National Formulary is in its early stages, changes in the drugs with volume commitments have not yet become a problem, but the VA has not evaluated the frequency or number of interchanges that are acceptable in the care of a veteran on long-term drug treatment in such instances. Therapeutic interchange standards should go hand in hand with an improved nonformulary exceptions process.

b. **Improvements in consistency and reporting of the nonformulary process should be made. The VHA should mount pilot tests of nonformulary exceptions processes that increase responsiveness and physician and patient acceptance.**

The nonformulary exceptions process is often informal and unrecorded in VHA national statistics, making it difficult to evaluate the process and to design improvements. Examinations of nonformulary request forms and anecdotal reports suggest that processes for obtaining nonformulary drugs differ across the VHA, as do associated delays and administrative burdens that in some cases may be problematic. A nonformulary exceptions process that is simple, fair, reasonable, and consistently applied could alleviate perceptions of restricted access to drugs, limited additions of new drugs, and dissatisfaction with therapeutic interchange. The focus should be on smooth and timely access, not barriers to needed drugs. The nonformulary process is an integral part of the National Formulary. It has important effects on many elements of the formulary and formulary system. Therefore, it, too, should be a uniform national entitlement. The relevant VHA directive (97-047) is not sufficient assurance of this.

3. **The VHA should improve acceptance of the National Formulary by its stakeholders, including members of the health professions and veterans. Improving acceptance might include representation in formulary discussions above the local P&T committee level, strengthened formulary committee participation by physicians, and a consistent policy of educating veterans about therapeutic interchanges and other formulary matters. Veteran consumers might be involved in input to the VA on the National Formulary, either in some advisory capacity, as is now required for the DOD Uniform Formulary, or as members of P&T or formulary committees.**

The IOM committee examined satisfaction with, or acceptance of, the National Formulary from both the physician and patient perspective. Physician satisfaction with, and participation in, the VA National Formulary and formulary system are not optimal as suggested by surveys and anecdotal data on complaints: 4 of 22 VISN committees have a majority of physicians, 5 VISN formulary committees have proportionately few or, in 1 case (VISN 6), no physicians. VISN committee pharmacist membership averages 52% and physician membership, 44%. The balance on many of these higher-level committees could be perceived to favor pharmacy budget priorities over prescriber views on medical factors in drug treatment.

Veteran complaints about access to drugs are relatively infrequent, amounting to 0.4% or less of all complaints to patient advocates or the Veterans of Foreign Wars. This indicates an apparent tolerance of the formulary system by veterans or suggests that dissatisfaction does not rise to the level of significant representation through the advocate reporting system. Nevertheless, there is evidence from a large multicenter survey of reactions to therapeutic interchange that some veterans do not feel adequately informed about some aspects of the formulary system. The committee notes that the Congress has required formal consumer input to the new DOD Uniform Formulary.

C. **With respect to quality of care, the IOM committee finds the following:**

Recommendations to assure quality are found under other related headings in this section. Although the VHA reports improvements in ensuring and assessing quality of veterans' health care in general, convincing reassurance regarding quality effects of the VA National Formulary requires data relating formulary and formulary system elements to veterans' health outcomes. With rare exceptions, such data are not available for either process or outcomes. On the positive side, the IOM committee did not identify drugs or combination drug products of questionable quality on the national list. The formulary appears to include numbers and varieties of drugs reasonably similar to other private and public-sector formularies. The quality of drag class reviews and guidelines is comparable to that in other systems. The VA has invested in expanded pharmacy programs with patient education and treatment monitoring activities, refleeting similar effective private-sector programs. The VA PBM, Medical Advisory Panel, and VISN Formulary Leaders Committees manage the VA National Formulary through scientifically appropriate drug class reviews and guidelines that focus on the quality of drug treatment for veterans.

D. **With respect to management and quality-of-care information, the IOM committee finds:**

As the manager of a national program, the VHA needs improved information on formulary system functions and their effects to ensure good management of the National Formulary. The VHA should also meet its responsibility to mount studies that illuminate quality implications of the VA National Formulary and formulary system. Congress should support the collection of data to improve National Formulary management and well-designed programs to inform formulary and drug treatment performance, quality, and cost.

Adequate medical data are an important structural guarantee of quality. The management of the National Formulary and formulary system depends on good data concerning system functions. Managers need to know the details of the nonformulary process and various restrictions and their effects. Patient-level drag tracking data can help to assess therapeutic interchanges. These and other reliable data on drug prices, utilization, and offsetting costs can help in assessing budgetary effects of the National Formulary. Deficiencies in data sets such as these were noted by the committee and are discussed in subsequent chapters of this report.

Although the committee appreciates the difficulty and cost of collecting patient care data to make quality assessments and recognizes that programs to do so are infrequent and incomplete in the private sector, improvements in VA data that assess particular programs are needed. Data on adverse drug events or reactions are insufficient to compare the VHA with other large health care systems. Data from drug utilization review (DUR) programs are collected almost exclusively at the local level and do not focus on National Formulary issues. Some promising VISN programs to enforce treatment guidelines have been implemented recently, and VISNs are beginning DURs relating to VISN formulary issues. There are few VHA attempts to design and carry out studies of the effects of therapeutic interchanges in suitably randomized, blinded, and monitored groups of patients in sufficient numbers to achieve statistical significance. An analysis of nonformulary use or an experimental approach to identifying outcomes of denials would be of value beyond the VHA. The need for studies that define this national program was noted elsewhere.

E. **With respect to effects on costs, the IOM committee finds:**

The VHA should continue to make careful choices among drugs, based first on quality considerations but with an understanding of cost implications, and should negotiate the best prices possible using the leverage of committed use and the ability to drive market share. The VHA should collect data to perform analyses addressing the question of offsetting expenditures and cost shifting. Continuation of the VA National Formulary is justified on the basis of cost savings, especially in the absence of data on adverse quality effects.

The closed and other classes with national committed-use contracts account for about 15% or more of the projected $2 billion in VHA drug expenditures in FY 2000, an annual expenditure of $300 million or more. The VA National Formulary and formulary system enable choice and volume commitments among members of restricted classes. This has resulted in 16 to 41% price reductions from manufacturers. The National Formulary and formulary system have been shown to have substantial, statistically significant effects on VA drug use, prices, and market share and to generate notable savings in closed-class outpatient pharmacy expenditures per outpatient veteran user by a conservative analysis.

The VA employs other prudent purchasing practices such as blanket purchase agreements, generic contracts, and bulk purchases. These provide valuable additional economies. At present, the VHA cannot provide cost and utilization data to allow a rigorous exploration of, or any conclusions about, potential off-setting of costs from the pharmacy budget to other VHA health care budgets. The committee performed an analysis of changes in inpatient discharges using available information, but this was not definitive. Absent the National Formulary, the VA would lose the ability to select drugs and negotiate price differentials below the Federal Supply Schedule—differentials that have probably produced aggregate savings approximating $100 million—and VHA drug costs would presumably escalate by this amount leading to equivalent reductions in other VHA services to veterans.

1

Introduction

LEGISLATIVE AND EXECUTIVE BRANCH HISTORY

House Report 105-610 outlined the basis for the Institute of Medicine (IOM) study of the VA National Formulary noting that:

> Serious concerns have been raised about the impact of the VA's new National Formulary. The Committee has learned that the formulary prevents physicians from meeting the unique health care needs of individual veterans and is overly restrictive. To address these concerns, the Committee directs the VA to contract with the Institute of Medicine to conduct an independent analysis of the effects of the National Formulary on the quality of care.
>
> Specifically, the study should be completed within 6 months and should provide the Committee with an estimate of potential costs to VA health care associated with the National Formulary for drugs, biologic products, devices, prosthetics and pharmaceutical treatment guidelines. The study should also include a comparison of the new VA formulary to private insurance formularies for drugs and devices and other government formularies, such as Medicaid.[1]

These four concerns—restrictiveness of the formulary, effect on quality of care, effect on costs, and comparison to other public and private-sector formularies—were expressed in the report that accompanied legislation from the House Committee on Appropriations that provided funding for the Departments of Veterans Affairs and Housing and Urban Development for Fiscal Year (FY) 1999 (Public Law 105-276, approved 10/21/98). House Report 105-610 also directed the Secretary of Veterans Affairs to report separately on the nonformulary waiver process operated by each Veterans Integrated Service Network (VISN, 1 of 22

---

[1] House Report 105-610.

regional VA health care systems comprising the national Veterans Health Administration [VHA]). The Secretary's response, submitted to Congress in February 1999, was based on a December 1998 survey of all 22 VISNs. It described basic features and statistics of the nonformulary waiver process.

The language of House Report 105-610 and of a Senate request to the U.S. General Accounting Office (GAO) (see below) was developed between January and June 1998. In preparation for the FY 1999 appropriations legislation, the House Appropriations Committee and both House and Senate Committees on Veterans Affairs, in hearings and in questions to the Department of Veterans Affairs (VA), identified a number of concerns regarding the National Formulary and the availability of pharmaceuticals to veterans. These dealt with issues such as the selection of drugs for the formulary, access of veterans to needed drugs, the effects of the formulary policy on quality of care to veterans, on costs to the VA health system, and on comparisons with other private or public-sector formulary systems. The VHA submitted detailed responses to the congressional committees' questions. These responses became part of the available record on the VA pharmacy benefit. The charge to the IOM committee on the VA pharmacy formulary analysis reflected the concerns expressed in this record and the House report.

On October 16, 1998, Senator Rockefeller, ranking minority member of the Senate Committee on Veterans Affairs, wrote to the acting Comptroller General formally requesting an examination of the VA National Formulary by the U. S. General Accounting Office. Noting that the language of House Report 105-610 had not been included in the House-Senate conference report, Senator Rockefeller asked the GAO, in addition to the IOM study, to compare the VA National Formulary to formularies of health maintenance organizations and Medicaid, to assess the fairness of the drug selection process and the timeliness and convenience of the nonformulary process, and to investigate whether the VA Medical Advisory Panel (MAP), the VISN formulary committees, and the VA Pharmacy Benefits Management Strategic Healthcare Group (VA PBM) were working together to the best advantage of veterans health care. The GAO initiated this study, structured as a program audit of the VA National Formulary system, in early 1999 and issued its first report on the audit late that year. Completion of the audit is anticipated shortly after release of this IOM report and should provide useful additional information about formulary systems in the VHA (see "VA's Management of Drugs on Its National Formulary," GAO, 1999).

History of the IOM Study

After unsuccessful efforts by VA pharmacy leaders in the fall of 1998 to persuade the House and Senate and VA leadership to consolidate the GAO and IOM assignments into one study (MAP/VISN minutes, Jan. 13, 1999), a draft statement of work for the IOM study was prepared by the VA. In meetings in January 1999 between VA PBM staff and GAO and IOM, the problems of the 6-month timetable for the IOM study and the similarity of the two projects were discussed. Consultation with Congress ultimately resulted in the structuring of the GAO study as a program audit of the National Formulary system, as noted above, and in an extension of the timetable and definition of the IOM study as described below (VA PBM/MAP minutes, Feb. 3, 1999).

A January 26, 1999 VA task order to the IOM outlined a report addressing the four essential questions, that is, restrictiveness, effects on quality of care and costs, and comparison to other formulary systems. The task order stated that VA pharmaceutical costs were experiencing double-digit inflation, that the VHA budget was "straight lined through the fiscal year 2002," and that management of the pharmacy benefit in terms of cost, adverse drug reactions, and clinical outcomes was key to continuing to treat the same or more veterans within the planned budget. (Ultimately, the VHA appropriation was increased for FY 2000). The task order also stipulated that an analysis of the VA system was to consider the nonformulary process a part of pharmacy benefits. The VA formulary system was understood to mean the National Formulary, VISN formularies, VA medical center formularies, and the nonformulary process as well as drug treatment guidelines. The IOM was to work with and have unimpeded access to VA PBM members to obtain relevant data and information in a timely manner. The 6-month timetable was deleted.

The final IOM-VA contract, effective April 12, 1999, included deliverables responding to the following questions and designed to implement the original language of congressional concerns from House Report 105-610[2]:

- "Is the National Formulary overly restrictive and does it prevent physicians from meeting the unique health care needs of veterans?
- What are the potential costs to VA health care associated with the National Formulary for drugs, biological products, devices, prosthetics, and with pharmaceutical treatment guidelines?
- What are the effects of the National Formulary and related policies on quality of care?
- How does the VA National Formulary compare with private insurance formularies for drugs and devices and with other government formularies (e.g., Medicaid)?"

A prepublication report was scheduled for release in the 13th month of the project and a final National Research Council (NRC)–IOM peer-reviewed report by the 15 month. The report was to be book length, address the four defined questions, and include the IOM committee conclusions and recommendations. In a subsequent action, Congress specified July 11, 2000, as the delivery date for this final report (House Report 106-379, Conference Report to accompany H.R. 2684, a bill which became P.L. 106-74, the appropriation for the VA

---

[2] This contract reflects the agreement between the VA and the IOM, resulting in minor differences between its language and the House report language quoted on the first page of this introduction.

[and other agencies]). An interim report at month 6, was to address the issue of how the VA National Formulary compares with private insurance and government formularies. The format of the interim report was left to the IOM committee. The committee decided it should be a short document, which would not require NRC–IOM peer review, accompanied by a detailed briefing. The interim report and briefings were delivered on January 28, 2000, by the IOM committee chairman, Dr. David Blumenthal, to the VA, the Senate and House Committees on Veterans Affairs, and Congressman Frelinghuysen of the House Committee on Appropriations. The interim report is reproduced in Appendix A of this final report.

The IOM Committee

As specified in the IOM plan of action, a committee of 14 members was assembled to carry out the IOM-VA contract. Because of the subject matter of the study, the organization of the VHA, and the demographics of the veteran population, certain disciplinary backgrounds and areas of experience and expertise were sought. Two members with extensive knowledge of, and experience with, the veteran population were selected. They worked for the Disabled American Veterans (DAV) and the Paralyzed Veterans of America (PVA), two veterans service organizations (VSOs) that are particularly suitable because they represent significant numbers of veterans, especially those with service-connected disabilities who are intensive users of, and dependent on, the VHA.

Veterans who use the veterans health care system are disproportionately minorities and more likely to be old, sick, and disadvantaged. The VHA is emphasizing primary and ambulatory care (Fonseca et al., 1996; Hisnanick and Gujral, 1996; Kazis et al., 1998; Kizer, 1999; Wilson and Kizer, 1997). For these reasons, committee members with expertise in clinical medicine and nursing who had backgrounds in geriatrics and general medicine and experience in caring for minority populations were appointed. Among these members were directors of major academic units or departments of clinical epidemiology, clinical pharmacology, general medicine, nursing research, and health care policy. Some of these experts were also leaders of their institutional or managed care organization pharmacy and therapeutics (P&T) committees.

Some members of the IOM committee were selected because of experience working in managed care organizations (MCOs) with formularies and pharmacy benefit plans. Their experience was especially relevant to understanding VISNs, which are essentially regional veterans MCOs, and to comparing the National Formulary with private-sector formularies. Committee members from national pharmacy benefits management (PBMs) organizations were appointed for similar reasons. With the help of these individuals, the IOM identified elements of restrictiveness for a national survey carried out in early 2000 by the Academy of Managed Care Pharmacy.

Several members of the committee were senior members of the U.S. academic or commercial pharmacy community with wide experience in P&T committees and the profession of pharmacy, at both the practicing and the leadership levels. The IOM committee also included a member with national Medicaid drug benefit and drag utilization review (DUR) experience and current experience with private-sector DUR and drug standards at the U.S. Pharmacopoeia, as well as a senior health economist and professor of health policy and management.

The IOM contractual agreement with the VA authorized a subcontract to assist the committee in assessing the effect of the VA formulary system on costs, one of the major deliverables of the project. The IOM determined that the Department of Health Care Policy of Harvard Medical School had the necessary expertise and experience to carry out this work. Two health economist members of the department, with support from other departmental staff, became official consultants to the IOM and submitted an analysis of the National Formulary's impact on health care costs. The agreement also provided support for a paper on formularies used by MCOs and Medicaid to assist the committee in comparing the VA National Formulary with formularies in these other systems, another major deliverable of this project. The IOM decided that this task should be carried out by an experienced Ph.D. graduate student from Brandeis University studying in this area. He also became an official consultant to the IOM.

The IOM committee met three times to review information, identify and discuss issues, and review drafts of the interim and final reports. These meetings consumed a day and a half each time—September 30 and October 1, 1999, December 13 and 14, 1999, and March 8 and 9, 2000. At the first meeting, the committee was briefed on the National Formulary system by the VA PBM staff and representatives of the VHA MAP and by GAO staff responsible for its program audit of the VA National Formulary. A member of the IOM committee and IOM staff attended an August 1999 meeting of the VA MAP and PBM in Chicago and reported back to the committee. The committee also spent additional days reading the medical and pharmacy literature; assimilating data from the consultants, the VHA, the VA National Formulary, and other systems; and preparing this report. The committee enjoyed good cooperation and responsiveness in the provision of data from the VA PBM, both from the central office in Washington, D.C., and from the operational VA PBM headquarters located outside Chicago. Members of the MAP and other individual staff from VA facilities around the United States also contributed much useful information. Where data that could have allowed better analysis, or firmer, more extensive conclusions were not available or were incomplete, this is noted in the relevant chapters of this report.

FORMULARIES AND FORMULARY SYSTEMS: HISTORY AND DEFINITIONS

Traditionally, formularies were lists of remedies and their formulas (Weintraub, 1978), that is, books containing medicinal substances with specific formulas for converting raw materials into finished dosage forms, especially for individual consumption (Rucker, 1988). A Sumerian tablet discovered in Nippur, dating to about 3000 B.C., is the oldest known example of a formulary (Sonne decker, 1972). European examples date from Florence in 1498. Many early formularies were called pharmacopoeias (literally, a book to make remedies). The term had not yet taken on its present meaning of a compendium of drug standards for purity and strength. The first formularies in the United States were issued in the eighteenth century. These included the *Lititz Pharmacopoeia* (1778) used by the American continental army's military hospitals and *Coste's Compendium Pharmaceuticum* (1780) used by the French forces supporting the American Revolution. These were followed by the *Pharmacopoeia of the Massachusetts Medical Society* (1808), *Seamans Pharmacopoeia Chirurgica* for the New York Hospital (1811), listing 145 agents; the *Pharmacopoeia of the New York Hospital* (1816), which for the first time attempted to incorporate the opinions of the medical staff and listed 430 items; and the *Pharmacopoeia of the United States* (USP) (1820), listing 217 drugs, primarily from the Massachusetts formulary. In the ensuing years, hospitals and localities continued to issue formularies or phamacopoeias—for example, Bellevue Hospital (1868), the cities of New York and Brooklyn, the State of Kentucky, the Commonwealth of Pennsylvania (the late 1800s), German Hospital (1902), Syracuse University Hospital (1925), and the USP convention about every 10 years after 1820. The Syracuse University Hospital formulary was notable in that it involved a formulary system in which 45 physicians and 1 pharmacist established a scientific basis for drug control and elimination of duplication in a drug therapy program (Dillon, 1999).

From the seventeenth through the nineteenth centuries, crude preparations (e.g., decoctions, extracts, and infusions) of natural substances, called galenicals, were removed from formularies. Beginning in the late nineteenth century, purification and standardization of the potency of active ingredients began to be represented in formularies as a result of improved chemical manufacturing and the introduction of pharmacology as a medical school discipline in the 1890s. The *Formulary and Therapeutic Guide of the New York Hospital* (1933) included selection and regulation of drugs for a facility and preferential generic nomenclature. Secret remedies, drugs differing only in name, and exaggerated claims were eliminated, and the formulary was used as a tool for improving the economics of drug prescribing and use in the hospital, as reported by Hatcher and Stainsby (1933). At about that time, the American College of Surgeons (1936) adopted and issued the first "Minimum Standard for Pharmacies in Hospitals" by Western Reserve pharmacists Spease and Porter. The American Society of Hospital (now Health-System) Pharmacists (ASHP), the American Pharmaceutical Association (APhA), the American Medical Association (AMA), the American Hospital Association (AHA), and others issued standards and policy statements beginning in 1959. In that year, the ASHP also published the American Hospital Formulary Service, a loose-leaf binder containing clinical, technical, and dosing information to serve as a reference on all drugs for pharmacists and other heath care professionals. Other standards and policy statements have followed at intervals (see American College of Physicians [ACP], 1990; AHA, 1974, 1975, 1999; AMA, 1994; ASHP, 1981, 1983, 1988; ASHP et al., 1964; Francke, 1967; Hoffman, 1984; King, 1987; Sonnedecker, 1972, 1976; Wein traub, 1978). These statements supported formularies in principle, but also staked out the prerogatives and responsibilities of the several issuing professional organizations.

Advances in the science of medicine and pharmacology allowed improvements in the quality of formularies (Rucker, 1982, 1986; Rucker and Visconti, 1978). Coincident with this evolution, the Veterans Administration implemented formularies in its hospitals and considered systemwide standardization of some pharmaceuticals by the 1950s (VA M-2, Professional Service, 1955). In the 1950s, the Joint Commission on Accreditation of Hospitals (then JCAH; as of 1987, Joint Commission on Accreditation of Healthcare Organizations [JCAHO]) encouraged hospitals to form P&T committees and establish formularies (Goldberg, 1997). The JCAH and the Medicare program made guidance of drug use by P&T committees a requirement for U.S. hospitals in 1965 and 1966. In 1986, Medicare Conditions of Participation explicitly required formularies for hospitals wishing to participate in Medicare (and Medicaid) (Liang et al., 1987). By the 1970s, 60% of large, mostly academic hospitals (Rucker and Visconti, 1978), and 82% of Medicare-approved community hospitals (Rolands and Williams, 1975) had formularies. Continued surveys documented this growing use over the next several decades (Rascati, 1992; 96.2% of 130 community hospitals).

In the 1970s also, formularies began to be applied beyond the confines of the inpatient hospital sector in significant numbers. Initially, these formularies in staff or group model HMOs were similar to hospital formularies in control and standardization of drugs. They reflected staff and P&T committee views on drug use. Many states operated formularies of several different types in managing their Medicaid programs, with varying success (Meyer et al., 1974; National Pharmaceutical Council [NPC], 1973). Particularly after the stimulus of the federal HMO Act of 1973 (42 USC, 300 et seq.), which supported HMOs, new forms of MCOs such as independent practice association (IPAs) and network models, were developed, and many of these, including some very large managed care health systems, began to use formularies to control their inpatient and outpatient pharmacy benefits (Dillon, 1999). This trend continued during the 1980s and 1990s. Use of formularies by HMOs to help manage drug benefits grew from 39% in 1989 to 67% in 1992, to 80.6% in 1994, and to 92.9% in 1997.

These trends led to considerable state (Herstek, 1999; and see Chapter 5 of this IOM report) and federal (Omnibus Budget Reconciliation Act [OBRA], 1990, 1993) legislative activity to require public disclosure and limit formulary restrictions among other things. Over the same period, a number of foreign countries, including Germany, Canada, and Australia, established national or regional formularies—some limiting the numbers of drugs, others enforcing the formulary with differing levels of strictness. This brief history traces the steps in the development of formularies from their original status as lists of formulas for medications to their much more complex current forms and purposes. Facility,

TABLE 1.1 Potential Advantages and Disadvantages of a Formulary System

Advantages	Disadvantages
• Educates physicians and patients about drugs • Can reduce adverse drug events • Can enhance cost-effective prescribing • Can increase quality of care through evidence-based management of disease • Can assure use of quality drug products	• Administrative burden and inconvenience to participants • May not be an effective drug list for 100% of the population served • Can decrease quality of care by denying access to needed medications • May cause unwanted or unexpected outcomes due to discontinuation of drug therapy

health system, local, or national formularies are not new inventions. They have an extensive history in the United States and elsewhere.

Modern Formularies and Formulary Systems

A modern formulary is a continually revised compilation of pharmaceuticals that meet pharmacopoeial standards. The IOM committee decided to start with this simple definition of a formulary and then, in defining and describing a formulary system, to identify the elements that a system might employ in managing a formulary to achieve policy objectives. As a practical matter, most modern hospital settings use formularies and formulary systems. Historically, formularies have served ancient societies, city states, and other political jurisdictions, the American revolutionary army, and professional groups, among others. Today, formularies and formulary systems affect most of the 76.6 million Americans enrolled in HMOs and the more than 230 million covered by PBMs and other drug management systems (Cook et al., 2000; Novartis, 1998, 1999). They should be considered, then, as operational components of organized health care delivery systems. As care is increasingly managed and more attention is paid to quality and cost, formularies and evolving formulary systems have played important roles in the pharmacy benefits of delivery systems, whether they are hospitals, clinics, HMOs, PBMs, or others (ASHP, 1988). The committee recognizes both the benefits and the risks of implementation of a formulary and formulary system (see Table 1.1). Any formulary requires careful implementation to maximize the benefits while minimizing the risks.

A formulary system is a method whereby the medical management or administration of an organization, working through a P&T committee or an equivalent group (or groups) of physician and pharmacy experts, objectively evaluates, appraises, and selects from among numerous available drug entities and drug products, those that are considered most useful in patient care. The pharmaceutical products, listed with nonproprietary and proprietary names, are those that are preferred for use or, in some cases (for example, in health plans), for coverage or reimbursement (AHA, 1974; Nash et al., 1993). Involved, knowledgeable physicians make clinical decisions and, together with system managers, may provide information on procedures, safety, and efficacy and systematic drug evaluations based on contemporary treatment guidelines and pharmacoeconomic principles. These are the critical elements of a formulary system that define its function as a standard of care for drug therapy. Simply stated, the P&T committee should select items for the formulary based on an objective evaluation of their relative therapeutic merits, safety, and cost, minimizing duplication of the same basic drug type, drug entity, or drug product (ASHP, 1992).

Economic Focus of Formularies

Prescription drug costs outpaced the growth in overall health care costs in the 1990s (Levit et al., 1999). Although estimates may vary, they all show an increase in trends for drug costs. According to data provided by the Health Care Financing Administration (HCFA), drug expenditures increased by 9% in 1994– 1995, while total health care costs increased only 5.3%. In 1997, total health care costs increased 4.8%, but prescription drug costs rose 14% (Iglehart, 1999). Total prescription drug retail sales for 1999 are estimated at $121.6 billion for 2.97 billion prescriptions, 18% higher than in 1998 (www.nacds.org/news/ releases/ nr_082999_projections.html). As noted elsewhere, VHA drug expenditures have experienced double-digit annual increases in recent years. Disproportionate increases in drug expenditures reflect increases in drug utilization and higher prices of newer drugs. Reacting to these trends, more and more formulary systems are performing economic analyses (Glennie, 1993; Mannebach et al., 1999; Roberts and Summerfield, 1986; Segal and Pathak, 1988). Compared with more traditional formulary systems, recent systems emphasize the economic efficiency of different drugs and include disease management as well as drug selection strategies. These revised formulary systems typically include integrated drug utilization review, nonformulary exceptions procedures, and the use of treatment guidelines to assist in containing costs.

Types of Formularies and Their Restrictiveness

As noted above, almost all organized health care settings or systems use formularies to serve various objectives,—quality drug treatment, cost control, drug price negotiation, among others. Formularies differ, therefore, but fundamentally they are lists of drugs that may be "open,"—that is, they contain many drugs and drug products, and those that are not listed are generally available and reimbursed,— or "closed" (in whole or in part),—that is, they contain fewer drugs and drug products, and those that are not listed are generally not available nor reimbursed. Management of access to, and reimbursement of, drugs is more pervasive in closed formularies. Elements of restrictiveness, controls, or other modifications comprise the formulary system that is employed in the management of access and reimbursement to achieve the objectives for the pharmacy benefit of a health care system. These elements can include, for example, genetic substitution, therapeutic interchange, tiered copayments, and preferred or excluded drugs, among others. Some pharmacy benefit controls, such as limits on number, value, or frequency of prescriptions, are also elements of restrictiveness used in parallel to a formulary and are considered relevant to the question of restrictiveness raised by the Congress and the VA. In the remainder of this section, the committee expands this basic description and provides further details on formularies, formulary systems, and relevant controls.

Open formularies may include a great variety of drugs and drug products, and not place limits on, or require clinical justification of, drugs that are approved, prescribed, or stocked. They generally do not require generic substitution or therapeutic interchange.[3] Coverage, approval, and reimbursement of drugs and drug products are explicit for entities listed and generally assumed for those not listed. In some cases, an open formulary is termed "intermediate" or "mixed" if it allows or encourages generic substitution. In other cases, some drugs or drug products listed in the formulary are promoted as "preferred" to prescribers (sometimes called an "incentivized" or "managed" formulary when preferred products are promoted by economic rewards for the payer). In some circumstances, certain drugs are available only after a trial of another drug, a step protocol (Goldberg, 1997; Kreling et al., 1996; Nash et al., 1993).

Current formularies are often closed; that is, the drugs and drug products listed are limited, and entities that are not listed are not covered, approved for use, or reimbursable except through a prior authorization, nonformulary exceptions, or waiver process. Drugs require clinical justification for inclusion in such a formulary, and generic substitution and therapeutic interchange of formulary for nonformulary drugs are encouraged or required. The smaller number of drugs and drug products in such formularies (generally from 300 to 1,000 drug dosage forms [Goldberg, 1997]) means limitations on the number of drugs in therapeutic classes. If a formulary is partially closed, it is restricted in one or more ways for some drugs and drug products and open for others.

Closed or partially closed formulary systems employ a variety of management features. Only a few representatives from one or more therapeutic classes

---

[3] Generic substitution is the exchange of drug products that have the same, chemically identical, active ingredient(s) and are identical in strength, concentration, dosage form, and route of administration to the drug prescribed. Therapeutic interchange is the authorized exchange of various therapeutic alternates by pharmacists under arrangements between pharmacists and authorized prescribers who have previously established written guidelines or protocols within a formulary system. Therapeutic alternates are drug products of different chemical structures that are of the same pharmacologic or therapeutic class and can be expected to have similar therapeutic effects and safety profiles. See later sections of this chapter for details.

may be selected, and the remainder of the class members excluded. One or more entire therapeutic classes may be eliminated in rare instances. Some classes may be allowed only with prior authorization or use of a step protocol (occasionally also referred to as a "managed" formulary). Drugs may be accepted on a restricted and temporary basis to allow their evaluation. Only one brand of dual licensed products may be approved for use. Potentially toxic or expensive drugs or drugs for specific indications may be restricted to prescribers with special experience or expertise, to particular settings (specialty services or inpatient care), or to use in relevant diagnoses or stages of disease for which the drug is approved and clinically indicated. These latter evidence-based restrictions can improve patient care and educate prescribers. Evidence-based restrictions can also promote cost-effective use of certain drugs in some classes, when clinically appropriate. Limits may be set on the number of prescriptions, quantity of drug, or day's supply per prescription, or caps may be enforced on dollar value, quantities, and the like. These latter restrictions are often considered benefit controls.

Generic substitution and therapeutic interchange are tools used within a formulary system to gain enhanced compliance with formulary or preferred formulary products. A nonformulary process of some type is also considered essential to allow products that are not on the formulary to be dispensed and reimbursed. Formularies may be either positive—drugs and drug products are explicitly listed for coverage or approved for use or reimbursement—or negative—drugs are specifically identified for exclusion, which is often the case in Medicaid (Goldberg, 1997; Lyles et al., 1997; NPC, 1998; Rucker, 1999; Shepard and Salzman, 1994). Drugs or drug classes that are specifically designated as excluded in a formulary (for example, cosmetic, life-style, or contraceptive drugs) are not covered or dispensed through that formulary—that is, not only are they nonformulary, but they are not available through any drug exceptions process. They must be purchased at retail, out-of-pocket expense by the patient.

Formulary Control

Pharmacy and therapeutics committees are responsible for formularies and formulary systems in most organized delivery systems. P&T committees began in the 1930s, reportedly at Western Reserve University (Weintraub, 1978). Their role in evaluating drugs for inclusion in hospital formularies was described in 1959 by the AHA and ASHP (Summers and Szeinbach, 1993). They took on important regulatory and legal status in 1965 when they were required by the JCAH for hospital accreditation. Thereafter, the Medicare program ruled that only those inpatient drugs in official compendiums or approved by a P&T committee would be reimbursed (Weintraub, 1978). Medical, hospital, and pharmacy professional groups and organizations have described policies for the structure and function of P&T committees (ASHP, 1992).

A P&T committee is recognized as an advisory committee to the medical staff that represents the official line of communications and liaison between the medical staff and the pharmacy department. It is typically composed of an organization's physicians, pharmacists (who tend to be the most influential on drug matters [Ascione et al., 1998]), and additional members of the health professions such as nurses, administrators, quality assurance coordinators, and others as appropriate. A physician usually is the chair of the committee. A pharmacist acts as secretary (ASHP et al., 1992). Among other things, the P&T committee must evaluate the medical usefulness and cost of pharmaceuticals and recommend for the formulary those which are most useful and cost-effective in patient care (AMA, 1997; ASHP, 1964). The committee may develop policies and procedures on therapeutics and pharmacy services. It may also play an educational role within its organization. Some organizations appoint outside physicians to their P&T committees, although concerns about the independence of these professionals have been expressed. Formularies developed with little input from practicing professionals may not be effective. Acceptance, and therefore effectiveness, of formulary systems may be jeopardized if P&T committees are perceived not to represent an organization's staff of prescribing physicians (AMA, 1997; Carroll, 1999).

In the academic hospital sector, P&T committees preside over formularies that usually are closed and practice generic substitution (Mannebach et al., 1999). Therapeutic interchange with the prior consent of the authorized prescriber is common also (55%) (Ascione et al., 1998; Nash et al., 1993). The same is true in the managed care sector. Of the plans surveyed in 1997, almost all (92.9%) used formularies: 38.1% were closed, 34.1% were partially closed, 63% required generic substitution, and 35.2–56.5% allowed therapeutic interchange (Gold et al., 1989; Hoechst Marion Roussel, 1998; Kreling and Mucha, 1990; Novartis, 1998). The 1998 figures from Novartis (1999) were 26.9% closed and 45.4% partially closed, figures that vary by the year and by the cohort of MCOs surveyed. These P&T committees are important in evaluating and promoting drug efficacy and cost-effectiveness, monitoring safety, and providing for an appropriate nonformulary process (American Association of Health Plans [AAHP], 1998; AMA, 1997; American Society of Health-System Pharmacists [ASHP] et al., 1964; ASHP et al., 1991; Hanson et al., 1992; Hazlet and Hu, 1992; Shea et al., 1998). As the primary medical advisor, the P&T committee plays a lead role in clinical decisions and works with other managers to structure and implement the elements that a formulary system may employ to realize pharmacy benefits and health system objectives (ASHP, 1998). The P&T committee, chaired by a physician and representing the medical staff, is an important element in the legal authorization of formulary system actions that could affect clinical care, such as therapeutic interchange (Liang et al., 1988).

GENERIC SUBSTITUTION

Pharmaceutical equivalents are defined as drug products that have the same active ingredient(s) in the same dosage form, route of administration, and strength or concentration (FDA, 1999a). However, pharmaceutical equivalents may not always have the same therapeutic effect or safety profile. Other factors, such as compounding technology, bioavailability, and patient acceptance or compliance, may be important. Potential problems with substitution of nonproprietary or generic versions of "innovator," "pioneer," or "brand name" products among themselves or for the branded, proprietary product were reviewed by Strom (1987). Advances in pharmacological science, changes in federal and state law, and issuance of therapeutic equivalence evaluations by the Food and Drug Administration (1999a), however, have made the practice of genetic substitution routine in public and private-sector formulary systems (Kreling et al., 1996). Reasons for the increased availability of generic drug products and the greater acceptance of generic substitution were described by Nightingale and Morrison (1987).

> **Generic Substitution:** The substitution of drug products that contain the same, chemically identical active ingredient(s) and are identical in strength, concentration, dosage form, and route of administration to the drug product prescribed.

Occasionally, P&T committees conclude that a brand name product and its generic pharmaceutical equivalents may not have reliably similar clinical effects even though they are approved for genetic substitution and listed as therapeutically equivalent by the FDA (1999a). The VA National Formulary identifies several such instances (carbamazepine, digoxin, phenytoin, warfarin). These and a few others have achieved some currency (Covington and Thornton, 1995; Spencer and Crouse, 1999), but the FDA does not agree that there are such problems with generics (see www.fda.gov/CDER/news/ntiletter.htm). Some of these drugs, for example, warfarin, were reviewed by the VA PBM recently and changes made as described in Chapter 3 of this report. Some pharmaceutically equivalent generic drug products may be known not to have the same therapeutic effect. The VA National Formulary includes such an instance (disulfiram). In general, however, academic hospital and other private-sector MCO and PBM formularies identify drugs by their nonproprietary as well as their proprietary names. They require genetic dispensing or provide economic disincentives to the use of more expensive branded products when suitable therapeutically equivalent generic products are available from the FDA list (AAHP, 1998; Hoechst Marion Roussel, 1998; Kreling et al., 1996; Nash et al., 1993; Novartis, 1998, 1999; Sax and Emigh, 1999).

If generic drugs are almost universally less expensive than their brand name counterparts (see Figure 2.6), and if they have the same therapeutic effect, they represent more cost-effective drug choices. As a result, genetics currently comprise about 47% of national prescription drug volume and about 8% of dollar sales (Barents Group LLC, 1999a). The policy of generic dispensing is more effective than would appear from this percentage, given that only about half of drugs in the market have genetic equivalents. Experience with genetic substitution provides reassurance that safe and effective clinical care can be obtained with suitable therapeutically equivalent genetic drug products. Laws and regulations that recognize this in one way or another have been enacted in virtually every state. The 1984 federal Drug Price Competition and Patent Term Restoration

Act required the FDA to publish and update periodically its evaluations of generic drugs (in the "Orange Book"), although the agency had first issued its final version of the list of approved drugs with their therapeutic equivalence determinations in 1980 (FDA 1999a; 44 *Federal Register* [FR] 2932; 45 FR 72582). In general, these evaluations are categorized as: either single source drugs considered to have the same therapeutic effects as other pharmaceutically equivalent products because there are no known or suspected bioequivalence problems (for example, designated AA, AN, AO, AP, or AT, depending on dosage form); or because actual or potential bioequivalence problems have been resolved with adequate *in vivo* or *in vitro* evidence (for example, designated AB); or as single source drugs that are not considered to have the same therapeutic effects as other pharmaceutically equivalent products (for example, designated BC, BD, BE, BN, BP, BR, BS, BT, BX, or B*, depending on dosage forms, status of review, among others) (FDA, 1999a). The FDA has recently reconfirmed the reliability of generic substitution of its designated equivalent drugs in all therapeutic drug classes, including drugs or classes with narrow therapeutic indices or ratios (that is, with toxic and effective doses that are close together, as defined in 21 CFR 320.33[c]). Generic substitution should no longer be controversial; it should require additional tests or precautions only with very rare exceptions, and it is reliable for all classes of drugs when they are approved for bioequivalence by the FDA (FDA, 1998; Nightingale, 1998; www.fda.gov/CDER/news/ntiletter.htm). The Congressional Budget Office (1998) estimated that generic substitution saved $8 billion to $10 billion on retail pharmacy drug purchases in 1994.

THERAPEUTIC INTERCHANGE

Therapeutic interchange involves substitution of therapeutic alternates, that is, replacing a patient's drug that is not on the formulary with one that is, in order to gain increased compliance with the formulary and its objectives. Therapeutic interchange can be an important part of formulary systems. It is at the core of many of the criticisms of hospital and health plan formu laries and formulary systems. A number of terms that can be con fusing are used in describing therapeutic interchange. In the simplest terms, therapeutic interchange is the exchange of therapeutic alternates to achieve an equivalent drug treatment effect, or therapeutic equivalence. The relevant terms are defined and discussed further below.

> **Therapeutic Alternates:** Drug products of different chemical structure but the same pharmacological or therapeutic class.
> **Therapeutic Equivalents:** drugs containing the same active ingredient and expected to have the same clinical effects.

Therapeutic alternates are drug products (as a practical matter, generally brand name drugs) with different chemical structures that are of the same pharmacological or therapeutic class. This means that, as members of the same drug class, they share similar structures, mechanisms of action, and indications for use (McAllister et al., 1999), and they can be expected to have similar therapeutic effects and safety profiles when administered to patients in therapeutically equivalent doses. They do not contain the same, chemically identical, active ingredient(s), that is, they are not pharmaceutical equivalents (AMA, 1997), as that term is defined in the previous section on generic substitution in this report.

Some commentaries on therapeutic interchange policies (American College of Clinical Pharmacy [ACCP], 1993; ASHP, 1998) refer to therapeutic alternates as therapeutic equivalents or use the term therapeutic equivalence in discussing both therapeutic interchange and generic substitution. The committee does not use the term "therapeutic equivalents" because this term is officially defined by the FDA (1999a) as meaning the same as "pharmaceutical equivalents" or genetic drugs that can be expected to have the same clinical effects and safety profile when administered to patients as specified in the labeling. To eliminate any possible confusion, the committee decided to accept this definition and refer to drugs with different chemical structures that are exchanged in therapeutic interchanges only as therapeutic alternates.

In developing its evaluations of equivalence in generic substitution, the FDA uses "therapeutic equivalence" to describe the clinical effects of interchange of pharmaceutical equivalents, that is, generic substitution, not the exchange of therapeutic alternates, that is therapeutic interchange (FDA, 1999a). In common usage, however, most people understand therapeutic equivalence to mean any drugs having the same clinical or therapeutic effects or properties. To avoid confusion, the committee decided in this case that it would be clearer not to use the FDA terminology and to use the term "therapeutic equivalence" in this broader, more inclusive way throughout this report.

Some policy statements differentiate between therapeutic interchange and therapeutic substitution. They define the former as the exchange of therapeutic alternates with the permission of the prescriber at the time of interchange, and the latter as exchange according to a previously established policy approved by a P&T committee and some, but perhaps not all, prescribers (Spencer and Crouse, 1999). Exchange without the approval of the prescriber is opposed by organized medicine (ACP, 1990; AMA, 1997), and it is not a common practice in formulary systems. In practice, exchange is often accepted in a tightly organized system where close patient monitoring is possible and likely, such as a hospital or staff model HMO. In these systems, all prescribers and the P&T committee are involved and have agreed to specific interchanges with the provision of an override mechanism. As implemented in less cohesive delivery systems, for example, IPAs, PBMs, or outpatient settings, exchange with specific prescriber permission at the time of dispensing is not opposed by organized medicine or other professional groups. In these less controlled settings, patient monitoring is looser, and P&T committees may be perceived as less representative of a diverse group of physicians. This results in less acceptance of interchange that is authorized by protocol or a P&T committee (ACCP, 1993; Academy of Managed Care Pharmacy [AMCP], 1997; ASHP, 1982, 1998; Carroll, 1999; Zellmer, 1993). Of course, from the perspective of patients, therapeutic interchange is sometimes involuntary and sometimes a concern.

Because VA data do not always allow certainty about the details of prescriber approval, the committee decided it would be simpler and less confusing to use the term therapeutic interchange only. Details of the interchange could be given when known or relevant. In the committee's view, therapeutic interchange usually means that specific prescriber approval exists before dispensing except in settings where exchange according to a collaborative practice agreement or a preapproved policy and protocol is practical and has been accepted by prescribers. Therapeutic interchange is allowed or encouraged by one-third to one-half of HMOs and PBMs, by the VA formulary system, and by most hospitals' formulary systems. Drug class reviews based on sound scientific data and analysis are generally carried out to support therapeutic interchange among therapeutic alternates in a drug class. The provision of a nonformulary exceptions process is the rule in formularies that are closed or partially closed and allow therapeutic interchange (Hoechst Marion Roussel, 1998; Kreling et al., 1996; VHA Directive 97-047). A smoothly functioning nonformulary exceptions process assists implementation of clinically appropriate exceptions to interchange, as noted below.

Although drugs in a therapeutic class share similar pharmacological and therapeutic properties, they are not identical, and their differences may cause problems when they are interchanged across a large group of patients, some of whom will inevitably have differing physiological and pathophysiological status. Differences may involve, for example, mode and extent of action, adverse effects, and potential interactions with other drugs (ACP, 1990; McAllister et al., 1999). An approved practice of therapeutic interchange can be supported in a number of ways. Education of physicians and patients and adequate advance notice with information and advice on relative dosing should be provided. Careful attention to potential effects on patient compliance is also useful. Adequate provisions for exceptions to conversion, nonformulary access to an alternative, or return to an original drug product, if indicated, are important. Follow-up to identify dosage problems, adverse drug events (ADEs), and other clinical results should be part of the program. Particular attention should be paid to those who are already stable on an original agent or taking multiple agents and those whose physiologic status is compromised. As noted, patient monitoring may be better on an inpatient service. Heightened attention to these considerations may be desirable in ambulatory care settings. Quality and cost considerations may not be significant enough in a number of drug classes to justify potential problems or the dissatisfaction of prescribers. For this reason, monitoring of true savings from interchange has been suggested (ACP in Zoeller, 1991; Carroll, 1999). Therapeutic interchange may be most effective, or cost-effective, when limited to classes having little pharmacological diversity among members, those having substantial diversity in price, or preferably both (ACP, 1990).

LOCAL VA FACILITY AND VISN FORMULARIES AND THE NATIONAL FORMULARY

History of VA Formulary Management Prior to the National Formulary

The Veterans Administration was established in 1930 to provide medical care to veterans in 54 hospitals. In 1946, the VA Department of Medicine and Surgery (which subsequently became the VHA) was created, and agreements between VA hospitals and medical schools were begun (Fonseca et al., 1996). As discussed earlier, P&T committees developed slowly beginning in the 1930s coincident with the American College of Surgeons' promulgation of standards for hospital pharmacy (1936) and the beginnings of modern hospital formularies in New York (1933). In the 1940s, formulary improvement continued in some U.S. hospitals with removal of outdated medications, but the relatively slow introduction of modern pharmaceuticals and the outbreak of World War II delayed complete formulary revisions (Weintraub, 1978). Indeed, as noted earlier, official pronouncements in this field from the AHA and ASHP did not occur until 1959. It is unlikely, therefore, that the first VA hospitals had much in the way of P&T committees or formularies.

In any case, data summarizing the status of formularies at VA hospitals or other local VA facilities in these early decades were not available to the IOM, although a VA manual, issued in 1955 and mentioned earlier, presumed the presence of a formulary (or the possibility of a formulary) at VA hospitals in the 1950s. VA facilities are not Medicare providers and therefore not required to comply with Title XVIII of the Social Security Act and its regulations on P&T committees, but VA hospitals participate in accreditation by the JCAHO and therefore have been covered by that organization's guidelines regarding P&T committees and formularies. Since the VHA is funded by congressional appropriation and not by third-party payments, which might be affected by facility accreditation status, JCAHO compliance may not have been as influential in encouraging implementation of formularies in the VA hospital system as in other health care systems. Nevertheless, the JCAHO, which has been accrediting VA hospitals since 1953, likely encouraged the installation of formulary systems in VA hospitals. Current VA policy requires VA hospitals to have a P&T committee that carries out at least those functions outlined in the JCAHO accreditation manual for hospitals[4] and the 1992 ASHP statement on P&T committees (VA Manual, M-2, Part 1, Chapter 3, Clinical Programs, Pharmacy and Therapeutics Committee, Dec. 13, 1993).

As noted earlier, a study by Rucker and Visconti (1978) of 52 large, mostly academic, private U.S. hospitals and 12 Medicaid programs found that about 40% of hospitals had no formulary whatsoever and that most of the formularies in use had significant deficiencies. This study did not include or refer to VA

---

[4] Currently the JCAHO does not require or regulate P&T committees, but the VA continues to use the standards set forth in earlier JCAHO accreditation manuals (1993).

facilities specifically. Nevertheless, there appears no reason to conclude that VA hospitals, many of which are also large and affiliated with medical schools, should have had a markedly better or worse record at that time. According to Kittel et al. (1978), the VHA hospital system at the time of their writing used the American Hospital Formulary Service published by the ASHP to disseminate drug information. This was supplemented by an index of drugs and dosage forms stocked by the pharmacy for each individual hospital. These authors described a project to computerize the formulary index at their VA hospital in a way that could be updated easily after each meeting of the P&T committee and could be used by all six VA hospitals in their district (1 of 29 VA hospital districts at the time). Continuing into the 1980s, VA P&T committees and formulary systems became widespread and firmly entrenched according to those involved with VA pharmacy and formularies during that period (Anonymous, 1988; M. Valentino, VA PBM, personal communication, 1999).

Reorganization of the VA

At present, the VHA consists of 146 medical centers or systems, including 172 hospitals, more than 600 ambulatory care and community-based clinics, 132 nursing homes, 40 domiciliaries, and a number of other programs (Kizer, 1999). The VHA is a unique health care system (and different from private-sector managed care) in terms of its size, cost, and budgeting; diversity of settings; geographic scope; role in the use and training of young physicians; and its permanently eligible patient population. In a 1993 survey of pharmaceutical services, 247 of 326 federal hospitals (76%) responded. The response rate from 156 VA hospitals that participated in this survey was 81% (127 hospitals). A P&T committee was present in 100%, prescribing restrictions in 94%, and a "well-controlled" formulary system existed in 90% of VA hospitals responding. Therapeutic interchange was reported in 76% of responding VA hospital programs. Since this survey heard from about three-fourths of all VA hospitals in operation at the time, it appears that by the early 1990s the VA hospital system was essentially 100% compliant with requirements for a P&T committee and a formulary system (Crawford and Santell, 1994). These results compare favorably with those of Reeder et al. (1997), who found 59.7% of 713 U.S. nonfederal hospitals with a well-controlled formulary and 74.5% with therapeutic interchange programs.

Although a group of VA facilities might decide to implement a formulary jointly (Kittel et al., 1978) or to have a multifacility core formulary (Lowe and Trilli, 1995), the control of formulary content rested with each facility's P&T committee at the time of the Crawford and Santell survey (1994). The local formulary, by agreement of the medical staff and P&T committee, shaped and to some extent limited drug use within a facility by imposing restrictions on the use of some drugs and by listing or not listing specific drugs, among other things. Since drugs could be added to the formulary at local option, limits on prescribing could be mostly temporary, however, lasting until the pharmacy added a new drug to inventory or purchased it from the VA prime vendor [5] or in the local private-sector market (Patterson et al., 1995). Drugs would also be available through the consolidated mail outpatient pharmacy (CMOP), which serves all VA facilities from six locations distributed across the country (OSDBU Fact Sheet No. 314, May 7, 1998). Presumably, drug use could also be influenced by marketing information from pharmaceutical sales representatives and by therapeutic guidelines or other educational efforts issued (and monitored) by the VA PBM. The relative effectiveness of the former and lack of effectiveness of much of the latter in the private sector have been discussed by Avorn et al. (1982) and Avorn and Soumerai (1983). This subject has also been reviewed more recently by Chren and Landefield (1994), who found that staff physician interactions with a drug manufacturer significantly influenced physician interest in adding products of that manufacturer to their hospital's formulary.

Impact of the VA Fixed Budget

The pharmacy budget is another significant influence on drug use. The total VHA budget was $17,057,396,000 in FY 1998 and in FY 1999, and $18,978,003,000 in FY 2000. Expenditures for pharmaceuticals were about 6% of the total budget from FY 1990 to FY 1994, or $715,879,000 to $924,482,000, but they had grown to $1,844,742,000 or 11% of the total VHA budget in FY 1999; in recent years, they have been escalating between 11 and 21% annually (GAO, 1999). Prices of pharmaceuticals in the VHA depend on a number of purchasing vehicles. These include the statutorily based Federal Supply Schedule which requires manufacturers to offer brand name products at 76% of the average manufacturer price (AMP). The National Acquisition Center, based outside Chicago, can negotiate contracts below this price or for some supplies and genetic drugs at good prices for VA (and other federal agency) use. VISNs and individual facilities can also negotiate lower prices through blanket purchase agreements (BPAs; see Chapter 5 of this report). Important price differences among brand name members of a drug class, between brand and genetic drugs, or among generic drugs of different manufacture can emerge from these acquisition processes.

Differences in drug acquisition costs presumably explain the presence of therapeutic interchange programs in 76% of VA hospitals. These exchanges are implemented to affect drug use and cost as reported by Crawford and Santell (1994). Individual examples of interchange among members of a particular drug class with significant differences in price at a VA hospital began to be reported in the early 1990s; for example, studies were carried out by Bartlett et al. (1996) in 1993 and by Kellick et al. (1995) in 1994. Other examples are reviewed in Chapter 2 of this report. Occasional restriction of a class and interchange of less expensive drugs from another class were also reported (Lederle and Rogers,

---

[5] The prime vendor, Amerisource, Inc., is a single organization that provides just-in-time drugs to all VHA facilities (and some other federal agencies) on a national contract.

1990). Therapeutic interchange is carried out in VA facilities following analysis and a decision by the P&T committee and notice to the medical staff, sometimes without obtaining case-by-case permission at the time of dispensing. In other cases, such permission is part of the interchange process. In either event, a record of the interchange is kept in the pharmacy and a notation made in the patient record. As a matter of policy, the central VHA office does not dictate how conversions are to be carried out. This is left to the individual VISNs (which also do not dictate conversion details) and facilities (VHA response to Item 5, personal communication to IOM, 1999).

Establishing the VA National Formulary

In late 1995, a reorganization of the VHA affected the status of all VA facilities and the relationships of the VA formulary systems, the control of drug use, and pharmacy operations. In October 1995, 22 VISNs were created—essentially 22 MCOs with their own capitation-based budgets. Each VISN on average encompasses 7–10 hospitals, 25–30 ambulatory care clinics, 4–7 nursing homes, 1 or 2 domiciliaries, and various other assets (Kizer, 1999). In the larger scheme of things, this reorganization was intended to promote decentralized management and improved care of veteran populations, to move toward enrolling all veterans with primary caregivers, to consolidate (and close) hospital beds, and to emphasize ambulatory surgery and ambulatory care. At the pharmacy level, VHA Directive 10-95-111, November 7, 1995, required each VISN to implement a VISN-level formulary process by November 15, 1995, and a VISN formulary by April 30, 1996. In part, the VISN formularies were to provide a uniform drug benefit and continuity of care in each network. They also were intended to be the foundation within a year or two for a National Formulary which would provide U.S. veterans with a single national entitlement to drugs and to medical and surgical supplies, supplementable at the VISN or local level.

Coincident with the formation of VISN formularies, the VA Pharmacy Benefits Management Strategic Healthcare Group was established in September 1995 and developed over the course of FY 1996. The VA PBM is located both in Washington, D.C., and outside Chicago and is staffed primarily by pharmacists. Its functions include data collection and analysis to monitor drug costs and utilization, selection and development of drug class reviews and therapeutic guidelines in conjunction with the Medical Advisory Panel, coordination of VISN pharmacy activities, guidance of the transition to a National Formulary, and management of the VA pharmacy benefit. At the same time, VISNs also formed P&T committees (called formulary committees), made up primarily of representatives from local P&T committees. At present, the composition of these committees (primarily pharmacists and physicians) varies widely, but on average, pharmacists predominate. A VISN Formulary Leader Committee of pharmacy leaders from each VISN and the MAP consisting of VA physicians interested in and knowledgeable about drug treatment, were established (VISN Formulary Conference Call Minutes, Jan. 26, 1996). Some members of these

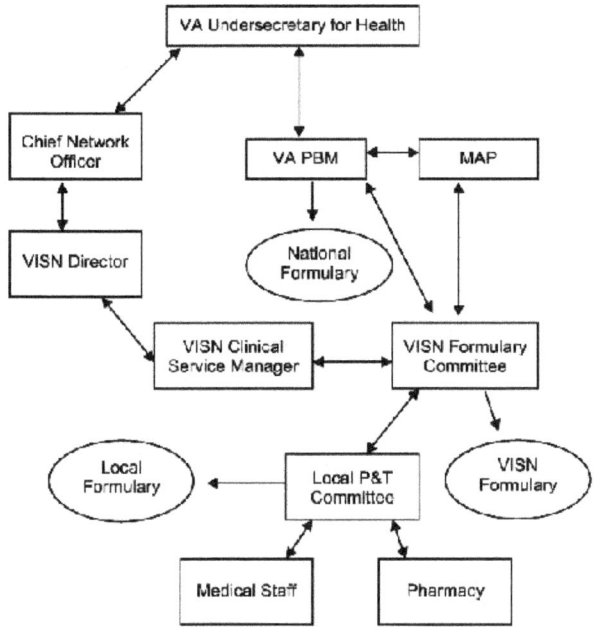

FIGURE 1.1 Reorganization of the Veterans Health Administration. MAP = medical advisory panel; PBM = pharmacy benefits management organization; P&T = pharmacy and therapeutics; VA = Department of Veterans Affairs; and VISN = Veterans Integrated Service Network.

two committees formed a VISN Research Steering Committee and a VISN Data Steering Committee. The first meeting of the MAP/VA PBM was held by conference call on April 3, 1996. Functions of the MAP are defined further below. Figure 1.1 summarizes this recent reorganization and its interrelations, although there are clearly informal ties and communication in addition to the formal ones.

Evolution of the National Formulary

Local formularies provided the foundation for VISN formularies. A formulary template was distributed to VISNs on March 11, 1996 to enable standardized submission of VISN formularies to the VA PBM to assist in development of the National Formulary (VISN Formulary Conference Call Minutes, April 22, 1996). The National Formulary, which presently consists of slightly more than 1,200 items —prescription and over-the-counter (OTC) drugs in 254 drug classes, as well as medical and surgical supplies—was issued in May 1997 (and has been modified several times since; for example, the original version omitted supplies that were added in December 1997). The official VHA Directive 97-047 followed on October 16, 1997. This directive requires a nonformulary process of each VISN and specifies criteria for granting exceptions. In therapeutic classes where national standardization or committed-use contracts are awarded (for example, any of four closed classes), additional items may not be listed, or listed items deleted, by VISN or local formularies. In other classes, additional items may be added to meet patient care needs as determined by the VISN or local facility. No items on the National Formulary can be made nonformulary at the VISN or local level, although local facilities may restrict National Formulary drugs to certain specialists, settings, or conditions. According to the VA, the objective of the National Formulary is to provide "high quality and best value pharmaceutical products while assuring the portability and standardization of the pharmacy benefit to eligible veterans" (VHA Directive 97-047).

By 1999, when VISN formularies were surveyed by IOM, the local formularies and the VISN formulary were the same in 16 VISNs. In four VISNs, there were differences in a few antibiotics and local restrictions; and in only two VISNs were there more numerous and significant differences among the formularies. Most VISN formularies were larger than the National Formulary, although in at least one instance the VISN formulary and the National Formulary were the same. Apparently, a policy of uniformity within regions is attractive despite the fact that, in theory, local formularies can deviate from the VISN-level formulary and differ among themselves. Of course, the listing of an item on a formulary may not guarantee that it is stocked, only that it will be made available. For example, facilities with patient populations that do not require certain items often do not stock them even though they are listed on the National Formulary (according to a 1999 IOM survey of local facilities). Special facilities such as spinal cord injury centers may have quite different policies from general care facilities on stocking drugs. Local facilities can still add items to their formularies and can request the addition of drugs to the VISN formulary, although such requests are not always granted. Each VISN is required to have an official nonformulary exceptions process based on uniform VHA criteria (VHA Directive 97-047), and some have a standard form for nonformulary requests. The nonformulary process is in part informal and personalized, however, so it is implemented variably depending on local factors, and the standard forms also vary (based on a 1999 IOM survey of local facilities in each of the 22 VISNs).

Despite the directive requiring conformity of closed classes in VISN formularies to the National Formulary, many VISN formularies were not in compliance when the IOM compared 19 drugs in closed classes across VISN formularies and the National Formulary in the spring and summer of 1999. VISN formularies ranged from 74 to 100% conformity; that is, in 16 of the 22 VISNs, from 1 to 5 of the 19 agents were incorrectly included, excluded, or restricted by the VISN formulary. There may be price differentials or local preferences among one or more members of a closed class listed in the National Formulary. In such cases, VISNs or local facilities may encourage the use of a particular member. The VA PBM does not object to this, although the practice does not explain why some class members are not listed on VISN or local formularies. Comparison of reviewed open or preferred classes also revealed that in about half of the VISNs, from 2 to 7% of the agents in these classes on the National Formulary were not included on the VISN formularies as required. Additions, which are permitted by the VA PBM as expressions of local autonomy, were also common, up to 24% in one case. Elsewhere, the committee comments on the problems inherent in divergence of the VISN or local formularies from the National Formulary.

Although local formularies were not reviewed by the IOM in a similar way, they likely were also not in compliance, since in most cases, all formularies in a VISN are the same. Some of this noncompliance probably stems from different schedules for formulary changes; some, from standardization contracts being established at various times; some, from the natural failures in any very large, complex, and changing system; and some, according to anecdotal reports, from disagreements between VISNs and National Formulary decision makers. It is unclear what implications, if any, minor noncompliance has for cost and quality of care. Enforcement appears to be relatively relaxed with some deference to local autonomy, however, as a matter of policy (M. Valentino, VA PBM, personal communication, 1999).

Medical Staff Input

The MAP works with the VA PBM and the VISN formulary leaders, and together they recommend additions and deletions to the National Formulary. National policy stipulates that new drug products cannot be considered for addition to the National Formulary until a year after FDA approval (except for FDA 1P drugs considered on a case-by-case basis). In this respect the MAP functions as a P&T committee, although it does not conform in structure or authority to ASHP (1992) descriptions of such committees. Its members are exclusively physicians. Appointments to the MAP are approved by the VA Undersecretary for Health on recommendation from the VA PBM and nomination by the VISN chief executives. Local facility P&T committees appear to provide greater opportunity for representation and influence of rank-and-file VA physicians on pharmacy benefit policy.

Although recommendations from the MAP, VISN formulary leaders, and VA PBM are routinely followed, authority to change the National Formulary rests formally with the Pharmacy Benefits Management Executive Steering Board. This board was established by VHA Directive 97-047, but to date has not been created. Decisions are currently made by the MAP-VISN-VA PBM consortium (answers to IOM questions by VHA, 1999). VISNs can request the addition of drugs to the National Formulary, and drugs that most—or many— VISNs add to their own formularies are also reviewed for addition to the National Formulary. Not all requests are granted, nor are all 1P drugs added (see Chapter 2 and Chapter 4 of this report).

Nevertheless, the MAP pursues many activities characteristic of P&T committees. It is made up of expert physicians from VA medical centers around the country, and it is assisted and staffed by the VA PBM. The MAP is charged with developing and coordinating disease state management practices that integrate quality clinical care and cost-effective drug therapy. By considering most frequently occurring conditions in the VHA and those with the top drug expenditures (which include hypertension, diabetes, coronary artery disease, hyperlipidemia, chronic obstructive pulmonary disease, congestive heart failure, prostate cancer, depression, psychosis or anxiety, and peptic ulcer disease, among others), the MAP established priorities for development of therapeutic guidelines and drug class reviews. Close to 30 drug classes have been or soon will be reviewed.

National Formulary Classes

Four classes are closed; that is, they have national standardization, or committed-use, contracts that provide volume-related low prices. Only a few members of the class are listed on the National Formulary. These members must be listed on VISN and local formularies, and other members cannot be listed on VISN or local formularies or dispensed except by nonformulary exception (although, as noted earlier, compliance with these requirements is not complete). These classes are angiotensin-converting enzyme inhibitors (ACEIs) to treat high blood pressure and heart conditions, hydroxymethylglutaryl coenzyme A reductase inhibitors (HMG CoA RIs) to control cholesterol, luteinizing hormone-releasing hormone (LHRH) analogues for treatment of prostatic cancer, and proton pump inhibitors (PPIs) for stomach ulcers and acid reflux. Two classes that were closed are now open, as products within one have become genetic and non-prescription (histamine$_2$ receptor blockers [H$_2$R blockers] for stomach ulcers and acid reflux), or the class has been made "preferred" (alpha blockers for treatment of high blood pressure or improvement of urinary flow in prostatic enlargement). Two classes are preferred, alpha blockers and calcium channel blockers (CCBs) for treatment of high blood pressure and heart conditions, that is, they are open, but they have national contracts that must be honored since prices depend on volume from exclusive use. Prescribing and utilization can also be affected by national usage criteria, or restrictions, which dictate drug usage based on treatment guidelines in classes that are otherwise open.[6]

When class reviews included specific consideration of closure, in six cases decisions were made to keep classes open or unrestricted (see Table 1.2). The great majority of classes (248) remain open, although closed classes accounted for about 16% of total drug costs in FY 1998 and 10% of total prescriptions and

---

[6] As work on this report was being completed, a fifth class, oral 5 hydroxytryptamine receptor antagonists for the relief of postoperative and cancer treatment nausea and vomiting, was closed. Because of a challenge to action, this closure and the selection of choice(s) in this class were not announced.

TABLE 1.2 Drug Classes That Remained Open or Preferred on Review

Drug Class	Reason from VISN Formulary Leaders☐ Minutes	Class Status
SSRIs	Medical staff advised against closing	Remains open, BPAs in effect
Angiotensin II inhibitors	Formulary leaders on review of utilization data felt the current arrangement was meeting VISN needs	Remains open, BPAs in effect
Fluoroquinolones	Sufficient competition was occurring and closing offered no advantage	Remains open, BPAs in effect
5-Hydroxytryptamine receptor antagonists (IV)	Anesthesiologists were against closing the IV class	Remains open
Ophthalmic beta-blockers	Drug products in class went generic	Remains open with a generic multi-source contract
Dihydropyridines	VISN formulary leaders, after review, felt that VISNs were already moving toward a preferred agent	Remains as a preferred class

NOTE: BPA = blanket purchase agreement; IV = intravenous; SSRI = selective serotonin reuptake inhibitor; and VISN = Veterans Integrated Services Network

13% of drug expenditures in FY 1999 (GAO, 1999). Some VISNs have purchasing agreements that influence prescribing and dispensing in addition to the obligations from the National Formulary listings and National Acquisition Center (NAC) contracting. Therapeutic guidelines have accompanied class reviews. Both the formulary status of members of a closed class and the contract prices negotiated by the NAC can have substantial effects on drug utilization as discussed later in this report.

Formulary Relationship to Pharmaceutical Companies

The relationship between buyers and sellers of products in a health care delivery system is a key issue for the VA National Formulary and any other formulary in an organized health care system. Organized buyers include, or have included, major federal government departments such as the VA or the Department of Defense, state programs, MCOs or HMOs, PBMs, group purchasing organizations, hospitals, and other health care facilities and systems. Members of all of these groups use formularies and formulary systems. Sellers are members of the pharmaceutical industry, and the products are pharmaceuticals.

As in any such relationship, prices depend on competition—the ability to choose among competitors, to purchase in volume, and to enforce compliance with market share agreements. By making choices and volume commitments, formularies and formulary systems are an important component in enabling prudent purchasing. If health care systems lose the ability to discriminate among pharmaceutical products, they will also be handicapped in negotiating prices and purchasing prudently.

Because pharmaceuticals are essential to health care, formularies and formulary systems must be controlled by experts in drug therapy, must safeguard the quality of pharmaceutical care, and must provide, through a waiver process, access to drugs deemed necessary by knowledgeable and informed prescribers. In this way, choices will be made wisely, and the quality of patient care will be protected. These and other objectives of a formulary system are described earlier in this chapter. A formulary system is not necessarily the only way to achieve all of them, but it is an integral part of price negotiation. The purpose of a formulary and formulary system is to achieve value in the purchasing and use of drugs.

REPORT OUTLINE

In subsequent chapters of this report, the concerns of Congress that define the four deliverables of the VA-IOM contractual agreement are considered, and the subject matter discussed in this introduction is expanded. In the final chapter, the committee draws together the material and evaluations from previous chapters in a review of the overall role of the VA National Formulary in veterans' health care. This review is more detailed than the short summary at the beginning of this report. The report concludes with the following material as appendixes: the committee's interim report, a survey carried out by the Academy of Managed Care Pharmacy, additional cost figures and tables, a glossary, and a drug list and drug index (the latter used to define terms and drugs used in this report).

To supplement the information here about the VA National Formulary, VISN formularies, and local formularies, or formulary systems, a detailed description can be found in the first GAO report on this subject, *VA's Management of Drugs on Its National Formulary* (GAO, 1999), which was requested by the U.S. Senate at the same time that House Report 105-610 requested this IOM study and that will be expanded in a subsequent companion GAO report. The subsequent report is projected to contain the first independent survey of physician perspectives on the National Formulary, which should be a useful addition to understanding the place of the National Formulary in the VHA. Based on the discussion and analyses in this IOM report, the committee comes to conclusions and makes recommendations for the consideration of policy makers in the Congress and the VA, which, it is hoped, may provide some guidance for constructive change in the National Formulary and formulary system. These can be found in the Executive Summary of this report.

2

Is the VA National Formulary Overly Restrictive and Does It Prevent Physicians from Meeting the Health Care Needs of Veterans?

To begin, the committee concluded that the answer to the question posed by Congress and the VA—whether the VA National Formulary was overly restrictive—was dependent, at least in part, on judgment. The restricted budgetary resources of the VHA that make veterans' health care a zero-sum game in which inflation in one sector obligates deflation in another will, of necessity, influence such a judgment. The IOM committee, as a panel of experts with broad experience, identified and evaluated the various elements, dimensions, or categories of restrictiveness as they are employed by the National Formulary and formulary system and compared them in pharmacy benefits of the VA, private-sector MCOs and PBMs, and two public programs, Medicaid and the Department of Defense. The information in Chapter 3 of this report supports an analysis of the economic factors that underlie some decisions on restriction. The central elements of restrictiveness of the formulary are also susceptible to independent analysis. Although there are deficiencies in the data, the committee found, in many instances, that there was sufficient information to support discussions, analyses and conclusions reached in this chapter.

BACKGROUND

Restrictiveness is a multifactorial attribute of a formulary and formulary system. At its root, the restrictiveness of the VA National Formulary, including the local, VISN, and national lists and systems, and the nonformulary exceptions processes, is a measure of the stringency of the controls on veterans' access to prescribed medicines at the appropriate times. Comparisons with other systems can influence judgments about such controls. *Nevertheless, if formulary structure or formulary system controls deny or significantly delay access to drugs that, in the reasonable judgment of medical experts, are clinically indicated, then the VA National Formulary meets a definition of "overly" restrictive.*

Such clinically indicated or medically necessary medicines are not necessarily those identified in television commercials or by pharmaceutical sales representatives, or those preferred by patients or physicians for other reasons. VA National Formulary treatment guidelines and drug class reviews are intended to improve prescribing decisions by caregivers. The evidence that there is room for such improvement is substantial. Physicians are often swayed by industry commercial messages when scientific data would indicate otherwise (Avorn et al., 1982; Avorn and Sounerai, 1983). Prescribers respond to patient pressure that may result from direct-to-consumer advertising (Barents LLC, 1999). Physicians also may provide drugs primarily for a placebo effect or to meet patient expectations for some sort of intervention (Schwartz et al., 1989). Prescribing errors are distressingly frequent throughout the U.S. health care system and have been shown in demonstrations to be correctable through consultation with clinical pharmacists or reengineering of systems of health care (Institute of Medicine, 1999; Leape et al., 1991, 1995, 1999).

Elements of Restrictiveness

The committee decided that the question of restrictiveness could be approached by examining several characteristics of the National Formulary and formulary system, both on their own merits and in comparison with other formulary systems. The elements of restrictiveness discussed in this chapter include the following: formulary size and coverage of agents in different therapeutic classes; timeliness of addition of new drugs or drug products and reappraisal of formulary listings; and appropriateness and responsiveness of the nonformulary exceptions process and access to nonformulary drugs. Restrictiveness also depends on therapeutic interchange policies and practices that are standardized and protect at-risk groups of patients from drug treatment misadventures. Coverage of nonprescription (over-the-counter [OTC]) drugs and generic substitution are also important. The committee concluded that the key elements in the VA National Formulary are the number of classes closed, number of drugs in closed classes, responsiveness of the nonformulary process, and sensitivity of the therapeutic interchange policy and

---

ELEMENTS OF RESTRICTIVENESS

- Formulary size
- Coverage of agents in different therapeutic classes
- Timeliness of addition of drugs newly approved by the Food and Drug Administration
- Reappraisal of formulary listings
- Appropriateness and responsiveness of the nonformulary process
- Access to nonformulary drugs
- Sensitivity of therapeutic interchange policy and procedure
- Over-the-counter coverage, generic substitution

procedure to patient risks and prescriber prerogatives. These are central elements in the implementation and management of the National Formulary, and revision of policies and procedures governing them will represent significant changes.

Criteria that the committee used for judging the restrictiveness of the attributes of the VA National Formulary include the following: how they compare to those of other organized private and public health care systems; how they compare to reasonableness standards in the literature or in the informed judgment of the committee; how they compare to objective standards where these are available; and how they affect the satisfaction and opinions of patients and prescribing physicians. The committee identified the elements of restrictiveness in the VA National Formulary and formulary system and, for comparison, in private-sector formularies and formulary systems. These are presented in Table 2.1. Private-sector data were collected through a special questionnaire (see Appendix B) circulated in January 2000 by the Academy of Managed Care Pharmacy (AMCP) to six major private-sector PBMs and two small MCOs covering in total about 176 million lives. Care should be exercised in interpreting these data in the sense that covered lives may be overstated due to double counting of two-wage-earner families. Also, some PBMs that provide claims services and not formulary management may have reported their own policies and not the actual client MCO formulary policies. Public-sector (Medicaid) elements are identified and discussed in Chapter 5 and summarized in Table 5.1 of that chapter. In all of these comparisons, clear differences in the involved health care systems in which the formularies are embedded suggest caution in drawing inferences, although the committee has attempted to limit the comparisons to the formularies and formulary systems not the health care systems.

Restrictiveness can be approached in another way. The use of restrictiveness elements or the characteristics of formularies and formulary systems that affect the availability of, or ease of obtaining, a drug in a health care system can be categorized, with the more severe limitations being those that absolutely deny access or limit access without medical need-based exceptions. Controls without need-based exceptions, such as absolute limits on numbers of prescriptions in some Medicaid programs, are rare in the private sector and are not part of the VA National Formulary. Box 2.1 lists such formulary limitations on receiving a safe, effective, and medically necessary drug, some with essentially no limit on access, others with complete inaccessibility. The committee concluded that the most important limits incorporated into restrictive designs were exclusions, volume or quantity limits that were unresponsive to medical necessity, drugs not being listed in a closed class, or not included or covered in the formulary, high copayments (these are also not related to medical necessity), and administratively and medically strict prior approval or nonformulary exceptions processes. Although this chapter is not organized by the listing in Box 2.1, an appreciation of these factors— their roles in, and contributions to, the availability or restriction of choice of drugs and drug products, is an important background to the committee's exploration of elements of restrictiveness of the VA National Formulary and comparison formularies. Formularies usually fall into one or more of the listed limitation categories and

SIZE AND COVERAGE OF THE NATIONAL FORMULARY

The VA National Formulary, dated July 1999, lists about 1,200 items, of which 133 are medical-surgical supplies. The nonsupply items are distributed in 254 classes and subclasses. Some of these classes are vitamins, dentals, vaccines, diagnostics, radiographic contrast agents, and intravenous (IV) or other solutions, that is, items that would not be considered typical pharmaceuticals and are often not included in other formularies. About 15 of the listings indicate that a drug class is under review without referring to any specific agent. Drugs needed in these classes will be found in VISN and local formularies until reviews are completed and national decisions made. About 170 of the items listed are OTC, such as nutritional supplements, vitamins, cough and cold remedies, simple ointments and other topicals, eye and nose drops, antacids and laxatives, and the like. Items such as these may be substituted for more expensive or risky prescription drugs. About half of the items in the VA classes are not separate chemical agents, but represent the same chemical entity in injectable, oral, or topical form. Dosage strengths are generally not identified. Drug dosages that are stocked and immediately available in VHA health care facilities are left to the discretion of each facility's management.

TABLE 2.1 Comparison of VA and Private Health Care

	VA (%)	Private Health Care (% of 176 million lives)
P&T committee composition		
Pharmacists	52[a]	32
Physicians	44	63
Others	4	5
Excluded		
DESI	100	10
Experimental	100[b]	99
Off-label use	0	36
OTC	0	9 0
Life-style	100[c]	92
Formularies		
Closed or partially closed		18
Open-preferred	100[d]	33
Open-passive		38
No formulary (PA)		13
No formulary (DUR)		1
No formulary (free access)		0

Closed formularies that contain only one drug in the drug class	100	3.5
Drug restrictions (specific prescribers, settings, disease conditions)	100	71
Required use of generic drugs	100	38
Nonformulary		
Coverage of nonformulary	100[e]	100
Copay to influence choice	0	100
Cost containment		
Limits on number of Rxs per patient at any time	0	23
Limits on refills	0	46
Limits on duration of use of some drugs	0	21
Limits on the supply of drugs per Rx	100	71
Presence of a PA process for some drugs	0	53
Waiting period requirements for new FDA-approved drugs	100[f]	6
Six months or more wait period	100[f]	1
Active monitoring of new FDA-approved drugs:		
Drugs for the treatment of AIDS or cancer	100	71
FDA "1P" drugs	0	34
Appeals process		
Internal appeals process for excluded drugs	100	47
Internal appeals process for nonformulary drugs	100	19
Independent external review of appeals process	0	7
Continuation of care		
Policy requires continuation of care for a few specific drugs	0[g]	3
Policy requires continuation of care for all drugs	0[g]	9

NOTE: DESI = Drug Efficacy Study Implementation; DUR = drug utilization review; FDA = Food and Drug Administration; PA = prior approval; 1P = FDA priority; P&T = pharmacy and therapeutics.

[a] Reflects the composition of VISN formulary (P&T) committees.
[b] The VA does not cover experimental drugs but it does not preclude the use of experimental drugs in its research programs.
[c] The VA does not exclude any class of drug, but if a specific agent is not on the formulary, it must be accessed by the nonformulary process.
[d] The VA formulary is a composite of a closed open–preferred, and open–passive formulary. The 100% for veterans should be compared to the summation of these three types.
[e] When medically justified.
[f] In some VISNs, drugs can be placed on the formulary earlier than 1 year.
[g] The VA does not have a specific policy for continuation, but a nonformulary drug can be continued if approved through the nonformulary process.
SOURCE: Private health care data from Academy of Managed Care Pharmacy.

Adequacy of the VA National Formulary

With respect to the adequacy of the VA National Formulary, the committee asked several questions. Is the overall size of the formulary reasonable? Are the closed classes limited to a reasonably small number for which economic and

---

BOX 2-1 FORMULARY AND FORMULARY SYSTEM LIMITATIONS OR OTHER RESTRICTIONS ON DRUGS IN A HEALTH CARE SYSTEM

1. Drugs are covered and listed in an open formulary or in an open class.
2. Drugs are not listed in the formulary, but the formulary is open. Coverage is assumed, or, at worst, a simple nonformulary or prior approval process is required.
3. Drugs are subject to mandatory generic substitution.
4. Drugs are restricted in some way:

   a. to a kind of prescriber or specialist,
   b. to certain conditions or diagnoses,
   c. to certain services or care settings,
   d. under a step protocol requiring a trial of another drug.

5. Drugs are preferred or encouraged in some way. Copayments, or copayments that vary in amount depending on the degree of preference, are required.
6. Drugs are not covered and not listed in a partially restricted or closed formulary; they are available

   a. by prior approval or
   b. by nonformulary exception.

7. Drugs are members of a closed class and are not listed: they are available

   a. by nonformulary exception or
   b. therapeutic interchange is required.

8. Drugs are subject to volume restrictions independent of medical necessity; there can be limits on:

   a. dispensing frequency,
   b. quantity dispensed,
   c. dollar value dispensed,
   d. number of prescriptions per unit time.

9. Drugs are listed as excluded or no-buy, or are members of excluded or no-buy classes. These are not available except by out-of-pocket, retail purchase by the patient.

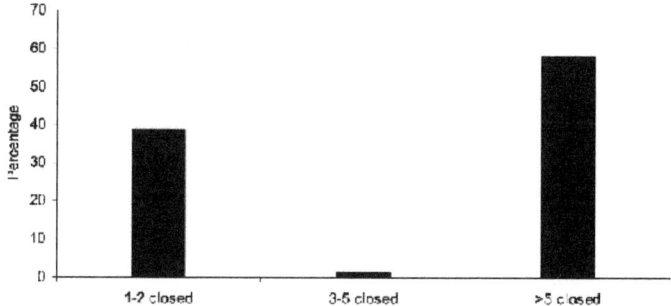

FIGURE 2.1 The number of closed classes in closed private-sector formularies by percentage of private-sector plans. SOURCE: Academy of Managed Care Pharmacy (2000).

therapeutic effects justify the effort (and possible inconvenience to prescribers and risks to patients) of managing that class? Are the numbers of members in a closed class listed on the formulary reasonable and sufficient, particularly in comparison with other formularies? The standard of reasonableness depends in part on the committee's professional judgment and experience with other formularies and in part on information in studies and reports in the scientific literature.

The overall size of a formulary is not necessarily a key characteristic. There is no standard that specifies a particular size for a given health care system. Large open formularies may contain from 1,000 to 3,000 drugs and dosage forms (Covington and Thornton, 1995). Those of the Mayo Clinic and the British National Formulary list more than 1,200 and 2,000 items, respectively. In 1997, most MCO formularies (60%) contained less than 1,000 items, and 37% were in the 750–999 category (Hoechst Marion Roussel, 1998). A majority of MCO formularies were closed or partially closed (Novartis, 1999).

A more open formulary that includes greater numbers of widely prescribed drugs does not automatically improve clinical practice. In studying Medicaid formularies after OBRA 1990, which traded drug rebates for abolition of restricted formularies, Walser et al. (1996) concluded that only 22% (4/18) of additions of top 200 drugs to state formularies conferred a net therapeutic benefit, that is, led to better patient compliance, were less expensive, or had greater effectiveness, according to panels of practicing physicians. The rest either were questionable or did not offer an additional benefit. The authors could not draw any policy conclusions from these data. Many drugs are widely prescribed because prescribers are influenced by industry sales techniques or for other non-scientific reasons (Avorn and Soumerai, 1983; Avorn et al., 1982; Schwartz et al., 1989), or because patient demand is generated by direct-to-consumer advertising

(Barents LLC, 1999a; www.imshealth.com/html/news_arc/06_07_1999_211.htm).

Rucker and Visconti apparently considered that a good-quality hospital formulary listed only about 450 single drugs, but their reports are dated, and in any case apply to a hospital, not a health care system (Rucker, 1982b; Rucker and Visconti, 1978). In 1986, Bakke reviewed the situation internationally and concluded that at that time, about 500 drugs should be available to deliver good care in most advanced countries (Bakke, 1986). This estimate is primarily of historical interest given its age and the fact that it was devised for countries not health care systems. Rhode Island Hospital, the principal teaching affiliate of Brown University, was reported to have 580 medications listed in its formulary in 1986 (Packer et al., 1986). In a review of survey data from 187 large, private, nonprofit, U.S. teaching hospitals, Mannebach et al. (1999) noted that most of their formularies were closed and that P&T committees tried, for the most part successfully, to limit the numbers of drugs listed in therapeutic classes.

The VHA allows VISNs (and local facilities) to add items that are not on the National Formulary. Therefore, choices actually available on these formularies (although the same in at least one instance, VISN 14) usually exceed those on the national list by a few to 544 items. VISN formularies frequently include about 10% more items. Precise formulary comparisons are difficult because the VISN formularies list multiple dosage forms and the National Formulary does not. One formulary for which precise figures were provided (VISN 19) contained 108 more drugs and a total of 615 different drugs.

> Prior to the VA National Formulary, some VISNs were functioning at 70% or less of the present National Formulary size.

Most VA local and VISN formularies had fewer listings before the national list was introduced in 1997. Some of these facilities were operating, apparently satisfactorily, with a formulary of 70% or less the size of the present National Formulary (VHA data provided to IOM, 1999). In view of the increase in drugs and drug products available to veterans since the introduction of the National Formulary and in comparison to MCO or hospital formularies, the number of items on the VA National Formulary seemed reasonable to the committee.

Closed and Preferred Drug Classes in the VA

The VA National Formulary's closed classes, the quality of the listings as affected by the quality of the input of P&T committees, the MAP, and VA PBM (see Chapter 4 of this report), and the access afforded through a nonformulary exception process are probably more important measures of restrictiveness than overall formulary size. Although dozens of therapeutic classes have been or are being reviewed by the VHA, only six classes (four at the present time) have been closed. Two classes are preferred, that is, they are open, but there are national contracts for one or more members of the class.

The closed classes, identified in this report's introduction, are (ACEIs), (HMG CoA RIs), (LHRHs), and (PPIs). They comprised about 16% of the prime vendor cost of drugs in 1998, and, because the VHA accounts for the great majority of prime vendor sales, probably about 16% of VHA drug costs in that year. According to GAO, they comprised 13% of drug costs in 1999 (GAO, 1999).* Because there are only about 20 chemical entities in these classes—that is, about 2% potentially (if expected new entries and different routes of administration and dosage forms are included), and less than 1% in reality, of the drugs on the National Formulary— these classes have an economic impact disproportionate to their numbers. This reflects their prices and the importance of their therapeutic effects; the prevalence of the conditions they can treat, especially in the older, almost all-male VA population; and the volume of prescriptions written for them. In fact, nationally, three of these closed classes were in the top five classes accounting for drug expenditure increases and the top seven in class cost in 1998 (Barents LLC, 1999a). According to the last Novartis (1999) survey of MCOs, gastrointestinal medications (such as PPIs), ACEIs, and HMG CoA RIs were in the top five classes by overall cost, number of prescriptions, and per-member per-year expenditures in managed care pharmacy benefits. The closed classes are clearly important, major classes (see also Figure 2.1 for comparison of number of closed classes in PBMs that close classes).

Preferred classes are also contributors to drug costs and utilization. As noted, there are two preferred classes (CCBs and alpha blockers), one of which (alpha blockers) was previously closed. The case for creating preferred classes may not be quite as persuasive as that for closed classes. In theory, more local options are provided in these classes because VISNs and facilities are free to supplement the national list. However, economics drive the choice to the nationally contracted drugs in the preferred class and may encourage changes in prescribing by physicians or initiate therapeutic interchanges. A previously closed class, (H2R) blockers, is open since some members are now generic and famotidine, cimetidine, and ranitidine are OTC. Price or cost control in this class is also exercised through contracting, which has a striking effect on utilization (see Figure 4.4, Chapter 4 of this report).

National usage criteria that generally depend on therapeutic guidelines or drug class reviews are also issued from time to time by the VA PBM. There were nine separate usage criteria in the fall of 1999 (http://www.dppm.med.va.gov/newsite/criteriadrop.html). These criteria may require certain patterns of prescribing or even therapeutic interchange. They may also dictate the ways in which nonformulary drug products (for example, new anti-inflammatory agents, such as cyclooxygenase-2 [COX-2] inhibitors), can be used acceptably for arthritis and other conditions. In encouraging such behavior, preferred classes, those with national usage criteria, or those with committed-use contracts are similar to closed classes, although they are officially open.

---

* Based on 1998 prime vendor purchase data, the projected fifth closed class (oral 5HT3 RAs) would account for less than 0.5% of the top 200 VA drug costs.

After VA drug class review, six classes that were reviewed for possible closure have not been closed, preferred, or subjected to restrictions at the national level, although they might have been. Such classes, which are often managed (closed, restricted, or subject to therapeutic interchange) in other health care systems, include some drugs (selective serotonin reuptake inhibitors [SSRIs], other antidepressants) used in mental health care or expensive antibiotics (for example, fluoroquinolones or cephalosporins) (Achusim, 1992, reviewed in Bootman and Milne, 1996; DeTorres and White, 1984, reviewed in Dunagan and Medoff, 1993; Dzierba et al., 1986; Edwards and Anderson, 1999; Guze, 1996; Kresel et al., 1987, reviewed in Mitchell et al., 1997; Nightingale et al., 1991; Reeder et al., 1997; Stock and Kofoed, 1994; Streja et al., 1999; Zhanel et al., 1989). MCO formularies also often restrict expensive, brand name products through higher copayments (Hoechst Marion Roussel, 1998; Smith, 1993).

Drugs in VA closed or preferred classes, although not chemically identical, are similar in therapeutic effect. Price differentials exist among class members. Generics are few or absent, and significant price reductions and aggregate savings through volume commitments are possible (see Chapter 3 of this report). These same classes are also subject to restrictions and therapeutic interchange in other (MCO) systems. Restriction to a few choices through closure or preference in each class is reported to be consistent with good care because class members are thought to be therapeutic alternates. That is, they have similar therapeutic effects based on the available medical evidence (see VHA class reviews and accompanying references at http://www.dppm.med.va.gov/newsite/reviews.html; see also Briscoe and Dearing, 1996; Gerbrandt and Yedinak, 1996; Hilleman et al., 1997; McMillan, 1996; Moisan et al., 1999; Oh and Franko, 1990; Petitta et al., 1997).

Potentially closed or preferred classes that are not economically significant, are low volume, have many generics, or have no comparatively substandard members may not yield economic or quality rewards from being designated as closed or preferred that are sufficient to justify the time, effort, and potential prescriber and patient dissatisfaction involved. Classes for which quality concerns would be raised by a designation as closed or preferred definitely should not be so designated (Carroll, 1999). These classes are not closed or preferred in the VA National Formulary.

Restrictiveness of Class Closure

The VA National Formulary has some classes with only a single agent, which is unusual in other formularies (see Table 2.1 and discussion of some MCO formularies and Medicaid in Chapter 5 of this report). These may be classes with only one or two members, such as chloramphenicol or PPIs (at the time of original listing). If the classes are open, facilities and VISNs are free to expand the listings. Listing only a single drug in a class is not prima facie evidence of excessive restriction, but it tests the ability of the nonformulary process to provide access to therapeutic alternates if medically needed. The absence of formulary alternatives (if such drugs exist) deserves examination. It is unlikely that a single member of a multidrug class will treat all patients for whom the class is indicated without exception (McAllister et al., 1999), and some investigators have reported that restriction of choice to a single agent compromises care and raises costs (Streja et al., 1999). Therefore, a smoothly functioning non-formulary process is important to preserving quality of care in this situation.

The listing of only one agent in closed classes, such as PPIs and LHRHs, results in almost all veterans being on the formulary agent lansoprazole or goserelin (see Figure 4.2 and Figure 4.3 in this report). All four potential choices (as of July 1999), including nonformulary omeprazole and leuprolide, are on the 200 top dollar expenditure list, however, so nonformulary costs are at least measurable. In general, VA nonadherence reports identify about 5% nonformulary dispensing in closed classes with a single formulary choice. Decisions on PPIs and LHRHs were made on the basis of good-quality drug class reviews (see Chapter 4 for analysis; for actual reviews, see http://www.dppm.med.va.gov/newsite/reviews.html). There is also a specific VA cost-effectiveness study that compares PPIs (Vivian et al., 1999). The VA nonformulary exceptions process is discussed briefly below and in Chapter 4 of this report.

In a lengthy review of restrictive formularies, many of which are also reviewed in Chapter 5 of this report, Levy and Cocks (1999) claimed that the VA National Formulary severely limits choice among brand name agents in six drug classes, three of them current VA National Formulary closed classes. These authors provided no evidence of effects on veterans' health outcomes by National Formulary restrictions in these classes. Although Levy and Cocks (1999) raised some interesting concerns, some of which are discussed further below, the committee concluded that they had not made a persuasive case for meaningful and severe limitation of choice in the six cited classes.

Median coverage by 13 Medicaid programs was 27 of the 27 brand name products in the six classes, and by the National Formulary, 8 of 27. It is not clear that these Medicaid programs are representative, and in any case, states must include in their Medicaid formularies all drugs that manufacturers list in the Federal Supply Schedule. Of four cited National Formulary classes with only one representative, three are either open or preferred so that VISNs and facilities are free to add drugs that are used and preferred locally. The other class, PPIs, which is closed, had only two brand name products (additional products have since been marketed) from which to choose, and they are considered therapeutic alternates (Chon and Suzuki, 1998; Vivian et al., 1999; see also the VHA drug class review and its accompanying references at http://www.dppm.med.va.gov/newsite/reviews.html). A VA drug class review recommended one nitroglycerin patch in that open class, based on cost and patient preference since available products are similar and, with the exception of a few high-dose patches, are rated bioequivalent by the Food and Drug Administration (FDA, 1999a). The other two classes (alpha blockers and H_2R blockers) are currently represented by two (prazosin, terazosin) and three members (cimetidine, famotidine, ranitidine), respectively.

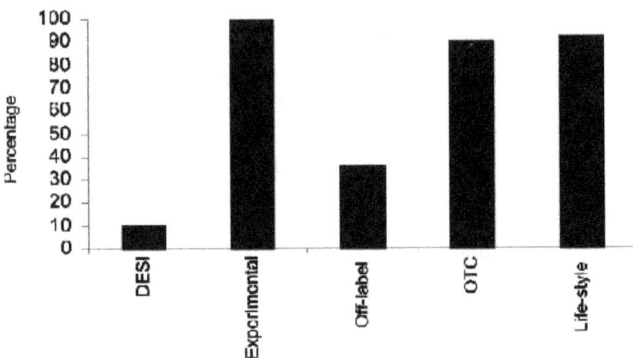

FIGURE 2.2 Drug categories excluded by percentage of private-sector plans. DESI = drug efficacy study implementation; OTC = over the counter.
SOURCE: Academy of Managed Care Pharmacy (2000).

Excluded Drugs and Other Limits

The VA, with extremely rare exceptions, does not use controls such as exclusions or volume limits, some of which, without medical necessity-based exceptions, are among the most restrictive (see Box 2.1). Although almost all state Medicaid formularies are open, they all exclude some drugs, for example, one or more of anorexiants, hair growth and other cosmetic drugs, fertility drugs, male impotence drugs, smoking cessation drugs, all or some OTC drugs, all or some drugs listed in OBRA 1990 (see Glossary), Drug Efficacy Study Implementation (DESI) drugs (see Glossary), and the like. States are free to make drugs subject to prior authorization, and most do to some extent. States also frequently restrict quantity dispensed, number of prescriptions per month, or number of refills, without providing exceptions for medical necessity (see Chapter 5 for details; see also National Pharmaceutical Council, 1997, 1998; Walser et al., 1996).

In general, the VA National Formulary is restricted in ways that support price negotiations and direct prescribing to the best-price drugs. This is true of MCO and PBM formularies too (although they also exclude certain drug categories as shown in Figure 2.2). Such restrictions are not as effective for Medicaid formularies or state policies because drug price discounts or rebates are already specified in federal statute. The congressional decision to require a relatively open Medicaid formulary (but allow prior authorization and exclusions) reflects the agreement on best-price manufacturer rebates rather than an analysis of the pros and cons of formulary structures (Walser et al., 1996). Medicaid formularies use restrictions to control expenditures not prices, as noted above, and they vary considerably from state to state.

National Formulary Effects on Drug Use

The VA National Formulary in closed classes and the national contracts in closed and preferred classes have marked effects on drug utilization. The use of VHA nonformulary or noncontract agents is close to zero in many cases (see, for example, PPI utilization data for omeprazole, Figure 4.2). In closed classes with national committed-use contracts, where Contract Adherence Reports identify that a VISN's nonformulary drug use is greater than two standard deviations above mean VHA nonformulary drug use, this is brought to the attention of the VISN. Apparently, VHA policy is to encourage corrective action through repeated contacts if adherence does not improve (VISN 13 P&T committee minutes, May 5, 1999). In the case of VISN 13, national use was 96.5% lansoprazole; VISN 13 use, 93.6%. A requirement that VISNs submit quarterly reports justifying nonformulary drug use (VHA Directive 97-047) was not implemented because the VA PBM decided that the value of these data was insufficient to justify the cost of gathering them given the high level of contract and formulary adherence. For their part, VISNs report that they do not have formal sanctions for nonadherence by local facilities. Their policy appears to be to bring this to the attention of responsible officials or physicians at the local facility and discuss plans for correction. This is reported to be effective. As noted elsewhere, the percentage of nonformulary drugs dispensed by MCOs with formularies is 10% nationally (Hoechst Marion Roussel, 1998).

Whether the VA National Formulary is overly restrictive relative to managed care experience probably depends on factors other than the actual size of the formulary or number of choices listed in important drug classes. These elements are not dramatically out of line with experience in other health care settings. Managed care systems use some controls not available to the VHA. The committee argued that the National Formulary, if supported by an administratively flexible and responsive nonformulary process, might be, in practice, less restrictive. Low-income veterans might have better access in such a system than in one that assessed financial penalties for the use of nonpreferred or nonformulary drugs.

The VA National Formulary serves numerous settings in addition to hospitals, so it is not strictly comparable to hospital formularies. However, it appears not to restrict choice in major or closed drug classes more than the average American hospital according to Mannebach et al. (1999). In 1995, these authors surveyed pharmacy departments in 187 large, private, nonprofit, U.S. teaching hospitals. Surveyed pharmacists were asked what drugs in three large popular classes (all three either currently or formerly closed in the VA National Formulary) were listed on their hospital formularies. On average, these formularies listed 3.3 ACEIs, usually captopril, enalapril, and one other; 1.8 HMG CoA RIs, usually lovastatin; and 2.3 H_2R blockers with no predominance of either cimetidine, famotidine, nizatidine, or ranitidine. Current National Formulary listings in these classes are very similar. They include captopril (as a generic), fosinopril, and lisinopril in ACEIs; lovastatin and simvastatin in HMG

CoA RIs; and cimetidine, famotodine, and ranitidine in H2R blockers. Therapeutic interchange programs in these classes are occasionally reported from nonfederal U.S. hospitals (Berkowitz, 1992; Briscoe and Dearing, 1996; Calvo et al., 1990; Fudge et al., 1993; Hilleman, 1997; McDonough et al., 1992; Oh and Franko, 1990).

As discussed earlier, the National Formulary's restrictiveness may depend, therefore, on the closed classes, national committed-use contracts, and the additional choices in open classes in VISN and local formularies. A smoothly functioning, responsive nonformulary exceptions process, especially for drugs in the closed classes in which most VISN formularies lost options in 1997, would substantially mitigate any untoward effects of these restrictions.

ADDITION OF NEW DRUGS AND FORMULARY REAPPRAISAL

National Policy Regarding New Drugs

Under current policy, drugs newly approved by the FDA are considered for addition to the VA National Formulary only after a 1-year delay, except in special cases of important new 1P category drugs, that is, new chemical entities classified for priority review by the FDA (VHA Directive 97-047). Formulary drugs should be selected with priority based on their relative therapeutic merits. The FDA is aware of the relative merits of drugs. The agency designates some drugs 1P for priority review because they are helpful in important diseases or conditions. The FDA also occasionally takes regulatory actions against misleading advertising claims of relative efficacy (Furberg et al., 1999). The agency, however, approves drugs based on their safety and efficacy, not their relative safety and efficacy compared to other available products. If there are a number of drugs in a class, P&T committees have an obligation, based on their best medical judgment, to select from among them those that are relatively as safe and effective as, or safer and more effective than, other members (much as those who sell drugs would like to see every possible member included). P&T committees also can take note of FDA 1P drugs in considering additions to formularies since these drugs may have particular importance, at least as seen by that agency.

In practice, the VA national policy has meant that new drugs for the treatment of HIV/AIDS have been added with less than a year lag, whereas other 1P drugs have been added only after a year or more, if at all. At present, these decisions are officially made by a consortium of the MAP, VISN formulary leaders, and the VA PBM. Although the final authority was vested initially in a VA PBM Executive Steering Board made up of officials from various units of the VHA central office, this board never became operational. As opposed to the policy of delay in additions of newly approved drugs, the committee did not find any policy of specified periodic internal review or external evaluation of the National Formulary.

The VHA policy of a 1-year waiting period is considered a safety precaution that allows evidence of adverse drug effects to accumulate during the interval. It also provides time to carry out studies comparing the safety, efficacy, or cost-effectiveness of new drugs with existing therapeutic alternates or drugs for similar indications. Such studies are usually not done during the FDA new drug approval process. Data, especially in the peer-reviewed open literature, to inform a decision on whether a new drug is an improvement over, or an addition to, existing drug therapies are generally not available until some time after release, if at all. In fact, Sloan et al. (1997) noted a dearth of phamacoeconomic or cost-effectiveness studies even beyond a year after market entry of new drugs. Waiting for a year does not guarantee that adequate comparative evaluations will be available (Lyles et al., 1997; Mather et al., 1999; see also VA drug class reviews at http://www.dppm.med.va.gov/newsite/reviews.html).

The VHA has cited reports of adverse effects and even FDA recall or restrictions that may occur with experience in the general population. Examples, such as troglitazone and mibefradil, which were not added to the National Formulary, have been given (VHA answers to IOM questions, 1999, but troglitazone was widely used in the VHA). According to the FDA (Federal Register 64[44], March 8, 1999; *Federal Register* 65[2], January 4, 2000), 15 agents were recalled in the 1990s, 10 of these since the National Formulary was implemented in mid-1997. Some of these drugs were not on the market, for example, antipyrine; were recalled much more than a year after entry, for example, terfenadine [Seldane]; were not 1P drugs, for example, fenfluramine (Pondimin); or were, in fact, on the National Formulary, for example, cisapride (Propulsid). Also, new drugs are generally more expensive. Therefore, in addition to safety considerations, there are significant budgetary implications in delaying the addition of new drugs to the National Formulary. For example, 1998 prices of drugs approved between 1992 and 1998 were significantly more than the 1998 prices of pre-1992 drugs (Barents LLC, 1999b; CBO, 1998; Levit et al., 1998).

VISN Addition of New FDA Approvals

New FDA approvals can also be added at the VISN level and, when local formularies are different, separately at that level also. VISN policies on adding new approvals vary but in general appear more permissive. For the most part, they do not require a 1-year waiting period, although a few do. Most VISNs await and react to activity at the local level. An occasional VISN reviews new approvals proactively if they are high-profile drugs. A few local facilities can add drugs and may also request their consideration for the VISN formulary. Prescribers can formally ask for additions, either of newly approved drugs or of existing drugs, to the local, VISN, or —through VISN formulary leaders—to the National Formulary. Many VISNs have standardized forms for such requests that require scientific analysis and justification. These requests are reviewed and approved or denied at the appropriate level. Drugs not reviewed at the VISN level because of a 1-year VISN waiting period for new approvals, may be added provisionally by local facilities in some regions. Drugs are always potentially available through the nonformulary process, and in such cases, access depends on the smoothness of this process. These data are summarized in Table 4.1 of this report.

The MAP, VA PBM, and VISN formulary leaders can bring up National Formulary changes on their own motion at any time. Important to this process are the drug class reviews on which approvals or disapprovals of many additions are based. As discussed in Chapter 4, these reviews are of good quality. Although they refer to cost or cost comparisons fairly often, they only occasionally (for example, SSRIs) have separate sections on pharmacoeconomics or cost-effectiveness. Separate pharmacoeconomic analyses are frequently not part of reviews in other settings either (Grabowski and Mullins, 1997; Gross, 1998; Lyles et al., 1997; Sloan et al., 1997).

Evaluation of the VA Process for Adding New FDA-Approved Priority Drugs

The committee reviewed the 42 FDA 1P drugs approved in 1996, 1997, and 1998. Ten of the 1P drugs that were introduced before the implementation of the VA National Formulary were included in the initial version. Four drugs were subsequently approved and added, primarily for the treatment of HIV/AIDS. By July 1999, the 28 remaining 1P drugs either had been reviewed and not approved (5), had not been reviewed (21), or were pending (2). The reasons for disapproving additions included "no advantages over contract agents," "evidence regarding efficacy was inconclusive," and "safety/cost concerns." At the same time, the FDA Center for Drug Evaluation and Research 1998 Report to the Nation (http://www.fda.gov/cder/reports/rptntn98.pdf) proposed that 1P drugs "represent an advance in medical treatment" and described a number of the drugs that had been disapproved or not reviewed by the VHA as "notable 1998 new drug approvals."

The MAP, VA PBM, and VISN formulary leaders must employ stringent evidentiary requirements for the addition of newly introduced drugs, since few are added to the National Formulary. As far as the committee could determine, however, there is no VHA policy or practice of identifying and reviewing new 1P drugs (for example, the 21 "not-reviewed" 1996, 1997, or 1998 1P drugs) or other new-to-market drugs in a systematic way. As discussed in the preceding chapter, VISN and local policies and practices, although variable, appear to be more permissive. Many decisions on drug class reviews, therapeutic guidelines, and formulary additions are made in the professional judgment of the MAP, VA PBM, and VISN formulary leaders and are memorialized in the minutes of their meetings. From an examination of these minutes and observation of a MAP/VA PBM meeting in August 1999 by the committee and IOM staff representatives, these groups appear to be appropriately expert professionals functioning in a thoughtful manner. Nevertheless, existing or newly introduced drugs are less likely to be added to the National Formulary than to the formularies of other organizations or to VISN or local formularies, and listed drugs are less likely to be deleted. One or more VISN or local formularies added 4 of the 5 disapproved 1P drugs and 4 of the 21 nonreviewed 1P drugs. In one case, 18 VISNs added clopidogrel (Plavix), a nationally nonreveiwed 1P drug. A decision was then made at the national level not to add this drug to the National Formulary, but it remained on VISN formularies.

Changes to these VHA formularies vary considerably from VISN to VISN. Obviously, as this continues over time, the role of the national list as a universal, uniform entitlement for veterans will be weakened while the role of the VISN list as an expression of local autonomy and choice is strengthened. This resolves the natural tension between a uniform, standardized national entitlement and local autonomy and flexibility, at least in part in favor of local preferences and loosened control. Of course, in theory, VISN or local formulary additions might not be needed given a very smooth, nationally consistent nonformulary process. The effect of VHA formulary management is a rather tightly managed national base of products and a more generous and decentralized drug policy at the regional and local levels. Inconsistencies in formularies (and other formulary system policies) also potentially expose veterans to inconsistent access and drug treatment in different VISNs.

The National Formulary disapproval of the (1998) FDA 1P drug sildenafil citrate (Viagra) for treatment of erectile dysfunction is undoubtedly an example of VHA concerns about cost. Although the committee did not carry out a detailed cost analysis, making this breakthrough drug available to veterans would clearly increase national VHA drug expenditures by tens of millions of dollars even at current federal supply schedule prices unless it was introduced with significant usage restrictions. Kaiser Permanente recently estimated that coverage of sildenafil would increase that health maintenance organization's (HMO's) drug costs by $100 million annually (Mehl and Santell, 1999). Although this large group model HMO has about twice as many covered lives (more than 7 million) as the VHA, it also has a younger population with a normal male–female distribution (Navarro and Cahill, 1999).

Not everyone agreed with this noncoverage decision. By December 1999, the VA had developed and implemented criteria for the use of sildenafil. Before then, a VISN (VISN 15) and a few facilities in VISN 9, in clear noncompliance with National Formulary policy, added this drug to their formularies. VISN 15 had many initial requests for sildenafil, but approximately 25% of these patients did not refill their prescriptions. The VISN is currently examining whether this was due to lack of effectiveness in these clinical situations or some other reason, although preliminary results indicate that treatment failure was usually associated with hypertension. Noncoverage of sildenafil citrate generated congressional and Veterans Service Organization questions about formulary policy. VA national coverage of other products related to human sexuality, for example, male and female condoms, oral contraceptives, and other technologies to treat erectile dysfunction, is broader than that of most other formularies.

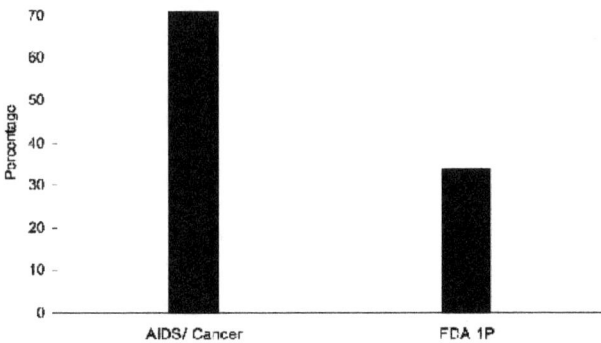

FIGURE 2.3 Percentage of private-sector plans having a mandatory policy of waiting before adding newly approved FDA drugs to the formulary. SOURCE: Academy of Managed Care Pharmacy (2000).

Addition of Existing Drugs by the VA

After the National Formulary was established, about 260 different, mostly existing drugs were added to VISN formularies, usually only to one or a few VISNs, so that individual VISN formularies expanded by around 15 to 20 drugs or occasionally as many as 80 items over and above nationally required additions. Very few changes were made to the National Formulary in its second year of operation. National changes were primarily the result of completion of class reviews. Four of the five SSRIs and a few CCBs were added. A number of oral contraceptives were changed to generics, some corrections were made, and the antimicrobial levofloxacin was added while ofloxacin was deleted. In total, by the end of 1999, 26 drugs had been added and 6 deleted from the National Formulary (GAO, 1999). Many VISN formularies originally listed quite a few drugs in addition to these on the national list. If they continue to expand—and especially if they add newly approved new chemical entities and 1P drugs and the National Formulary does not—at some point, veterans who move from one VISN to another may encounter drug access problems, as observed earlier. This might be mitigated if the nonformulary exceptions process is operating smoothly and uniformly. It also raises issues of equity and could lead to veterans visiting VISNs to get drugs, which may already have occurred with sildenafil.

HMOs are said to be cautious about adding newly approved drugs to their formularies, in part because of cost concerns and in part because of quality concerns about direct-to-consumer advertising-driven demand for drugs that may not be the most appropriate for patients' conditions. Nevertheless, 20% of

HMOs reported adding new drugs immediately, and 62% have an established review period for newly released drugs, which is usually (74.2%) 6 months (Novartis, 1998). In 1997, about half of PBMs were found to have partially closed formularies; about half of PBMs imposed a 3- to 6-month waiting period for addition of new FDA-approved drugs to their formularies, and the other half added new FDA approvals immediately (Novartis, 1998). Recent data from the AMCP survey indicate even fewer PBMs and MCOs with wait policies and an even higher likelihood of review, and presumably addition, of new drugs (Figure 2.4 and Table 2.1).There do not appear to be any VHA policies on periodic complete formulary reviews or external evaluations, although additions and deletions to the National Formulary are posted on the Internet several times a year. Review of MCO formularies is carried out quarterly by 48% of plans and at least annually by about 85% (Hoechst Marion Roussel, 1998). Although the committee does not have aggregate data on the thoroughness or quantitative results of such reviews, based on the experience of committee members, they are detailed and consistent with standards in the literature (ASHP, 1981; Langley and Sullivan, 1996, Lipsey, 1992; Majercik et al., 1985). Some have recommended a thorough hospital formulary review perhaps every 3 years and evaluation by an external expert group every 4 or 5 years (Rucker, 1988).

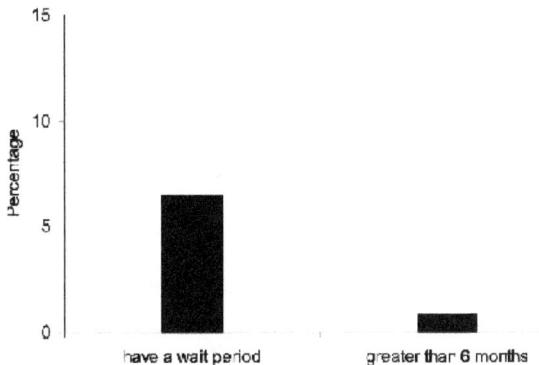

FIGURE 2.4 Percentage of private-sector plans having a mandatory policy of waiting before adding newly approved FDA drugs to the formulary. SOURCE: Academy of Managed Care Pharmacy (2000).

Addition of Newly Approved or Existing Drugs in Other Health Care Systems

The VHA policy of routinely waiting for 1 year after approval, the record of limiting expedited new National Formulary additions to HIV/AIDS drugs, and the addition of only 12.5% of new 1P drugs since inception of the National Formulary, is less generous than the policies and practices reported by private health care settings known to the committee (see Table 2.1 and Figure 2.3). Utilization management guidelines (UM 10 Procedures for Pharmaceutical Management) from the National Committee for Quality Assurance (NCQA) for MCO quality assurance require review of lists of preferred pharmaceuticals at least annually by actively practicing practitioners and, without waiting for requests, updating procedures as new pharmaceutical information is received. In discussing formulary decisions for a large and popular drug class in 38 HMOs, Bajpai and Pathak (1998) suggested considering formulary additions of new drugs 6 months after their introduction. Lyles et al. (1997) reported that more than half of the 51 HMOs they surveyed reviewed and assessed more than half of new drug introductions. In a smaller survey of HMOs with a 41% response rate, 29 HMOs reported that they covered on average 62% of 38 newly introduced drugs. Coverage was as likely to take place in the year of introduction as later on (Chinburapa and Larson, 1991).

A long lag in adding newly approved drugs and low percentages of these drugs added to formularies were not unusual in pre-OBRA 1990 Medicaid programs. An average lag of 20 months was reported by Grabowski (1988). Addition of newly approved drugs ranged from 19% to 73% between 1970 and 1980 (Schweitzer and Shiota, 1992; Schweitzer et al., 1985). One large program (California) required a 6-month wait at a minimum (Sloan, 1989), but this is no longer the case. Most state Medicaid formularies are now open. New drugs are added without much delay (as a result of OBRA 1990 and 1993), although prior authorization or other restrictions may be in force for some drugs. At present, Medicaid MCOs may add new drugs immediately. For example, the Common-wealth of Pennsylvania (HC-SW PH RFP No. 10-97), requires addition within 10 days of FDA approval (see Chapter 5 of this report).

In the survey report of Mannebach et al. (1999), hospitals added an average of 18.2 drugs in the 12 months preceding the survey and deleted 16.4. Included were both new approvals and drugs already on the market. These are more than were added to the VA National Formulary. They are consistent with the average changes in VISN and local formularies, however. In a much smaller (20-hospital) and older study, similar results were obtained. On average, 27 drugs were added to the formularies, and of 30 new FDA-approved unique chemical entities, 13 were added (Quigley and Brown, 1981). Most (78.4%) hospitals have formal procedures for formulary additions, although it is unlikely that many carry out a complete review each year (Rascati, 1992). Nevertheless, in a national survey of 103 (66% of 156 contacted) short-term, nonfederal hospitals, Sloan et al. (1997) found that more than 90% reviewed their formularies periodically for ineffective and obsolete drugs and for therapeutic categories with high risk, volume, or expense.

The committee agreed with the VHA that new drugs should not automatically be added to the National Formulary. On the other hand, as noted above, the committee found the evidence to support a blanket policy of an automatic interval of 1 year before such drugs were considered weak, and the results across the VHA and VISNs inconsistent, at best. At worst, this policy denies veterans access to some drugs the FDA finds significant, provides questionable protection from adverse events, and fosters a perception that it is a cost-based measure. Given that the VA has an expert MAP, a more thoughtful approach, in the committee's view, would involve a policy of a prompt and careful assessment for inclusion on the National Formulary by medically qualified VA reviewers of newly approved drugs on their merits for veterans.

THE NONFORMULARY PROCESS

The nonformulary process and the policy that underlies it are discussed at some length in Chapter 4 of this report. The discussion is taken up here as well, because access to nonformulary products is integral to the restrictiveness of the National Formulary. There is no dispute that an exceptions process is necessary—in fact, vital—to a properly constituted and operating formulary system. Provision for access to therapeutic alternates makes sense clinically. Policy statements consistently include a nonformulary process as an essential component of a formulary system (AAHP, 1998; ACP, 1990; AHA, 1974; AMA, 1994; ASHP, 1983). Francke (1967) expressed this clearly and succinctly more than 30 years ago. "Formulate procedures for obtaining nonformulary drugs which are simple, fair and reasonable, and do not involve needless delays and complicated technicalities." A nonformulary process is also required by accrediting bodies such as the NCQA (UM 10 Procedures for Pharmaceutical Management—"an easily understood process to request an exception . . . in a time frame that is appropriate") and the JCAHO.

The VHA has had nonformulary procedures in its facilities for many years. VHA Directive 97-047 set criteria for approving exceptions to the National Formulary and mandated that each VISN have a nonformulary process in place for VHA facilities in its region. The approval criteria include contraindications to, adverse reactions to, or therapeutic failure of the formulary on drug(s); lack of a formulary alternate; or previous response to, or stability of, a nonformulary agent. In 1999, based on its computer tracking of actual dispensing (which is likely to be accurate), the VHA reported that 3.45% of prescriptions were filled with nonformulary drugs (DVA, VHA Nonformulary Drug Use Process, 1999). Although the percentage contributions to expenditures of a number of popular nonformulary drugs in closed or preferred classes are on the FY 1998 list of top 200 dollar-expenditure drugs from the prime vendor (for example, omeprazole, pravastatin, atorvastatin, leuprolide, doxazosin), these do not add up to 3%, and it is likely that VHA nonformulary drug costs as well as volume represent less than 5% of total costs or volume.

These VHA nonformulary volume or cost data appear relatively restrictive in comparison to data from hospitals and MCOs. Sloan et al. (1997) collected information on hospital self-rating of formulary restrictiveness, expenditures on nonformulary drugs, and monitoring of prescriber performance. They proposed that the restrictiveness of a hospital's formulary was related, at least in part, to whether less than 5% of the drug budget was spent on nonformulary products (and to whether physicians were monitored for excessive use of nonformulary drugs). By this criterion, one of the few existing quantitative standards of restrictiveness, 60% of hospitals had restrictive formularies (Sloan et al., 1997). In MCOs, on average, 10% of prescriptions are filled with nonformulary drugs (Hoechst Marion Roussel, 1998).

In 1999, the VHA reported that the percentage of nonformulary volume in the VA National Formulary closed classes was between 4 and 6%. The just-noted lower overall nonformulary figure of 3.45% may therefore be somewhat misleading. It primarily reflects nonformulary use of the majority of drugs, which are in open classes where local preferences can influence expanded choice, and therefore lessened interest in nonformulary products at the VISN or local facility level. The 4 to 6% values presumably originate from contract adherence reports which show 5% or so nonadherence in some closed classes in some VISNs (see VISN 13 PPI nonadherence of 6.4% cited earlier, for example). These figures would be borderline indicators of restrictiveness by the Sloan et al. (1997) criterion.

In Chapter 4 of this report, the VA nonformulary process is reported to be often informal, unstandardized, and variable across VISNs and facilities. This assessment was based on one or more contacts to discuss nonformulary procedures and results with prescribing and/or pharmacy personnel in all 22 VISNs. VISN nonformulary request forms were examined when available. Nonformulary activity was described as often oral and unrecorded. The waiver request forms and processes were discovered to differ in administrative complexity in some VISNs. Not all VISNs had standard forms. The procedures for assessing and acting on a request appeared to require different amounts of time in different VISNs or facilities. A number of scenarios in which nonformulary drugs were prescribed or requested and no formal nonformulary record was likely to be maintained were explored with VISNs and facilities by IOM staff and confirmed. It was not possible to assess the frequency of any of these scenarios, however.

The committee appreciates that brief consultations between pharmacists and prescribers in clinical settings have ample historical and ongoing precedent (Gray, 1992). These consultations or informal telephone discussions with the pharmacy may represent the most rapid and efficient way to implement a nonformulary process and make nonformulary decisions for prescribers, pharmacists, and patients. Informal and unrecorded behavior may result in the distortion of VHA statistics and perceptions of uneven formulary enforcement, however. Such behavior is understandable in the case of discussions and advice in the clinic, perhaps less so when oral requests are refused, and questionable when nonformulary prescriptions actually reach the pharmacy. Accordingly, the committee had reservations about VHA data on the total number of nonformulary requests, the percentage request approval or denial, or the time parameters for processing requests. As noted earlier, the VHA did not implement quarterly VISN written reporting justifying nonformulary utilization in classes where national standardization contracts have been awarded. Those reports that are made are oral, so the committee was also handicapped in assessing reasons for nonformulary use or denial.

In addition, reporting in the VA 1998 survey that the nonformulary process was easy or difficult to use came from physician P&T committee chairs. Data were collected and facilitated through the VISN formulary leader. Since "easy" and "difficult" are subjective characterizations reported by participants in the nonformulary request process to their central managers, these descriptions may mean different things to different people. In terms of administrative ease or time to completion, the committee was as concerned that there might be patient care settings with significant delays in response to requests for nonformulary drugs as with average response time. In some cases, the nonformulary process includes review by the facility's P&T committee. This means that requests could take considerable time to be approved or denied.

Therefore, the committee was not comfortable comparing details of the VISN nonformulary process with experiences reported by other systems. Available non-VHA hospital data on the number of nonformulary prescriptions or requests and the percentage of approvals are quite variable; some hospitals exercise tight controls, others essentially allow unchecked nonformulary use (Casio and Williams, 1982; Jay et al., 1993; Packer et al., 1986; Sloan et al., 1997). Prior authorization for nonformulary drugs is employed by 69 to 82% of MCOs and, for all purposes, by up to 90% of MCOs (see Table 2.1 and Figure 2.5). Some MCOs do not have formularies (or their formularies are not restrictive)

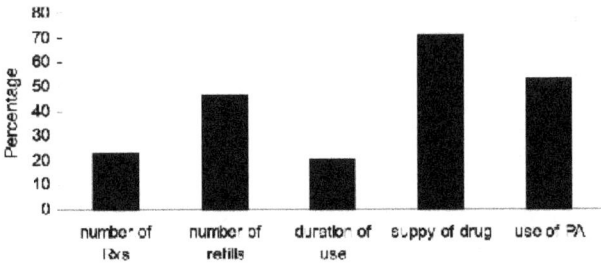

FIGURE 2.5 Limitations by percent of private-sector plans. NOTE: Number of Rxs = limits on the total number of prescriptions allowed per year; number of refills = limits on the number of refills per Rx; duration of use = limit on the length of time an Rx can be prescribed; supply of drug = limit on the quantity of drug the patient can have at one time (e.g., a 30-day supply); use of PA = requires prior authorization before drug can be prescribed and dispensed. SOURCE: Academy of Managed Care Pharmacy (January 2000).

however, and many also control physician prescribing indirectly through variable copayments (Hoechst Marion Roussel, 1998; Novartis, 1999). About 80% of MCOs allow prescribers to override the formulary in some circumstances, and MCO or Medicaid rates of approvals of nonformulary or prior authorization requests vary from 70 to 90% or perhaps slightly higher (Hoechst Marion Roussel, 1998; Jones, 1998; Kreling et al., 1996; Phillips and Larson, 1997; Schweitzer and Shiota, 1992; Sloan, 1989). For HMOs, the result of formulary systems is that 90% of all prescriptions are filled with formulary drugs (Hoechst Marion Roussell, 1998), as noted earlier. In the experience of some committee members MCOs and PBMs are known also to have informal systems for considering non-formulary drugs (see also Table 2.1).

The reported VHA rate of approvals, 88%, may not include an unknown percentage of informal nonformulary approaches and subsequent rebuffs, as previously stated. The reported individual VHA facility percentages vary from 50 to 100%, but IOM staff discussions with local personnel suggest that approval rates may be lower if oral refusals are counted and that 100% approval rates may sometimes reflect reporting artifacts. Recorded counts of requests in the VHA 1998 survey varied from 2 per month to 718 per month, probably due to differing sizes of facilities, real differences in request rates, and different counting customs (Chapter 4 of this report). The committee observed that coincident with implementation of a new nonformulary request procedure, the reported number of requests in the facility recording 718 requests per month was reduced by half. In the current nonformulary system, some facilities may be reporting substantial undercounts.

The character of these data and the incomplete data from other health care settings impair assessment of the contribution of the nonformulary process to the restrictiveness of the VA National Formulary or comparison to the restrictiveness of other formularies. Variation in the process probably depends in part on local custom. Tension between medical staff prescribers and those responsible for pharmacy who understand that expanding drug budgets may obligate difficult savings in other budgets probably accounts for another part. Medical practice patterns, pharmaceutical sales activities, patient demographics, and other factors likely also play a role. Evaluations of the effect of the nonformulary process on restrictiveness could be supplemented by examination of prescriber and patient opinions (and complaints) and of policies, procedures, and outcomes regarding formulary-driven therapeutic interchange. These are discussed below.

Changes in the nonformulary process should be considered with a view toward providing better program data, improving prescriber and patient acceptance of the National Formulary, and softening perspectives on its restrictiveness. This will not be easy. As the National Formulary matures, and if compliance remains at high levels or even improves, a policy of retrospective interventions might be entertained. At least some pilot tests as proposed in Chapter 4 of this report should be considered. This would entail budget assignments and feedback to prescribers or follow-up corrective education on retrospective review and identification of prescriber patterns of excessive or medically unjustified nonformulary use. Computerized data on drug utilization by prescriber could make this possible. This recommendation should not imply committee disapproval of reasonable formulary enforcement. Price negotiations will not be effective if prescribing is not directed to appropriately selected formulary drugs or drug products.

THERAPEUTIC INTERCHANGE

In managing the National Formulary and the pharmacy benefit, the VHA (with the National Acquisition Center) closes classes, and/or negotiates national standardized (committed-use) contracts or blanket purchase agreements with manufacturers for drugs in the classes or other classes, and/or issues national usage criteria or restrictions. In those situations, anticipated or promised volume supports better prices, which is, after all, one of the main rationales for the formulary. To achieve the promised volume (or market share) and realize the better price and, therefore, the savings, there is an expectation that VHA prescribers will discontinue using nonformulary or noncontracted drugs so that veterans are not started on these agents or that they may convert veterans from nonformulary or noncontracted drugs to the preferred or formulary agents. This expectation is no different than the expectation and practice in many U.S. hospitals and MCOs, as noted elsewhere. Interchange without individual prescriber permission at the time of dispensing is not uncommon in the VHA, however. Exchanges can be made by the pharmacy on authorization by the chair of the P&T committee without consulting each prescriber. The (prescribing and) dispensing by the pharmacist of a "therapeutically equivalent," pharmaceutically different drug than that prescribed for a patient by the physician (that is, therapeutic interchange with therapeutic alternates) is specifically authorized by the VA (VA Manual, M-2, Part 1, Chapter 3, Clinical Programs, Pharmacy and Therapeutics Committee, December 13, 1993).

Most therapeutic interchange in the VHA has been in closed classes or with a few popular drug products in other classes. These include situations in which there are price differentials, high volume, national contracts or usage criteria, current or former class closures, or VISN as well as national purchase agreements or contracts. In these situations the local facility, VISN, or VHA is anticipating target volume and target contract prices or responding to significant existing price differences to make savings in drug budgets (see reference to VHA reports below).

VHA investigators have published a number of reports describing therapeutic interchange programs in VA facilities in the 1990s. Additional reports have been presented at meetings but not published, and some less formal program data are also available. These reports often suffer from one or more of the following: small numbers, short follow-up, incomplete data and monitoring, and lack of controls, among others (Bartlett et al., 1996; Boston and Collins, 1995; Brunsting and Johnson, 1997; Cantrell et al., 1999; Desai et al., 1997; Edwards et al., 1998; Ganz and Saksa, 1997; Gray, 1999; Gustin et al., 1996; Ito et al.,

1999; Jones, 1999; Kellick et al., 1995; Kinnon et al., 1999; Lederle and Rogers, 1990; Lin et al., 1999; Lindgren-Furmaga et al., 1991; Minnich et al., 1997; Patel et al., 1999; Rindone and Arriola, 1998; Sprague and Gray, 1998; Stanaszek et al., 1997; Stock and Kofoed, 1994, Vivian et al., 1999). Therapeutic interchange in these reports, and in the VA in general, has been driven primarily by cost considerations (through contract and usage criteria adherence).

Some VA interchanges have been clinically successful (for example, see Boston and Collins, 1995; Cantrell et al., 1999; Ganz and Saksa, 1997; Jones, 1999; Kellick et al., 1995; Kinnon et al., 1999; Lin et al., 1999; Patel et al., 1999; Rindone and Arriola, 1998; Sprague and Gray, 1998: Vivian et al., 1999), but some have had clinical problems (for example, see Bartlett et al., 1996; Brunsting and Johnson, 1997; Desai et al., 1997; Minnich et al., 1997, Stanaszek et al., 1997; Stock and Kofoed, 1994). Economic outcomes have also been mixed because it may take time for the savings from a less expensive drug to pay back switching costs (Lindren-Furmaga et al., 1991), or savings from drug costs may have been offset by increases in other costs (Bartlett et al., 1996). On balance, however, most reports of therapeutic interchange have been encouraging, or at least reassuring, especially those describing more recent efforts.

A survey of 192 HMOs reported in 1988 that 30.5% used therapeutic interchange. Those that did not were concerned about physician dissatisfaction, interference with physicians' prerogatives to prescribe according to their best judgment, and the legality of substituting (Doering et al., 1988). Other surveys find that therapeutic interchange is an accepted practice in managed care that is becoming more prevalent each year. The Hoechst Marion Roussel survey (1998) reported 35.2% of plans allowing therapeutic interchange in 1997. Novartis (1998) reported that 47.7% of HMOs made use of therapeutic interchange in 1997; this survey projected an increase to 61.4% for 1999, and reported 56.5% of plans using therapeutic interchange in 1998 (Novartis, 1999). A survey of pharmacy benefits managers of employer plans in 1997 found 53.5% using therapeutic interchange (Wyeth-Ayerst, 1998).

The IOM committee noted that some of the VA drug classes involved in therapeutic interchange are also among those most often (more than 80%) subject to interchange in MCOs that practice interchange. These are antiulcerative (PPIs and H_2R blockers), antihypertensive (ACEIs, CCBs, and alpha blockers), and cholesterol-lowering drugs (HMG CoA RIs) (Hoechst Marion Roussel, 1998; Wyeth-Ayerst, 1998). Some classes that are commonly controlled through interchange in managed care, such as expensive antibiotics, are left to local discretion by the VHA. Patterns of use also reflect local microbial resistance patterns. Other commonly interchanged classes in MCOs, such as antihistamines and anti-inflammatories, are limited to a few members in the VA National Formulary but are open to respond to local preferences at the VISN or VA medical center level (Hoechst Marion Roussel, 1998). Many of these classes are also reported involved in interchange in hospital programs. The committee concludes that they are also classes that have therapeutic alternates and price differentials, where therapeutic interchange is both medically and economically reasonable, provided there is a provision for access to nonformulary therapeutic alternates when clinically necessary.

Therapeutic interchange has been carried out in hospitals for decades, and reports from hospital and other programs have been mostly supportive, reflecting experiences similar to those described by the VHA (reviewed in Achusim, 1992; Brown and Clarke, 1992; Bull et al., 1999; Green et al., 1989; Guastella, 1988; McAllister et al., 1999; Rich, 1989; Smith et al., 1989; Wall and Abel, 1996). Problems are pointed out in some of these reviews and elsewhere (for example, Barksdale AFB, 1998; Richton-Hewitt et al., 1988). Recent surveys, some of them quite extensive, find that therapeutic interchange is allowed or practiced in almost all U.S. hospitals (Nash et al., 1993 [76%, about two-thirds without notifying the prescriber]; Reeder et al., 1997 [74.5%]; Sloan et al., 1997 [79%]), and Mannebach et al. [1999] found that 69% of hospitals had formal therapeutic interchange policies).

Therapeutic interchange is supported by professional groups, provided the permission of the prescriber is obtained. As discussed earlier in this report, in hospitals and other well-controlled settings, such as some staff or group model HMOs, P&T committees in communication with the medical staff can design therapeutic interchanges. These interchanges are often implemented after advance approval by the P&T committee and medical staff, or they can be specifically approved by individual prescribers. In other health care systems, outpatient and less well controlled settings, PBMs, IPAs, and the like, the prescribers permission is almost always sought at the moment of interchange (ACCP, 1993; ACP, 1990; AHA, 1974; AMA, 1994; AMCP, 1997; ASHP, 1982; Lipton et al., 1999; Zellmer, 1994).

State laws on interchange vary in details to some extent. Washington is the only state that has specifically recognized therapeutic interchange, however, and has limited it to hospitals. States are consistent in requiring prescriber approval of therapeutic interchange. In controlled settings, this may be achieved according to protocols designed under collaborative practice agreements or other arrangements in which physicians are advised and approve (AMA, 1994). In hospitals, for example, physicians agree to abide by hospital policies and procedures when joining the hospital staff (Fink et al., 1998). MCO, PBM, and Medicaid providers must abide by state laws, but in a federal system like the VA, VHA policies on therapeutic interchanges (see below) preempt these state laws.

In theory, therefore, therapeutic interchange in the VHA does not appear restrictive in comparison to other health care systems. Interchange is a common practice. It is used in relatively few therapeutic classes in the VHA, and these classes are often subject to interchange in hospitals and MCOs and are medically defensible. Articles in the medical literature from the VHA or elsewhere do not report serious problems with most interchanges. On the other hand, there are no national VHA guidelines on therapeutic interchange, and the committee did not find any written policies at the VISN level. Although interchanges may be initiated and specified at either the national, the VISN, or the local level, they are designed and implemented at the local facility level. As such, they respond to local practices and need not be nor are they, consistent across the VHA. Some veterans subject to interchanges, when surveyed, report not having received adequate, or any, information on the replacement drug (see Chapter 4 ; W.N. Jones, personal communication, VISN 18, 1999). This suggests that informing veterans of interchanges could be improved even in VISNs that have experienced and thoughtful pharmacy leadership that tries to inform patients. Consideration might be given to having the responsible physician deliver the information in person.

Variation in some elements of therapeutic interchange to reflect local preferences and practice patterns may be desirable. Consistency in other elements might be important in ensuring program quality and patient and prescriber acceptance. In Chapter 1 of this report it was suggested that these elements might profitably include adequate advance notice and education on relative dosing and other factors for physicians and patients. Attention to patient compliance, provision for exceptions to conversion, and nonformulary access to an alternate or return to the original drug were also important considerations. Other elements included protections for at-risk patients, avoidance of frequent interchange or switching sick patients who were stable on a particular drug, and various methods of clinical and economic monitoring. The interchangeability of drugs in a class has to be evaluated with some care and expertise (McAllister et al., 1999). VA contracts are annually renewable. Drug prices, and therefore contracts, may change. At some point, the VHA will have to evaluate how frequently veterans taking a drug chronically should be subjected to interchange or the total number of interchanges that is reasonable in an individual patient. It is always important that interchanges may affect a stable drug treatment regimen, and from the veteran's perspective are involuntary and may not be well understood.

Lacking national or regional guidance or convincing evidence of a flexible and responsive nonformulary process, therapeutic interchange programs in facilities may appear inconsistent or restrictive to prescribers and patients regardless of where they originate. Concerns about clinical monitoring, compliance, economic data, assessment of patient satisfaction, dosing problems, and varying observation periods were expressed in some published or unpublished reports of VHA therapeutic interchange (Bartlett et al., 1997; Brunsting and Johnson, 1997; W.N. Jones; personal communication, VISN 18, 1999; Lederle and Rogers, 1990; Minnich et al., 1997; Rindone and Arriola, 1998; Vivian et al., 1999). For the most part, they were of minor import, and the overall conclusions of most of these reports were reassuring.

Patient and physician complaints about the National Formulary and access to needed, or at least desired, drugs are often related to therapeutic interchange programs and indicate a level of dissatisfaction. Patient complaints about access to drugs are a very small fraction (0.4%) of veteran complaints to patient advocates. Physician surveys tend to reinforce the concern that some therapeutic interchange programs may appear, or in fact be, restrictive from the perspective of prescribers. Interchange without individual prescriber permission may lead to patient or prescriber dissatisfaction unless the setting is controlled and those involved and affected have been adequately consulted and informed. These issues are discussed in Chapter 4 of this report and reviewed briefly below.

Much of the detail on therapeutic interchange programs and the nonformulary system is at the local level. Analysis of the restrictiveness of the National Formulary in comparison to other formularies and assessment of the contribution of therapeutic interchange to restrictiveness would benefit from data from the majority of the 172 VA hospitals. Time and resources did not allow the IOM to gather these data. Nevertheless, the committee found that some conclusions on this important issue were possible. The success of the National Formulary in providing leverage to negotiate low drug prices depends on the ability of the VHA to make choices among drug products and deliver volume, or drive market share as it is often described. Conversion of prescribing to the formulary or contract agent and actual interchange of drugs in existing treatment regimens support the responsiveness of the health care system to such choices and contractual terms. Restrictiveness will depend on how well the conversions are made. Factors include adequate access to original or other nonformulary agents when indicated, protection of at-risk patients who may not do well in interchange programs, and education of prescribers and patients among others. Concerns in some of these cases have been raised in the discussions above, and improvements suggested. On balance, however, the committee concluded that available information did not provide any convincing evidence that access to needed drugs is overly restricted.

OTC DRUG COVERAGE, GENERIC SUBSTITUTION, AND PHYSICIAN SATISFACTION

As noted earlier, there are 170 OTC listings on the VA National Formulary. These include nutritional supplements, ointments and lotions, nose drops and sprays, vitamins and minerals, laxatives and antacids, insulin and diabetic supplies, eye and ear drops and irrigating syringes, cough and cold remedies, analgesics and antipyretics, topical antibacterials, and antihistamines among others. The National Formulary also includes three H_2R blockers and nonsteroidal anti-inflammatory drugs (NSAIDs), but as the prescription not the OTC agents. There may be no price advantage to the OTC version for these drugs, given that they are mostly generic, and the OTC version is generally half the usually prescribed dose.

Coverage of OTC drugs is categorized as both a pharmacy benefit and a medical benefit in surveys of MCOs. Few HMOs offer OTC drugs as a specific pharmacy benefit, 7.3% in 1997 (Hoechst Marion Roussel, 1998) or 9.9% in 1999 (estimated) (Novartis, 1998). Nevertheless, OTC drugs in a number of therapeutic classes are often available in MCOs. The estimated percentage of HMOs including coverage in 1998 for insulin and diabetic supplies was 90.9%; for antihistamines, 50%; for H_2R blockers, 36.4%; for cough and cold remedies, 40.9%, for NSAIDs, 31.8%; and for vitamins, 22.7% (Novartis, 1998). In 1997, only 11% of employer pharmacy benefit plans excluded insulin and syringes, and 30% excluded prenatal vitamins (Wyeth-Ayerst, 1998). PBMs infrequently manage OTC benefits; when they do so, these are primarily insulin and diabetic supplies, but occasionally also cough and cold remedies and rarely H_2R blockers and antihistamines (Novartis, 1998). Recent data from a subset of PBMs and MCOs surveyed by the AMCP are consistent with low levels of PBM OTC coverage (Table 2.1).

About 12 state Medicaid programs cover very few or no OTC drugs. Most other states cover a majority or occasionally all of the listed categories of OTC drugs, sometimes with prior authorization, sometimes in institutions only. Usually only a limited number of drugs in a category are covered. Medicaid recipients in managed care would presumably receive the same OTC benefit package as those in fee-for-service Medicaid. Categories of OTC drugs variably covered by states include allergy drugs, cough and cold preparations, analgesics, antacids and H_2R blockers, topicals, feminine products, laxatives, vitamins, and a few others (NPC, 1997, 1998). The committee concluded that the VA National Formulary appears to be less restrictive in covering OTC drugs than MCOs or the Medicaid program.

Generic Substitution

The VA National Formulary uses generic terminology and practices generic substitution. Brand name drugs are used when there is no generic alternative, as nonformulary exceptions, and in five instances where there are concerns about the bioequivalence of generic versions of the drug (although some of these are under review). Standardized national contracts or local purchase agreements are available for some generics when good prices can be negotiated from a single generic manufacturer. This process is simply another form of generic substitution and, therefore, unexceptional. Generic prescribing and generic substitution are reasonable from a medical, pharmacological, and economic standpoint. They constitute a near-universal practice, sanctioned in state law and by the FDA (FDA, 1999a). The use of generics in the VHA exceeds that in the private sector or health care generally. The VHA in the four quarters ending in July 1999 purchased from the prime vendor 64% generics and 36% branded products amounting to 9% of total expenditures for generics and 91% for branded product (VHA data submitted in response to IOM questions). Comparable U.S. figures, cited earlier, were 47% of volume and 8% of dollar sales (Barents LLC, 1999a).

Generic substitution was described as an accepted practice in the introduction to this report. In hospitals, it is usually automatic, that is, carried out on dispensing regardless of the specification on the prescription (for example, 94% of hospitals in the survey reported by Sloan et al., 1997). About half of the states require dispensing of the genetic drug, if there is one, in their Medicaid programs (NPC, 1998), and all states have laws addressing this issue in varying ways. In 1997, 97.7% of MCOs made use of generic substitution, and 43.8% of prescriptions were for a generic drug (Novartis, 1998). In 1998, HMO generic product utilization was 45.6%, accounting for 21.9% of drug expenditures (Novartis,

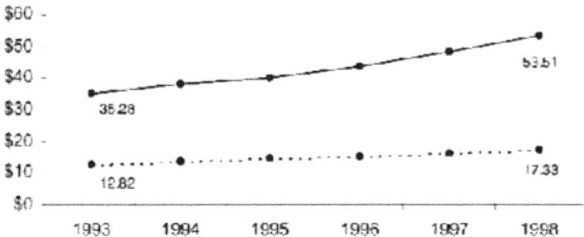

FIGURE 2.6 Average prices per prescription are lower for the generic version. SOURCE: Generic Pharmaceutical Industry Association.

1999). All PBMs have genetic substitution programs, and 50% of employer plans use these (Novartis, 1998). Mandatory substitution was reported for 38% of the covered lives in the recent AMCP survey (Table 2.1). Hoechst Marion Roussel (1998) reported that 63.8% of HMOs required genetic substitution in 1997 and 43.8% of prescriptions were filled generically. The committee concluded that generic prescribing and substitution have no implications for the restrictiveness of the National Formulary. Cost savings are undoubtedly realized (Smith, 1993), given the known differences between average prescription prices for generic and brand name drugs (see Figure 2.6).

Veterans' Complaints

Complaints from veteran patients collected by the VHA patient advocates and the VSOs are reviewed in Chapter 4 of this report. Patient complaints are anecdotal self-reports. Lacking a denominator (that is, a defined group at risk) except for the total population of users of VHA facilities, they are numerator data only. As collections of incidents, representing an unknown percentage of an unknown relevant population, they can function only as generators of hypotheses about the subject matter of complaints, not as scientifically valid evidence. To become evidence, data on events described in complaints would have to be gathered in careful surveys of scientifically selected representative cohorts, validated by chart review or patient examination, and analyzed statistically in comparison to a control group. In any case, veteran complaints about access to drugs comprise only about 0.4% of total complaints and overwhelmingly concern nonformulary drugs, the largest category (about 10% of drug-related complaints) being about access to sildenafil. These data suggest that some veterans believe they are not getting the drugs they need (or want) or that their physicians think they need and are prescribing. Complaints also suggest that veterans feel inconvenienced.

The committee concluded that these data were consistent with taking a closer look, as noted earlier, at some aspects of the formulary process including addition of new existing and new FDA-approved drugs, the nonformulary process, and programs of therapeutic interchange. Action to change or improve these elements of the national formulary system would then be based on such analyses, not on complaints or anecdotes. However, if the numbers of complaints are any guide, these issues are not major concerns of veterans at present. The committee recognizes that as a practical matter, the VHA cannot routinely investigate issues based on complaints that amount to less than 1% of total complaints. These issues merit the attention of the VHA for the reasons cited in this IOM report. They are also concerns of a significant minority of VA physicians, have political salience and wider health care implications, and are part of a new clinically and economically important process, the National Formulary, that should be evaluated like any significant change.

VA Physician Satisfaction

In 1998, 1 year after implementation of the National Formulary, the VA PBM in consultation with the RAND Survey Research Group surveyed 4,536 VA physicians, more than half of them general internists, and received responses from 2,952, or 45.2% (Glassman et al., 1999). The objective of this survey was to evaluate the effect of the National Formulary on access to drugs, quality of care, and physician efficiency as seen from the perspective of VA physicians caring for veterans in the VHA. Although most VA physicians (82%) were aware of the formulary, only 32% had actually referred to it, according to the survey. Most clinicians agreed that they could prescribe the drugs needed for their patients, but 29% felt that the National Formulary impinged on quality of care and 37% felt it was more restrictive than formularies in the private sector. Overall, most VA physicians were either neutral or positive about the effects of the VA National Formulary on care to veterans.

Somewhat similar results emerged from a much smaller January 1999 telephone survey. Yankelovich Partners (1999) completed interviews of 418 VA physicians from a sample of 2,810 who could be reached or agreed to respond. The total available cohort consisted of a privately generated roster of 6,288 physicians in a wide variety of specialties. This survey, in part designed by and wholly financially supported by Pfizer, Inc., found fewer VA physicians very familiar with, and more with negative experiences or perceptions regarding, the National Formulary (Yankelovich Partners, 1999).

The committee noted problems with the RAND study, some of which had also been identified by the VHA. The sample was drawn from subscribers to a VA journal, and it was not clear whether this was, therefore, a random sample or whether it was a group of physicians especially interested in VA matters. Less than half of those contacted responded, which represents an insufficient response rate. Respondents were allowed to report whether the formulary improves care or access, not whether it reduces quality or access, a serious flaw. Minority, but still substantial, percentages of respondents reported they could not prescribe needed drugs (29%) and that their workload had increased (34%). This seemed a high number and was of concern to the committee. Some VA physicians might have confused the national list and system with VISN or local formularies and systems. For the purposes of this report, as defined by the terms of the VA agreement with the IOM, all formularies are considered part of the National Formulary, but identification of the exact locus of problems would be important in considering solutions. In any event, the committee concluded that this survey supported taking a closer look at certain aspects of the National Formulary, among them the nonformulary process, therapeutic interchange programs, and the relationship between VISN or local activities and National Formulary policies and procedures. Similar conclusions were reached by the authors of this survey report (Glassman et al., 1999).

The committee noted that the Yankelovich study was also unpublished and not peer reviewed. It suffered from small numbers. Only 14.8% of those who were reached ultimately completed the interview, an inadequate sample. This study asked respondents about negative effects and so could be expected to have results less supportive of the National Formulary and formulary system (Yankelovich Partners, 1999). Truly credible surveys of VA physicians await the design and implementation of such instruments by completely independent experts in a process independent of the VA or any other parties at interest. A survey currently being carried out by GAO for the second report on the VA National Formulary could satisfy this need.

A few additional surveys of physician satisfaction were available to the committee. Others have observed that if prescribers report that a formulary does not impair quality of care, there may be less reason for concern about a formulary and formulary system (Gross, 1998). Furthermore, it is generally agreed, and the committee concurs, that "physician support is essential to the success of a formulary, and refusal by doctors to cooperate with formularies may greatly reduce anticipated savings" (Nash et al., 1992). In 1990, Nash et al. (1992) sent a short, 20-question survey to 5,000 primary care physicians involved in managed care and selected randomly from a list of 51,000 national MCO physicians. Only 9.96% of those contacted returned usable surveys. This survey found high rates (49%) of negative opinions and concern that formularies address costs only, although most respondents reported that formulary compliance required little effort.

A 1997 report described a survey of New York physicians' opinions on managed care formularies also with a very low (17%) response rate (Green, 1997). This and an accompanying pharmacist survey found substantial dissatisfaction with formulary choices and therapeutic interchange. The low response rate in these two surveys prevents drawing any reliable conclusions, although the results may help to identify areas that are in need of further examination. Black et al. (1988) carried out an informal survey of opinions of physicians in an IPA about a newly introduced formulary with more than 1,300 choices. Among 179 (35.8%) of 500 physicians surveyed, 49.7% found the formulary somewhat or very difficult to work with, 59.8% found it somewhat disruptive of prescribing practices, and 24% indicated that the quality of patient care was reduced or (1.1%) greatly reduced. Many physicians reported that the formulary was too restrictive in some (39.7%) or all (3.9%) areas. These physician surveys suggest that physician acceptance of formularies is an area that warrants continued attention.

It is generally accepted that patient (and likely provider) satisfaction is an indicator of quality of care. A national survey of consumers found that they usually did not perceive their physicians' prescribing to be limited by prescribing restrictions. Only 15.6% overall, and 21.7% in managed care, knew of some restrictions (Novartis, 1998). However, consumers also rated prescription drug coverage as one of the top three reasons for selecting an HMO, and what they liked best about the pharmacy benefit was low prices, that all their prescriptions were filled, and that they received the drugs they wanted (Copyright © CareData Reports, Inc., in Wilson and Burke, 1999). Surveys like this and experience from the VHA, in times of rapidly escalating drug costs, indicate that the pharmacy benefit is important to enrollees in managed care and veterans using VA health care (Novartis, 1998). It is clear that there is a direct relationship between restrictions on how services are provided and received and provider and patient satisfaction (Navarro and Cahill, 1999). The committee appreciates this normal human tendency to want unfettered access to all available benefits without economic or other restriction. Nevertheless, VA patient complaints and VA (and other) prescriber dissatisfaction should be taken seriously. They suggest that some elements of formulary design and implementation in health care generally and in the VHA specifically should at least be reviewed.

SUMMARY

As is almost always the case in public policy, data to inform and support conclusions and recommendations about the National Formulary are incomplete. Nevertheless, the committee concludes that the information in this chapter and other chapters of this report is sufficient to suggest directions and could be usefully considered by the VHA and congressional policy makers in evaluating possible decisions about the VA National Formulary and formulary system. All of the questions that Congress asked the IOM committee to consider are highly relevant and important. This chapter on restrictiveness defines and addresses one key overall effect of the VA National Formulary. This was first among the effects or issues raised in House Report 105-610 and the VA–IOM contract. In discussions here, the committee has described how formularies, or lists of drugs, can be managed through the use of elements of restrictiveness and other management approaches, to affect access to and cost of a pharmacy benefit. The restrictiveness of the formulary can be assessed, admittedly to some extent as a judgment, but also by objectively evaluating what controls are employed, how they are used, and how they compare to restrictions and controls used in managing other formularies, public and private. In analyzing the National Formulary and formulary system in this way, the committee found that it had characteristics that were sometimes more but often less restrictive than other formularies and formulary systems. The committee has used the information and analyses here to support its conclusions and recommendations. They can be found in the Executive Summary of this report, beginning with the overall conclusion that the National Formulary does not meet the committee's definition of overly restrictive. The committee hopes that the information, analyses, conclusions, and recommendations here might also guide policy evaluations by others.

3

What Are the Potential Costs to VA Health Care Associated with the National Formulary for Drugs?

INTRODUCTION

The VHA is one of the largest purchasers of pharmaceuticals in the United States. Under a decentralized system where VA facilities made local formulary decisions, the VHA was unable to take advantage of its potential bargaining power with manufacturers, particularly for classes of drugs used commonly by the veteran population. Among the stated objectives of the VA National Formulary are standardization of the pharmacy benefit and increased portability across the country. In addition, the National Formulary should help to consolidate the bargaining power of the VHA with pharmaceutical manufacturers, with one result being lower prices and reduced pharmaceutical spending relative to what spending would have been in the absence of this policy intervention. This chapter examines the effect of the National Formulary on pharmaceutical costs for the VHA.

The National Acquisition Center (NAC) negotiates and administers contracts for pharmaceuticals (in addition to other items used by the VHA). The NAC reports substantial savings resulting from implementation of the National Formulary and all its other contracting responsibilities for the VHA over the past 4 years. As of February 11, 2000, total pharmaceutical savings (including savings on pharmaceutical supplies) associated with the full range of NAC activities are estimated by the NAC to be at least $572,521,352 for the period FY 1996 to FY 2000. The NAC defines savings as the difference between its estimate of actual spending and what it estimates would have been spent on the affected pharmaceuticals in the absence of these activities.[1]

---

[1] This estimate includes savings achieved from generic drug contracts but does not include savings achieved through all blanket purchase agreements (BPAs). Only savings accruing from BPAs for alpha blockers and for selective serotonin reuptake inhibitors are included. The estimate is calculated by multiplying the price change for a given item resulting from NAC contracting activities by the quantity of that item used in the previous year.

The estimate includes savings accruing to the VHA for a variety of items including drugs in closed and preferred classes on the National Formulary; blanket purchase agreements (BPAs) (described below) for selective serotonin re-uptake inhibitors (SSRIs) and alpha blockers; exclusive contracts for generic drugs (that is, a contract purchasing all units of a generic drug from a single manufacturer); and bulk purchase of pharmacy-related supplies (for example, vials, sponges). The NAC estimate also captures any savings from the expiration of patents and subsequent generic competition. Although each of these items may have generated reductions in prices for the VHA, many (for example, brand patent expirations) are not attributable to the implementation of the National Formulary. In examining the cost impact of the VA National Formulary, this IOM analysis focuses narrowly on savings associated with prices negotiated for closed and preferred drug classes. As a result, this analysis produces a conservative estimate of the effects of VHA bargaining power associated with the National Formulary and national purchasing.

In this chapter, VA National Formulary savings in pharmaceutical expenditures are estimated as any reductions in pharmaceutical expenditures attributable to the National Formulary using a pre-/post-design that controls for changes in the size and characteristics of the veteran user population over time and across VISNs. This analytical approach allows an accounting of changes in both price and quantity resulting from adoption of the National Formulary. It focuses on the cost effects of the closed and preferred classes, the heart of the VA National Formulary. Because BPAs are sometimes used to forestall class closure (as described below), savings on selected BPAs could arguably also be attributed to the National Formulary. In part because the IOM committee could not assess the effect of BPAs on the decision to close classes, the committee's estimate represents an underestimate of the savings resulting from the National Formulary.

The committee addressed four primary questions in assessing the effect of the VA National Formulary on VHA costs: (1) How does the National Formulary affect prices for closed and preferred classes? (2) How does the National Formulary affect prescribing patterns within closed and preferred classes (that is, what is the level of compliance with the National Formulary for closed and preferred classes)? (3) How does the National Formulary affect pharmaceutical spending per veteran user for closed and preferred classes? and (4) Is there evidence that changes in formulary policy result in increased utilization elsewhere in the VHA system?

THE VHA NATIONAL FORMULARY AS IT AFFECTS COSTS

Background

The VA National Formulary uses a combination of formulary and contracting approaches, including closed, open, preferred, committed-use, and other contracts, and blanket purchase agreements. These different approaches can be considered along a continuum with respect to their influence over pharmaceutical decision making, with open classes exerting the least influence and closed the greatest. For open classes, the formulary places few restrictions on which drugs are preferred for VHA users. The vast majority of pharmaceutical classes on the National Formulary, 248 out of 254, are currently open (see Chapter 1 of this report). Prices for drugs in open classes are taken from the Federal Supply Schedule (FSS), a standard negotiated price schedule administered by the NAC and available for use by all federal agencies (unless a BPA offering a discounted price is in place, as described below).

In contrast, for closed classes, only a limited number of drugs in a class are included in the National Formulary. Other drugs in the class may not be listed on VISN or local formularies, and committed-use contracts are signed with the manufacturers that produce the selected National Formulary drugs. These class members must be used systemwide. Committed-use contracts are 1 year in duration with four optional 1-year renewals. As of February 2000, 4 of the 254 pharmaceutical classes on the National Formulary were closed (HMG CoA RIs, LHRHs, PPIs, ACEIs).[2] Two other classes were closed in the past but have since been reclassified. H_2R blockers were designated as open in August 1998, and alpha-blockers were designated as preferred in June 1998. Although the four closed classes represent a small fraction (<2%) of the total number of drug classes on the National Formulary, they account for 13% of all VHA pharmaceutical expenditures (GAO, 1999). In closing a drug class, the Medical Advisory Panel (MAP) decides that drugs within the class should be considered therapeutic alternates permitting therapeutic interchanges. Nevertheless, as described elsewhere in this report, a nonformulary exceptions process is administered at each VA medical facility to permit the use of nonformulary agents in closed classes if medically necessary.

In preferred classes, a limited number of drugs within a class are listed as preferred agents on the National Formulary. However, other agents in the class are available for use depending on VISN or local decisions. In designating a class as preferred, the MAP decides that drugs in the class are therapeutically interchangeable for the majority of patients. Typically, there is a significant

---

[2] The MAP has recommended closing two additional classes, but these closures had not been implemented as of February 28, 2000. A closed-class contract is expected to be awarded for the oral 5-hydroxytryptamine agents imminently. Although the MAP recommended closing the nonsedating antihistamines, a legal challenge from the manufacturer of one of the agents has delayed the awarding of contracts.

price differential across agents in classes considered for preferred status. In exchange for preferred status on the National Formulary, which in theory could change prescribing behavior, manufacturers have been willing to negotiate prices below the FSS. Currently, two classes, alpha blockers and calcium channel blockers (CCBs), use preferred contracting arrangements.

The VHA uses special contracting vehicles referred to as BPAs for a number of drug classes. Under BPAs, the NAC is able to extract some benefit beyond that derived from using the FSS (usually a lower price). Unlike committed-use contracts, BPAs can be terminated by the manufacturer at any time with 30 days notice. BPAs are desirable to manufacturers because they may lead to greater market share and, in fact, often link VHA market share and price. For example, the NAC uses a tiered contracting arrangement for felodipine, a CCB. The price paid by the VHA drops as the market share for this CCB increases.

Manufacturers may also sign a BPA in an attempt to prevent class closure or other threats to market share of their drug. One example is the case of Coumadin, an anticoagulant commonly used in the treatment of atrial fibrillation to prevent emboli. Although Coumadin was no longer under patent protection, the generic pharmaceutical equivalents, even though officially bioequivalent, were considered unsuitable for substitution by the VHA due to the narrow therapeutic index of the drug, despite Food and Drug Administration (FDA) findings of their suitability for substitution (FDA, 1999a). As a result, Coumadin was the dominant drug product in its class used by the VHA. Because of significant price differentials between the brand and generics, the VA PBM restudied this drug, considered a change to generic competition, and proposed an award to the lowest-price generic manufacturer. In response, the manufacturer of Coumadin (DuPont) agreed to a significantly lower price through a BPA, thereby fore-stalling this contracting shift.

In addition to BPAs, committed-use contracts like those used for closed classes are sometimes used for drugs in open classes as well. Under these arrangements, the VHA agrees to purchase a particular drug (for example, nifedipine, a generic CCB with many manufacturers) only from the contractor in exchange for a lower price. These arrangements are particularly common for generic drugs (that is, the NAC will contract with a single manufacturer to supply all units of a particular generic drug). Like BPAs, these contracts result in lower prices for the VHA and occur because of VHA bargaining power. BPAs and committed-use contracts for open classes differ with respect to contract terms, contract duration, and what the VHA promises in return for the lower price. BPAs typically link the price for a drug with its market share within the entire class. Such market share objectives can foster therapeutic interchanges with the BPA drug.

Since the National Formulary's adoption, the MAP has conducted 14 drug class reviews in order to decide whether to change the status of a class on the National Formulary from open to closed or preferred (see Table 1.2). Of these 14 classes, 6 have been closed to date. The status of two of these (H_2R blockers and alpha blockers) was subsequently changed as many of the class members became generic and OTC providing low-cost alternates. The MAP has also recommended closure of two of the other eight classes reviewed (oral 5-hydroxytryptamines 5[HT_3s] and nonsedating antihistamines). In most of the six classes that the MAP decided not to close, it felt that class members were reasonable therapeutic alternates based on analyses of safety and efficacy data. However, a decision was made that closure was not necessary because sufficient competition could be achieved by BPAs and genetic single-source contracts (see, for example, SSRIs at www.dppm.va.gov/newsite/reviews.html).

Basic Economics of the VA National Formulary

Consumers of prescription drugs within the VHA do not pay out-of-pocket for prescription drugs prescribed by VA physicians. VA physicians, who are central to decisions made about the use of prescription drugs, are typically salaried and face no direct financial incentive linked to pharmaceutical expenditures on their patients. The VHA uses another, less direct mechanism, common in the private sector, to affect prices paid for drugs—that is, a formulary to create market incentives for manufacturers to compete on price.

The VA National Formulary employs clinical knowledge about the safety and effectiveness of various prescription drugs to bolster the buying power of the VHA. Like most private-sector PBMs, the VHA buys generic drugs when they are available. When there are a number of therapeutic alternates within a class, the VHA can make choices and use this bargaining power to obtain favorable prices. In economic terms, the aim of the National Formulary is to make the demand for specific prescription drug products more responsive to price than might have been the case otherwise. It is the price response of the demand for specific products that confers bargaining power on a purchaser, or in industry jargon, it is the ability to "move market share" that leads to price concessions by manufacturers.

Formularies have become central to the pricing of brand name prescription drugs in the United States. Formularies increase a buyer's bargaining power, enabling buyers to be more aggressive in price negotiation. The ability to exclude certain products entirely or to shift demand significantly between competing products allows the buyer to present a seller with a more elastic (price-responsive) demand, thereby inducing a lower price. The greater the ability by buyers to direct the volume of prescriptions among competing products, the more elastic will be the demand for the product, and this results in enhanced bargaining power for the buyer. The basic economics of formularies has been recently summarized in the *Minnesota Prescription Drug Study* (Schondelmeyer, 1993). The VA National Formulary enhances the VHA's bargaining power in several specific therapeutic areas. The National Formulary has specific features that serve to move market share and, as a result, may enhance the VHA's bargaining position with manufacturers of prescription drugs. The presence of the National Formulary and the enhanced bargaining power it confers on the VHA may also affect, to some extent, classes of drugs that are neither closed or preferred.

Features of the National Formulary

The VHA represents a different type of health system compared to those under private insurance arrangements in the United States. The regional health systems of the VHA, known as VISNs, operate under fixed budgets. If the medical staff of a VISN make choices that forgo the opportunity to purchase supplies, devices, or pharmaceutical products at the most advantageous prices, the VISN budget will be less able to accommodate the needs of veterans in the region. Also, physicians are primarily employees of the VHA and obtain their patients almost exclusively through the VHA. For this reason they are likely to be more responsive to directives regarding prescribing policy than similar physicians in the private sector who contract with a number of health plans.

As discussed above, there are several specific features of the VA National Formulary that are used to move market share and enhance the VHA's bargaining power with manufacturers of prescription drugs, including closed classes, preferred classes, and BPAs. Because no other drugs can be added to local formularies for closed classes, and an exception must be granted to use a nonformulary drug, the closed classes in the VA National Formulary represent strong administrative directives to affect prescribing behavior. Any burden associated with a medical exceptions process also serves to encourage compliance with the formulary. Scientific drug class reviews justifying the closed classes and feed-back to clinicians provide education about use of the formulary. The VHA also shares information with VISNs on prescribing patterns and compliance with the National Formulary for both closed and preferred classes.

Preferred classes represent a weaker form of administrative directive. Under preferred classes, compliance with the formulary is encouraged through drug usage criteria and information about the preferred drugs and the conditions under which therapeutic interchange should take place.

The third main mechanism for moving market share is the BPA. VISN participation in BPAs is voluntary (although some BPAs are associated with official drug use criteria, CCBs), but they have a strong incentive to do so because of the lower prices typically offered through BPAs. VISNs may negotiate similar or better prices on their own, so the price for a given pharmaceutical in an open class may vary across VISNs. There is an implied threat that the VHA may close classes under a BPA if adequate performance (primarily in the form of low prices) is not realized. As noted earlier, BPAs are sometimes used by the VHA instead of closed or preferred arrangements. In these cases, the VHA's market power is strong enough that the mere threat of class closure can lead to significant price discounts from manufacturers.

Each of these mechanisms should produce three desirable results: (1) shifts in prescribing toward the closed or preferred products; (2) price concessions relative to open-class products and compared to the pre-National Formulary period; and (3) lower spending levels per veteran user for the classes of drugs subject to these management methods than would have occurred absent the policies of the National Formulary. The effects presumably will be strongest for the closed classes.

VISN Implementation Issues

Although the VHA uses a National Formulary, the formularies guiding prescribing decisions by physicians arc not uniform throughout the VHA system. Most of the 22 VISNs and 172 local hospitals continue to maintain a variably different formulary. For the four closed classes, the VA National Formulary and VISN or local formularies are exactly the same, although, as noted elsewhere, compliance with the national listings is not perfect. For all other classes, however, VISNs and medical centers are free to add agents to provide flexibility to respond to the needs of their regional or local populations. Although the VA PBM does not explicitly track differences in formulary content across VISNs and medical centers, the PBM estimates that the 22 VISN formularies include approximately 5,500 separate forms and dosages of pharmaceuticals that are not on the National Formulary (GAO, 1999).

VISNs and medical centers arc prohibited from altering the closed classes, but they have some flexibility in how quickly they implement national class closures. For the six classes that have been closed at any time, implementation of a national class closure at the VISN level has occurred anywhere from immediately to as long as 6 months after the national implementation date (see Table C.1 in Appendix C). Although there arc no explicit penalties for VISN or local failure to comply with VA National Formulary requirements, compliance (that is, use of the formulary agent) is greater than 90% overall for closed classes. This may flect local interest in achieving projected savings in drug spending.

Other Influences on VHA Pharmaceutical Spending

In the period spanning the development and implementation of the National Formulary, there have been a number of other possible influences on VHA pharmacy expenditures. First, there has been a shift away from inpatient care toward the use of outpatient services over the past few years (GAO, 1999; Kizer, 1999), a trend that likely increased the use of outpatient pharmacy. Second, the number of veterans accessing the VHA has been increasing (see VA Annual Reports). Pharmaceutical coverage outside the VHA has become more limited, especially for older age groups (Cook et al., 2000). As a result, the increase in VHA users may be disproportionately affecting the pharmacy budget. Veterans with other health care coverage may use the VHA system for their pharmaceuticals, although VHA policy is not to fill prescriptions written by other than VA prescribers. Also, VHA pharmaceutical spending has likely been affected by nationwide changes in drug treatments, as new, expensive drugs have become available and become an integral part of the treatment of chronic illnesses (GAO, 1999; Levit et al., 1998). To accurately estimate the effect of the VA National Formulary on pharmacy costs, the effects of these changes and trends must be separated from the effect of the National Formulary and formulary system.

ANALYTICAL FRAMEWORK

In estimating the cost impact of the VA National Formulary, the IOM committee focuses on the effect on expenditures for drugs of designating classes as closed or preferred. Using VHA data, changes were examined in pharmaceutical prices, market share for products within a drug class, and outpatient pharmacy spending per veteran user before and after implementation of closed and preferred classes for the National Formulary. Regression analyses were conducted to estimate the impact of the National Formulary on outpatient pharmaceutical spending per VHA user for closed and preferred classes, controlling for changes in the VHA system and its user population over time. Finally, the committee explored whether changes in formulary policy resulted in an increase in utilization elsewhere in the VHA system by studying discharge data for diagnoses of conditions likely to be affected by drugs in closed or preferred classes.

DATA

To assess the impact of the National Formulary on VHA expenditures, person-level data (including data on inpatient, outpatient, and pharmaceutical utilization) should be used to compare per-person expenditures for 1 to 2 years before and 1 to 2 years after National Formulary implementation. With person-level data on utilization across the VHA system, changes in pharmaceutical spending and in overall health care spending associated with National Formulary adoption could be examined. Consequently, whether changes in the National Formulary resulted in cost shifting from the pharmaceutical budget to the rest of the VHA budget could be assessed. If drug class closures that lead to favorable drug prices result in additional hospital admissions for complications resulting from a therapeutic interchange, total VHA expenditures might be increased even though VHA pharmacy expenditures decreased.

Because person-level utilization data for pharmaceuticals and other VHA health care services were unavailable until FY 1999 (2 years after National Formulary implementation), this analysis focuses instead on aggregate-level drug utilization data by month at the VISN level for each drug used in the VHA. The utilization data provided by the VA PBM were limited to the outpatient sector only for the period FY 1994 through July 1999. Data on 14 classes of pharmaceuticals were examined, 6 of which have been classified as closed or preferred at some point since National Formulary implementation (ACEIs, alpha-blockers, H_2R blockers, HMG CoA RIs, PPIs, and CCBs) and 8 that have remained open (atypical antipsychotics, SSRIs, beta-blockers, nonsedating antihistamines, NSAIDs, oral diabetics, inhaled antiasthma agents, and antiemetics). Utilization data on one closed class, LHRHs, were not available.

To create VHA pharmaceutical expenditure data at the month and VISN level, the average purchase price for each VA product in a given VISN and month was multiplied by the number of units of the product dispensed in that month and VISN.[3] Because the purchase price data that were provided covered the period January 1, 1995, through November 30, 1999, and the utilization data covered the period October 1, 1994, through July 31, 1999, the expenditure data are limited to the period of overlap between these two data sets, January 1, 1995, through July 31, 1999.

The VA PBM reported utilization data by VISN for 39 pharmaceutical products for which price information was not provided. (For the purposes of this analysis, a "product" refers to a particular dosage form of a drug, for example, cimetidine, 100-mg tablets.) Average monthly consolidated mail outpatient pharmacy (CMOP) prices (that is, prices from the VHA's seven automated mail order pharmacies) were available for four of these drugs.[4] For the remaining 35 products lacking price information, CMOP price data were also missing. Utilization data for these 35 products (representing a total of 5,121 prescriptions during the study period, or 0.005% of the total [97,619,839] prescriptions for the study period) were dropped from the analysis of expenditures. In addition, price data for 481 products were missing for a subset of VISN months for which utilization was reported. For these products, prices were imputed for the missing months by taking a moving average of prior and subsequent month's prices for the product.

To control for changes in the VHA user population over time, data by month by VISN were requested on the following: number of VHA pharmacy users (to calculate changes in pharmaceutical spending per user), age and gender distribution of users, and information on the severity of illness or case mix of the user population. The following information was provided: (1) the number of outpatient VHA users (the number of VHA pharmacy users was not available) and (2) the age and gender distribution of all VHA users. Information on case mix or severity of illness was not provided.

The committee explored the possibility that the National Formulary led to shifts in service utilization in other parts of the VHA. Aggregate data on the total number of inpatient discharges were collected. Data on the number of discharges for selected diagnoses that might be treated by drugs in certain closed or preferred classes by month by VISN for FY 1994 through July 1999 were examined. Analyses to assess relationships between discharges and VA National Formulary activities were performed and are discussed below.

---

[3] There will be some noise in an estimate produced using this approach because all products purchased in a given month are not necessarily used in that month. However, since prices do not typically change each month and most VA facilities do not stock large quantities of pharmaceuticals for long periods of time due to the relationship with the VHA's prime vendor (an exclusive contract with a single wholesaler), any bias resulting from this is likely to be small.

[4] At the suggestion of PBM staff, the average price across the seven CMOPs was used for four of the products for which purchase price information was unavailable.

EMPIRICAL METHODS

Trends in outpatient pharmaceutical prices, utilization, and spending per veteran outpatient user by month across VISNs were analyzed. These trends are presented in Figure 3.5, - Figure 3.25 and in Appendix C. Regression analyses to control for secular trends not related to National Formulary implementation, time-invariant unmeasured differences between VISNs, and changing demographics of the population were conducted. Two regression models were estimated, each with different dependent variables: (1) the natural logarithm of outpatient pharmacy spending per outpatient VHA user and (2) the natural logarithm of discharges for selected diagnoses potentially linked to closed or preferred classes divided by the number of veteran outpatient users.[5] The unit of observation for each model was a VISN-month. Independent variables in the models include VISN dummy variables, a quadratic time trend, gender distribution, age distribution, and an indicator representing the change in status for each class.

RESULTS OF THE IOM COMMITTEE ANALYSIS OF COST EFFECTS

How Have the VHA and the Veteran User Population Changed During the Study Period?

As noted above, both the size and the characteristics of the VHA user population changed during the study period. As seen in Figure 3.1, the number of outpatient users increased 43%, from 1,018,250 in October 1993 to 1,460,019 in October 1999. During this same period, the total number of inpatient discharges decreased 32%, from 73,660 in January 1994 to 50,000 in December 1999, as shown in Figure 3.2.[6] The veteran user population became slightly younger on average during this period. The proportion of users age 65 or older decreased from 50.1% in FY 1994 to 43.9% in FY 1999, as seen in Figure 3.3. Figure 3.4 shows that the gender distribution of users remained constant during this period, approximately 90% male.

How Has the National Formulary Affected Prices for Closed and Preferred Classes?

To explore the impact of enhanced bargaining power conferred by the National Formulary, price reductions resulting from National Formulary implementation

---

[5] The natural logarithm of the dependent variables was used because a proportional effect (as opposed to a linear effect) was expected and to address skewness in the distribution of the dependent variable.

[6] These numbers represent both discharges from VHA facilities and discharges of VHA users (paid for by the VHA) from non-VHA facilities. Non-VHA discharges are approximately 2 to 3% of total discharges for the VHA population.

TABLE 3.1 Price Changes for Most Commonly Prescribed Drugs in Closed Classes After National Formulary Class Closure

Drug (class)	Percentage Change
Lisinopril 10-mg tablets (ACEI)	41 ↓
Terazosin 5-mg capsules (alpha blocker)	27 ↓
Famotidine 20-mg tablets (H$_2$R blocker)	32 ↓
Simvastatin 10-mg tablets (HMG CoA RI)	25 ↓
Lansoprazole 30-mg capsules (PPI)	16 ↓

of closed and preferred classes were studied. The committee examined the average price change per pill across VISNs for the most commonly prescribed product in each affected class. To calculate the change in price for each product, the pre-National Formulary price calculated as the average VISN price over the 3 months before National Formulary adoption was compared with the post-National Formulary price calculated as the average VISN price over the 3 months after National Formulary adoption.

Figure 3.5, through Figure 3.10 illustrate the changes in price per pill after National Formulary implementation for the most commonly prescribed product in each closed or preferred class (the spike in Figure 3.10 was smoothed out in the regression analysis to eliminate any effect on the expenditure estimate), and Table 3.1 shows the percentage change pre- versus post-National Formulary for the most common products in closed classes. The price per pill dropped after class closures were implemented for each of the five closed classes, but the magnitude of the price decrease varied across the closed classes from 16 to 41%, as shown. In contrast, the price per pill for the most common product form of the preferred agent (felodipine, 10-mg tablets) among the CCBs, a class with preferred but not closed status, remained constant after implementation of the National Formulary (Figure 3.10).[7] Of course, increased relative utilization of a low-cost preferred drug might confer a savings even though there was no price decrease.

How Has the National Formulary Affected Prescribing Patterns Within the Closed and Preferred Classes?

After examining the effect of the National Formulary on prices, the committee assessed the effect of the National Formulary on market share for

---

[7] The most commonly prescribed product among CCBs was not the preferred agent (felodipine), but diltiazem, 60-mg tablets.

WHAT ARE THE POTENTIAL COSTS TO VA HEALTH CARE ASSOCIATED WITH THE NATIONAL FORMULARY FOR DRUGS?

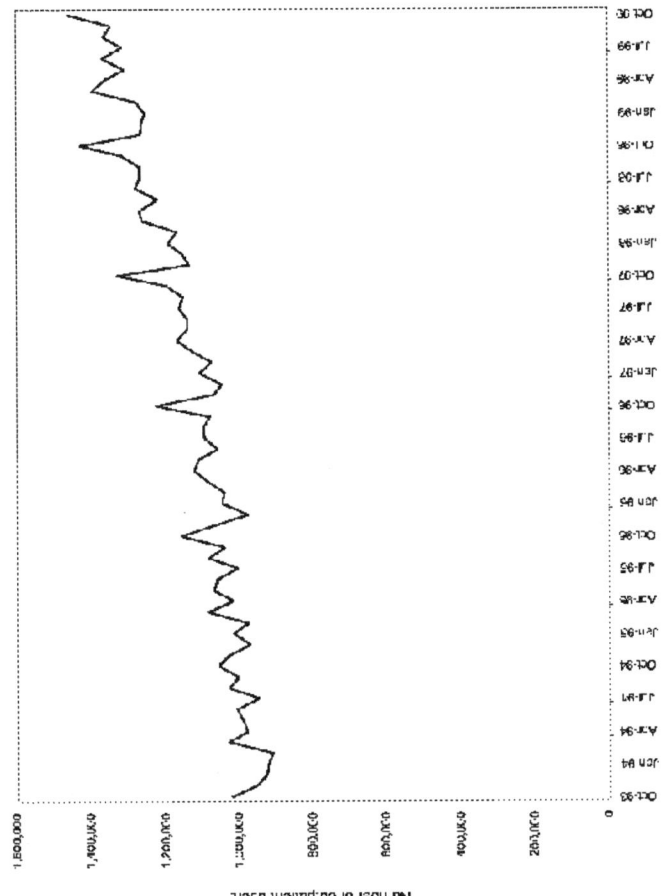

FIGURE 3.1 Total number of VA patients utilizing its outpatient services.

WHAT ARE THE POTENTIAL COSTS TO VA HEALTH CARE ASSOCIATED WITH THE NATIONAL FORMULARY FOR DRUGS?

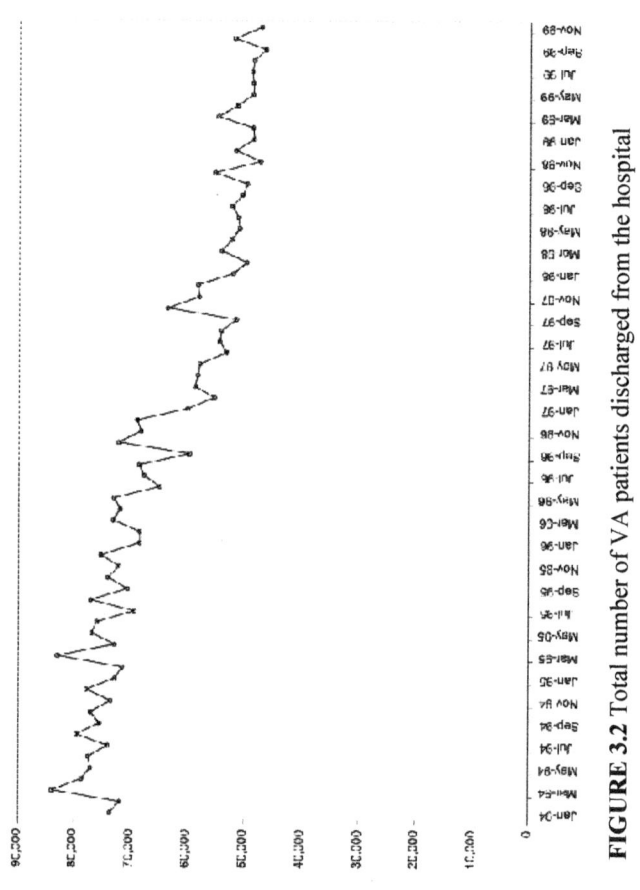

FIGURE 3.2 Total number of VA patients discharged from the hospital

WHAT ARE THE POTENTIAL COSTS TO VA HEALTH CARE ASSOCIATED WITH THE NATIONAL FORMULARY FOR DRUGS?

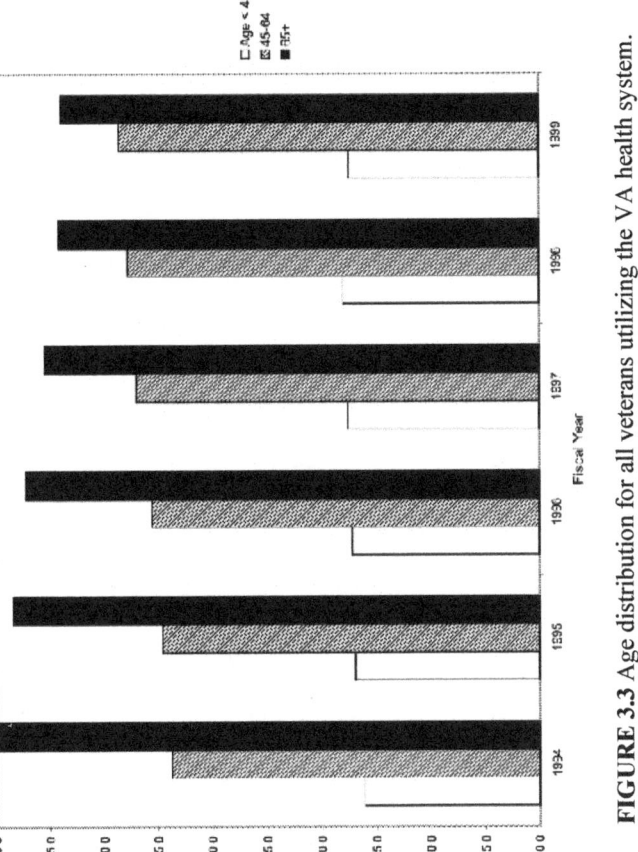

FIGURE 3.3 Age distribution for all veterans utilizing the VA health system.

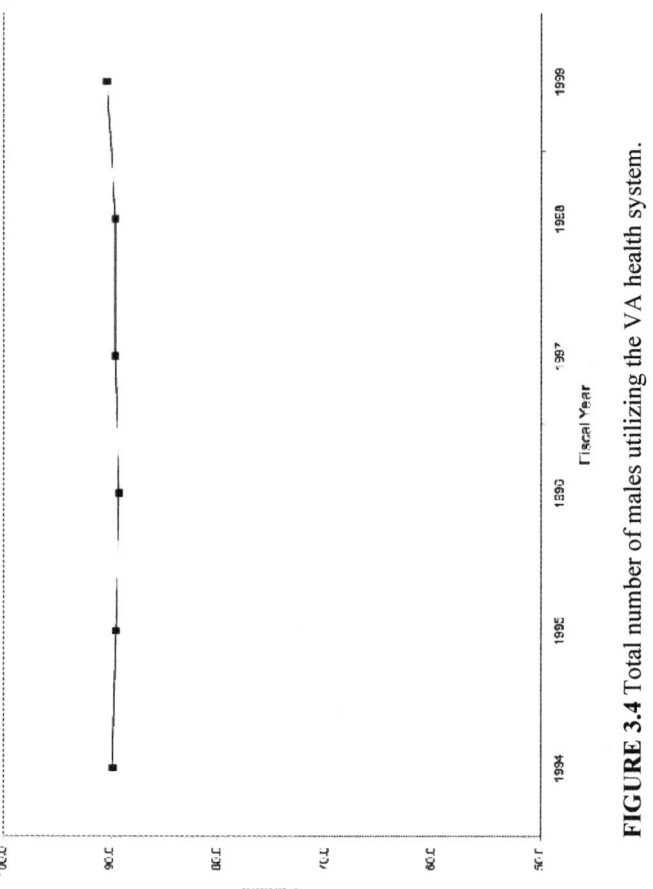

FIGURE 3.4 Total number of males utilizing the VA health system.

WHAT ARE THE POTENTIAL COSTS TO VA HEALTH CARE ASSOCIATED WITH THE NATIONAL FORMULARY FOR DRUGS?

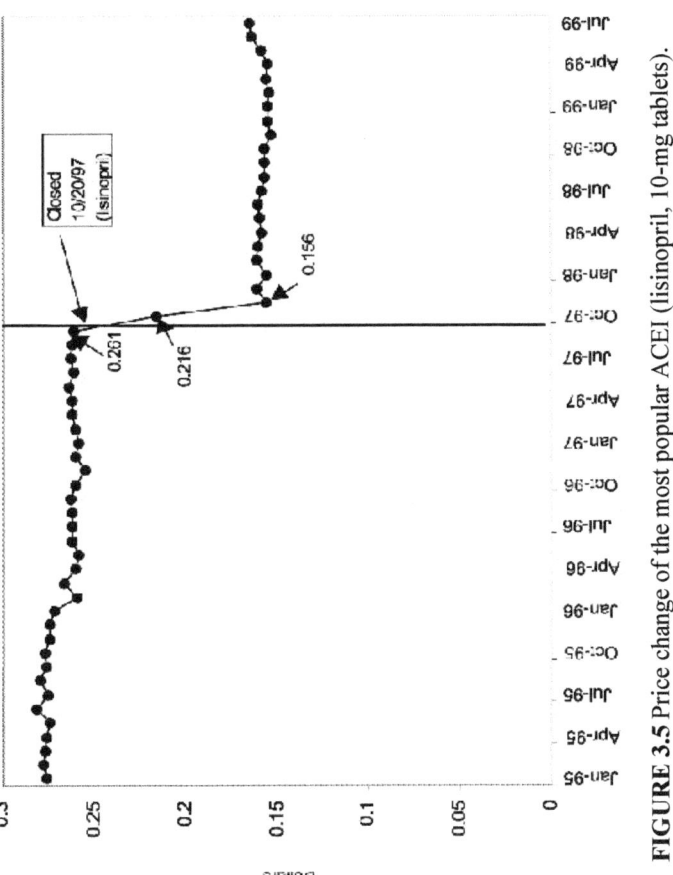

FIGURE 3.5 Price change of the most popular ACEI (lisinopril, 10-mg tablets).

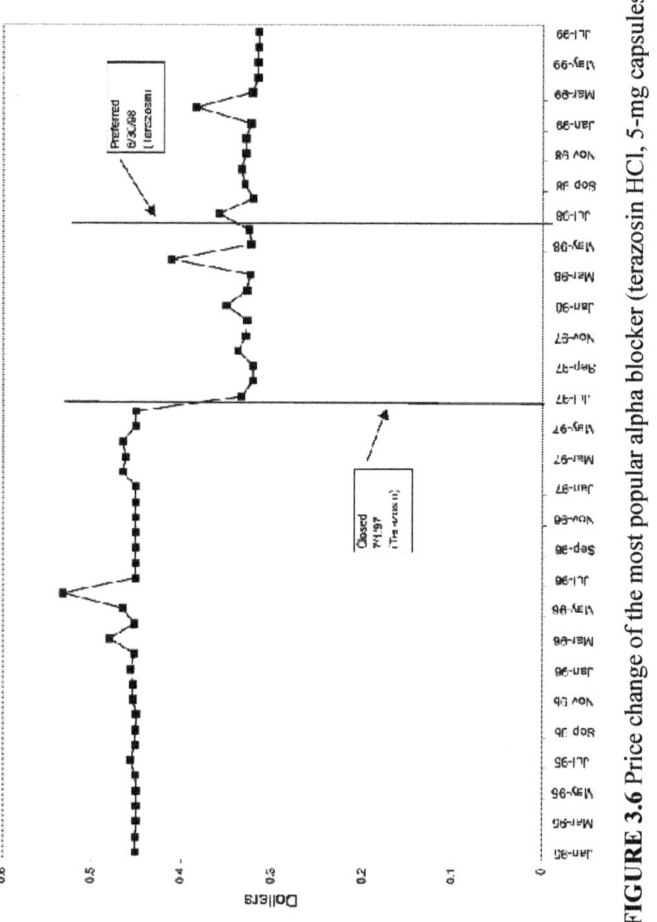

FIGURE 3.6 Price change of the most popular alpha blocker (terazosin HCl, 5-mg capsules).

WHAT ARE THE POTENTIAL COSTS TO VA HEALTH CARE ASSOCIATED WITH THE NATIONAL FORMULARY FOR DRUGS?

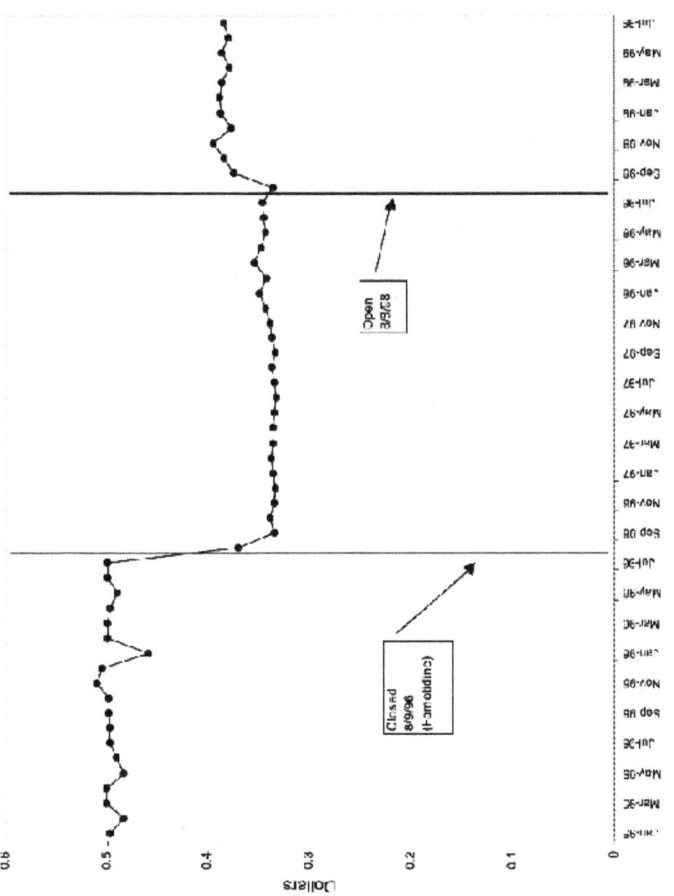

FIGURE 3.7 Price change for the most popular H_2R blocker (famotidine, 20-mg tablets).

WHAT ARE THE POTENTIAL COSTS TO VA HEALTH CARE ASSOCIATED WITH THE NATIONAL FORMULARY FOR DRUGS?

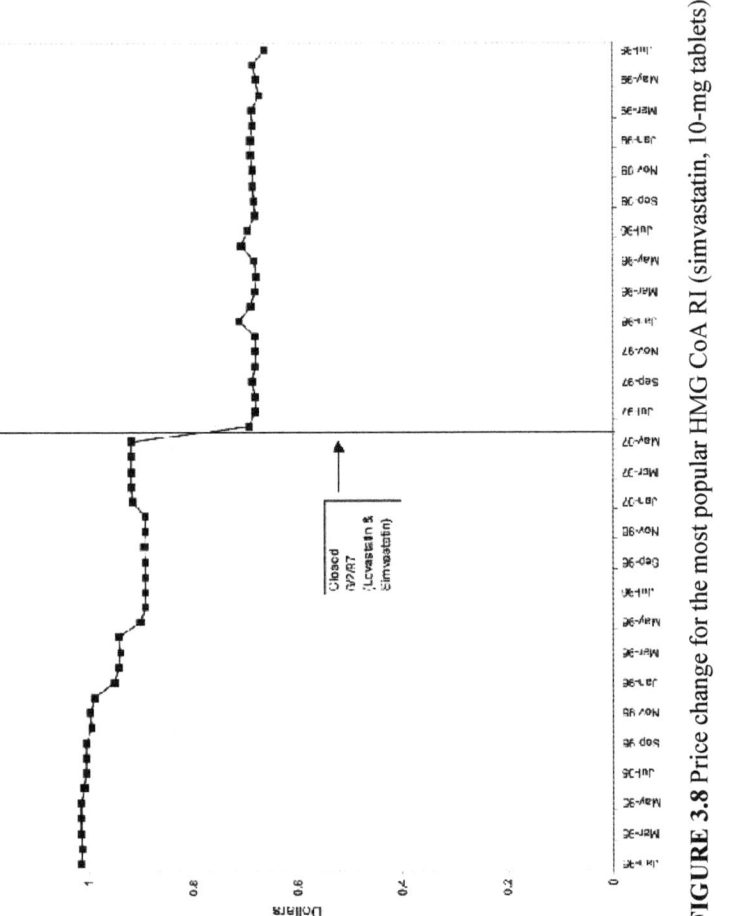

FIGURE 3.8 Price change for the most popular HMG CoA RI (simvastatin, 10-mg tablets).

WHAT ARE THE POTENTIAL COSTS TO VA HEALTH CARE ASSOCIATED WITH THE NATIONAL FORMULARY FOR DRUGS?

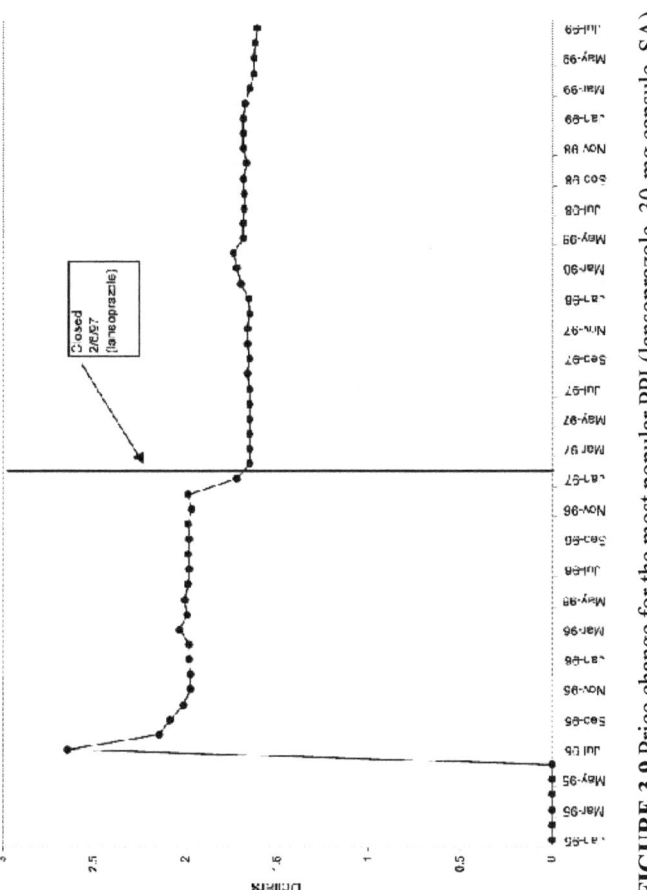

FIGURE 3.9 Price change for the most popular PPI (lansoprazole, 30-mg capsule, SA).

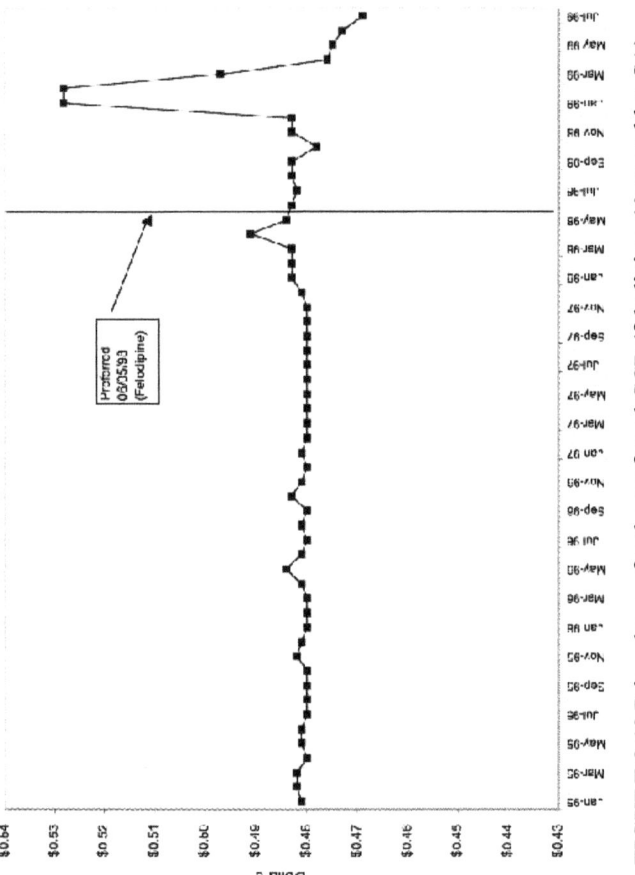

FIGURE 3.10 Price change for the preferred CCB (felodipine, 10-mg tablet, SA).

TABLE 3.2 Compliance with National Formulary

Drug Class	Compliance as of July 1999 (%)
Closed	
ACEI	85.1
HMG CoA RI	94.9
PPIs	96.5
LHRHs	Data not available
Preferred	
Alpha blockers (originally closed)	77.1
CCBs	23.2

each agent within the closed or preferred classes. The level of compliance with the National Formulary in terms of prescribing behavior and the utilization shift to the closed or preferred agents were considered. Figure 3.11, through Figure 3.16 illustrate changes in market share for the closed or preferred agents in the National Formulary. Appendix C includes similar graphs for classes that remained open during the study period (Figure C.1, and Figure C.8). Table 3.2 shows the percentage of utilization within each closed and preferred class that is in compliance with the National Formulary. Market shares for lisinopril and fosinopril (ACEIs), terazosin (alpha blocker), famotidine (H_2R blocker), simvastatin and lovastatin (HMG CoA RIs), and lansoprazole (PPI) increased approximately 35, 62, 42, 75, and 80 percentage points, respectively, on class closure and national contracting, as shown in the figures.

In contrast, market share for the preferred agent among CCBs, the only class that has had preferred status without ever being closed, did not change as dramatically. Felodipine's market share was approximately 15% before the drug was made the preferred agent. After this designation, the market share for felodipine increased to approximately 24%, still a relatively small share of the total market for CCBs (see Figure 3.16). However, it is important to note that there is greater heterogeneity within the CCB therapeutic class than within any other drug class studied by the committee. The class contains three distinct chemical species, and its members are used for a number of different indications, for example, angina, hypertension, and cardiomyopathy. Consequently, it is not surprising that the preferred agent has a relatively low share of the CCB market.

These figures show large changes in market share toward closed drugs in response to National Formulary implementation. As shown in Appendix C, (Figure C.1, through Figure C.8) similar increases in market share are not seen in classes that remained open during the study period, with the exception of classes in which a breakthrough drug entered the market during this time. For example, for the atypical antipsychotics, market share for olanzapine increased steadily beginning in 1996 and reached approximately 43% by June 1999, an increase that was not limited to the VHA and is not linked to the VA National Formulary

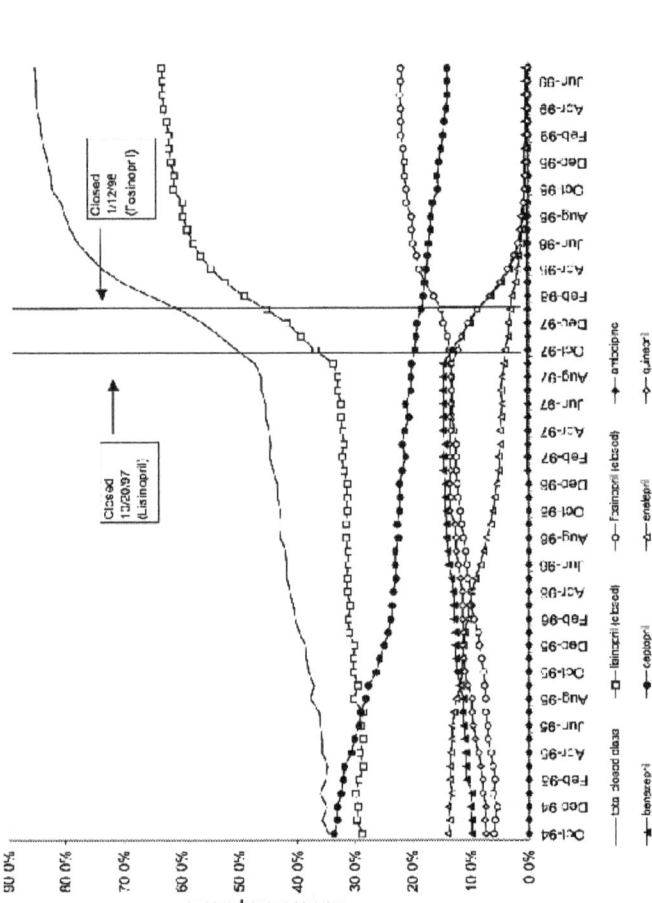

FIGURE 3.11 Market share of the angiotensin-converting enzyme inhibitor pharmaceutical class (closed class). NOTE: Some drug products (moexpril, quinapril, ramipril, and trandolapril) had negligible market share and were removed for clarity.

WHAT ARE THE POTENTIAL COSTS TO VA HEALTH CARE ASSOCIATED WITH THE NATIONAL FORMULARY FOR DRUGS?

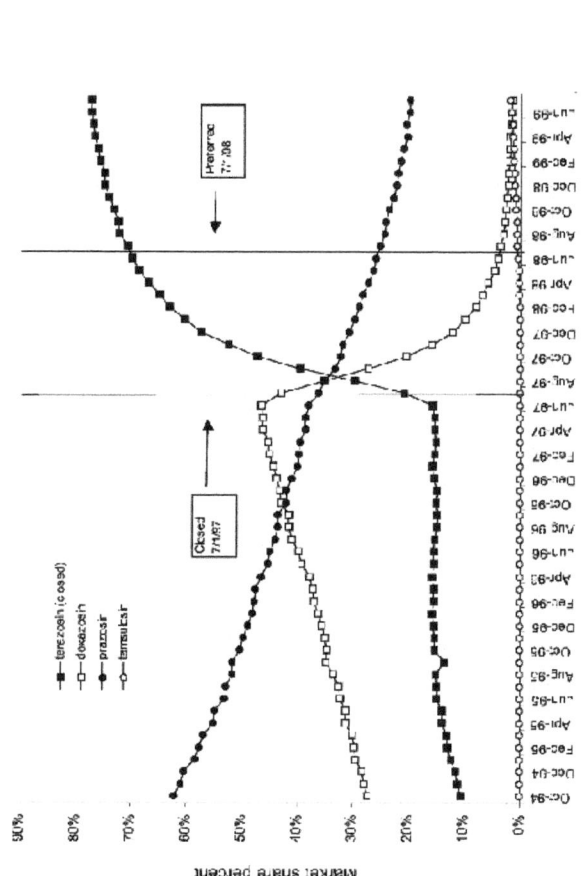

FIGURE 3.12 Market share of the alpha blocker pharmaceutical class (initially closed class).

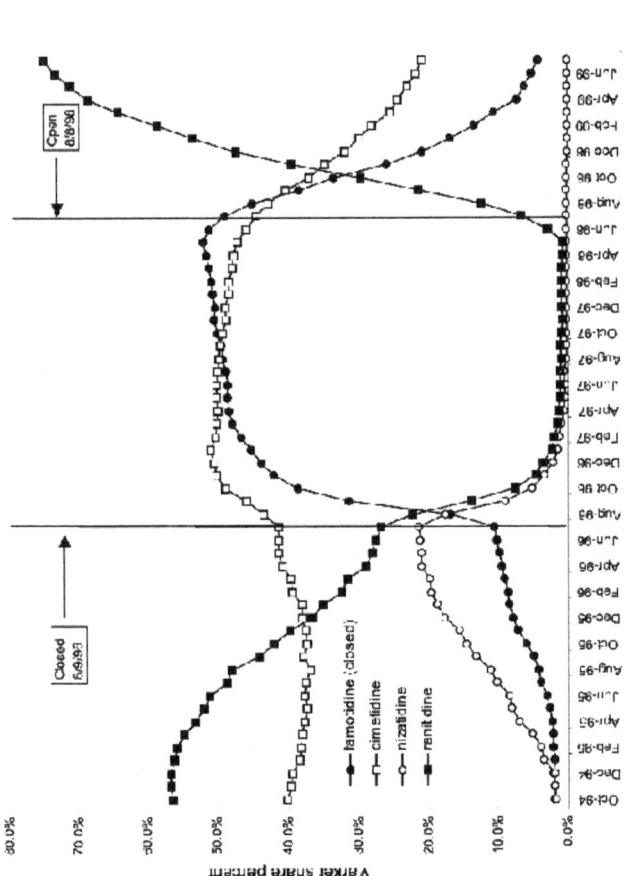

FIGURE 3.13 Market share of the H_2R blocker pharmaceutical class (initially closed class).

WHAT ARE THE POTENTIAL COSTS TO VA HEALTH CARE ASSOCIATED WITH THE NATIONAL FORMULARY FOR DRUGS?

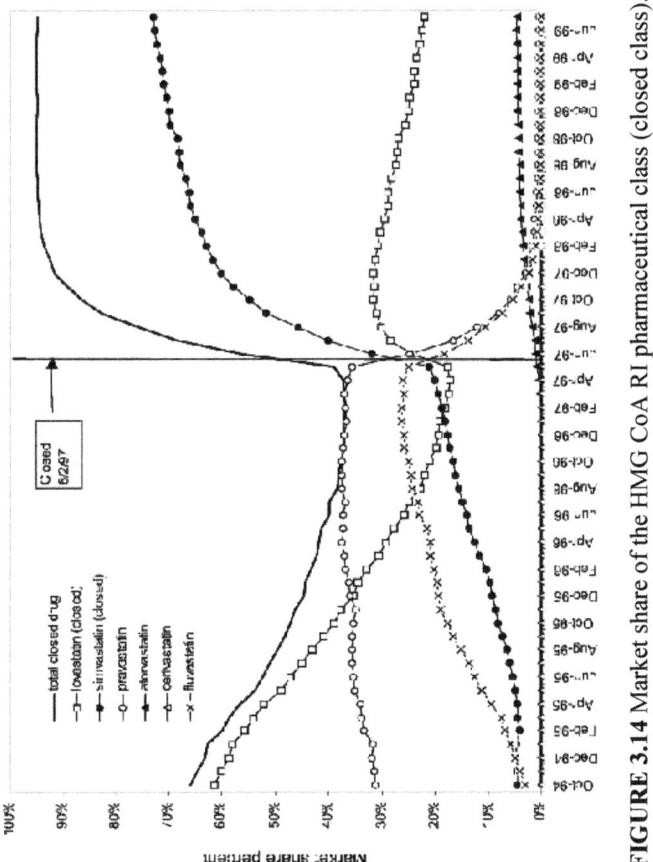

FIGURE 3.14 Market share of the HMG CoA RI pharmaceutical class (closed class).

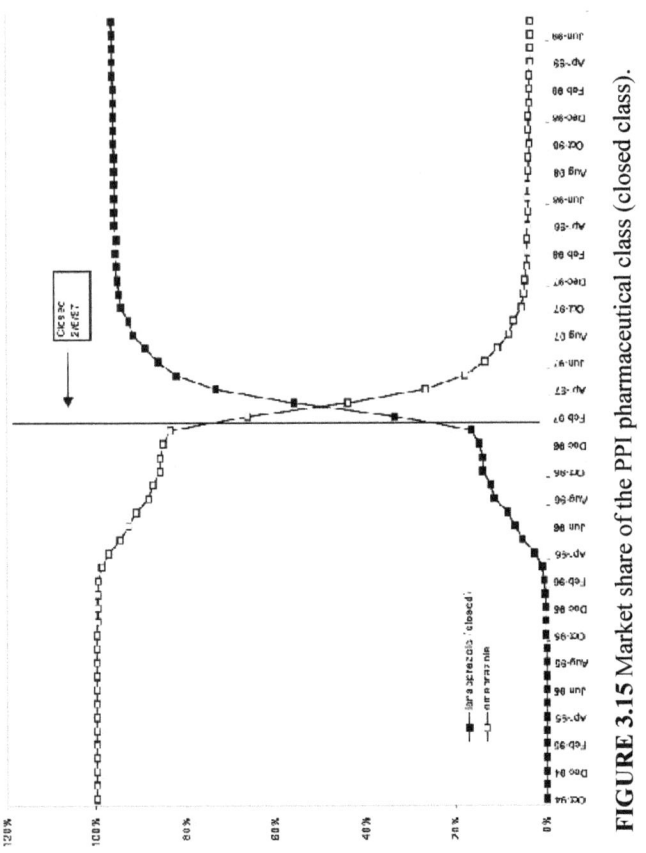

FIGURE 3.15 Market share of the PPI pharmaceutical class (closed class).

WHAT ARE THE POTENTIAL COSTS TO VA HEALTH CARE ASSOCIATED WITH THE NATIONAL FORMULARY FOR DRUGS?

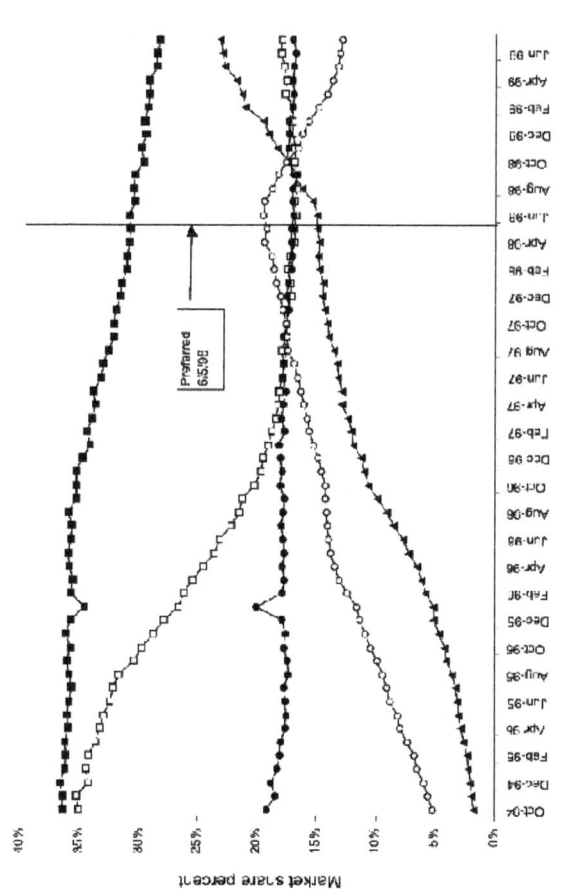

FIGURE 3.16 Market share of the CCB pharmaceutical class (preferred). NOTE: Agents that had a low percentage of market share were not included to improve the clarity of the graph.

(see Figure C.2) (Frank et al., 1999). The National Formulary seems to have been successful in moving market share toward closed-class agents for which sizable price discounts were negotiated.

How Has the National Formulary Affected Pharmaceutical Spending per Veteran User for Closed and Preferred Classes?

Trends in average outpatient pharmacy spending per outpatient VHA user are presented in Figure 3.17, and Figure 3.22 for the closed and preferred classes. Trends for two additional classes that remained open throughout this period, SSRIs and beta-blockers, are provided in Figure 3.23, and Figure 3.24 for comparison. Appendix C includes similar figures, Figure C.9, and Figure C.14, for six other open classes. The trends in average outpatient pharmacy spending per outpatient user over the study period vary substantially across classes. For three of the closed classes (ACEIs, H_2R blocker, and alpha-blockers), implementation of the National Formulary appears to be associated with a decrease in what average spending on the given class per outpatient user would have been had the preformulary time trend continued (see Figure 3.17, and Figure 3.19). On the other hand, for PPIs and HMG CoA RIs, average spending per outpatient user continued to increase throughout the period (see Figure 3.20 and Figure 3.21). During this time, the average number of prescriptions per user was increasing steadily for these classes, which is responsible for the increases in outpatient pharmacy spending per outpatient user. For CCBs, average spending per outpatient user remained fairly constant after National Formulary designation as a preferred class (see Figure 3.22).

Table 3.3 displays results for the key coefficients of interest for assessing the spending effects of the VA National Formulary. A separate regression is estimated for each closed or preferred class. Each regression model was specified so that the dependent variable was measured as the logarithm of spending per out-patient VHA user in a VISN in each month from January 1995 through July 1999. Several independent variables were included in the model. Two variables representing the age composition of the population (that is, the percentage of a VISN's user population under age 45 years and the percentage age 45 to 64) were included to account for changing health needs. The percentage of users that were males was included to account for changes in utilization and spending attributable to demographic changes. A quadratic time trend was entered into the model to account for overall trends in pharmaceutical prescribing and spending within the VHA system. The key variables of interest are a set of indicators about the open, preferred, or closed status of specific drugs during a given month. Finally, a set of dummy variables was included for each of the VISNs to control for time-invariant, unmeasured characteristics of the VISNs and their user populations. The need for a time dummy was accommodated by the quadratic time trend. The complete regression results are reported in Appendix C (Table C.2 and Table C.3).

WHAT ARE THE POTENTIAL COSTS TO VA HEALTH CARE ASSOCIATED WITH THE NATIONAL FORMULARY FOR DRUGS?

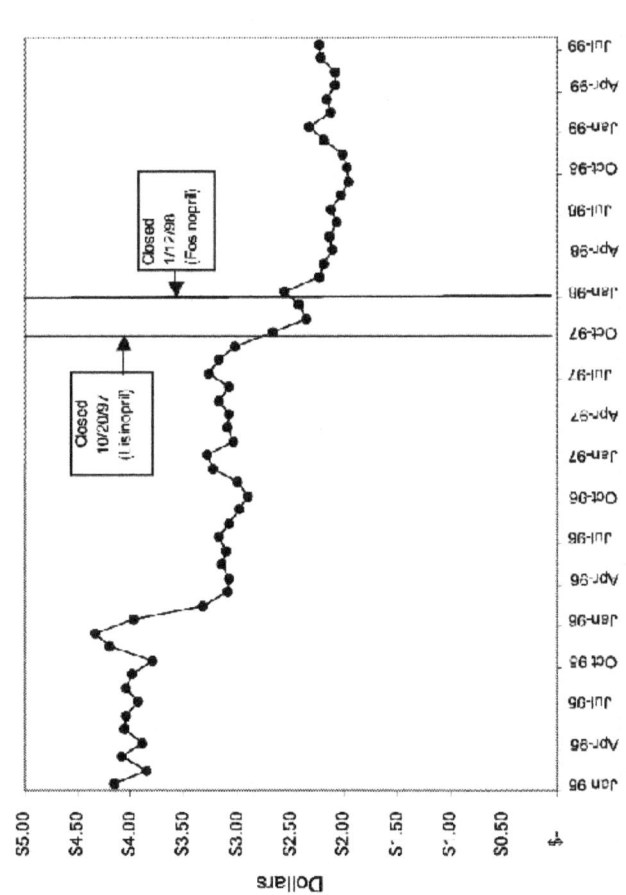

FIGURE 3.17 Average outpatient pharmacy spending per outpatient user by month on angiotensin-converting enzyme inhibitors.

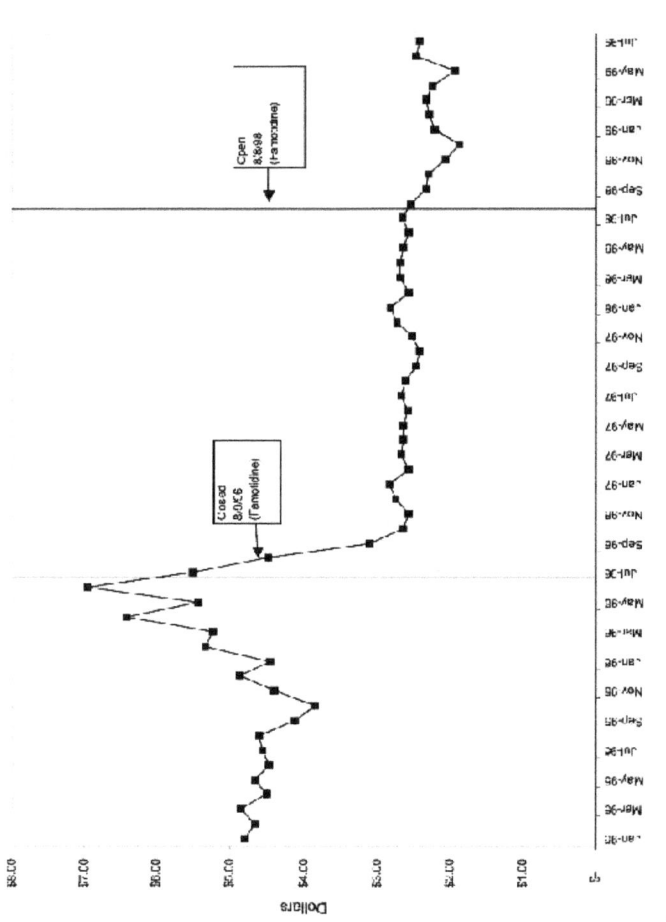

FIGURE 3.18 Average outpatient pharmacy spending per user by month on H_2R blockers.

WHAT ARE THE POTENTIAL COSTS TO VA HEALTH CARE ASSOCIATED WITH THE NATIONAL FORMULARY FOR DRUGS?

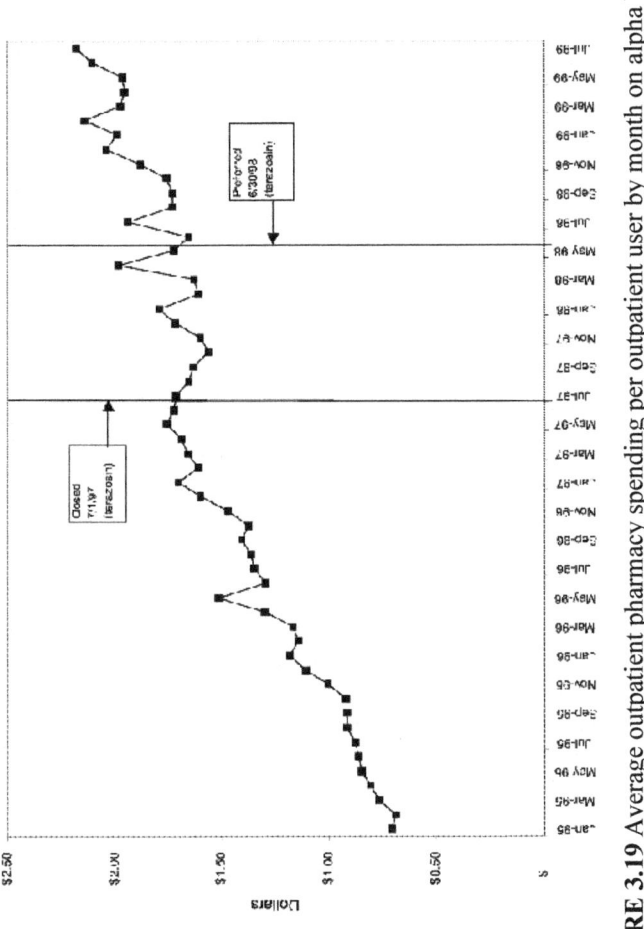

FIGURE 3.19 Average outpatient pharmacy spending per outpatient user by month on alpha blockers.

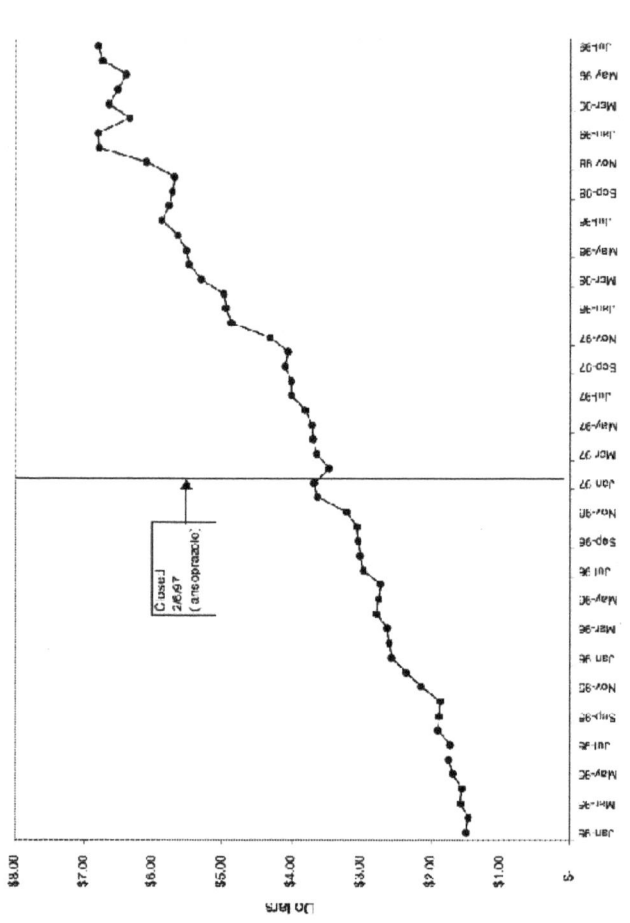

FIGURE 3.20 Average outpatient pharmacy spending per outpatient user by month on PPIs.

WHAT ARE THE POTENTIAL COSTS TO VA HEALTH CARE ASSOCIATED WITH THE NATIONAL FORMULARY FOR DRUGS?

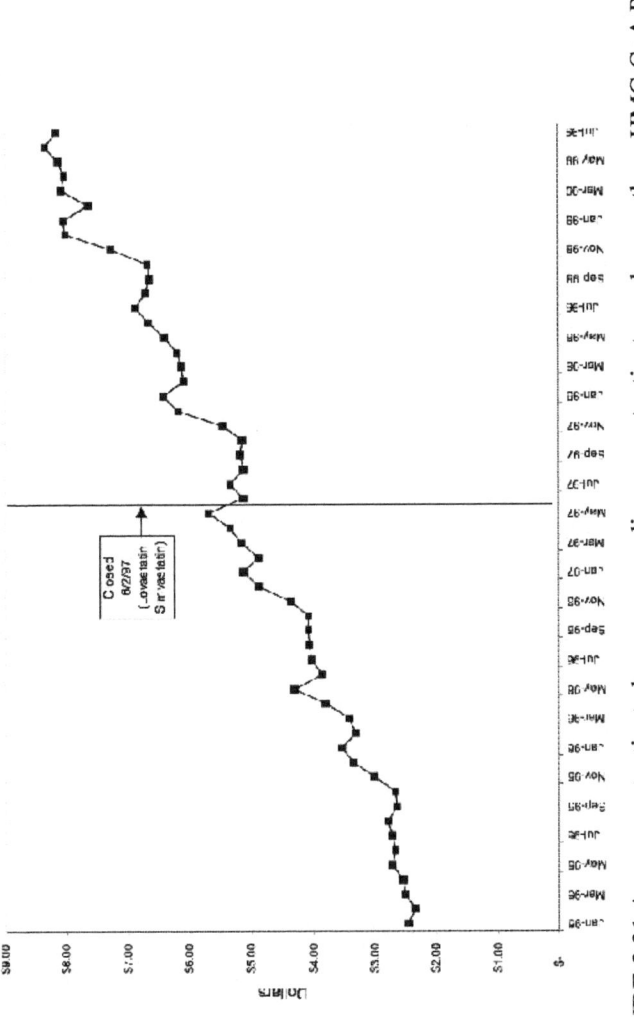

FIGURE 3.21 Average outpatient pharmacy spending per outpatient user by month on HMG CoA RI.

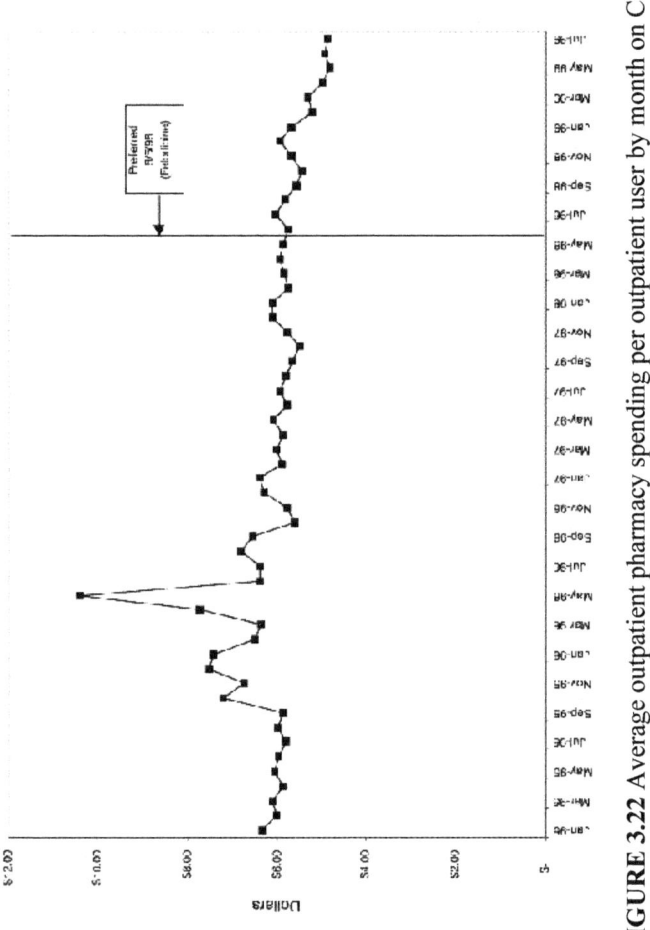

FIGURE 3.22 Average outpatient pharmacy spending per outpatient user by month on CCBs.

WHAT ARE THE POTENTIAL COSTS TO VA HEALTH CARE ASSOCIATED WITH THE NATIONAL FORMULARY FOR DRUGS?

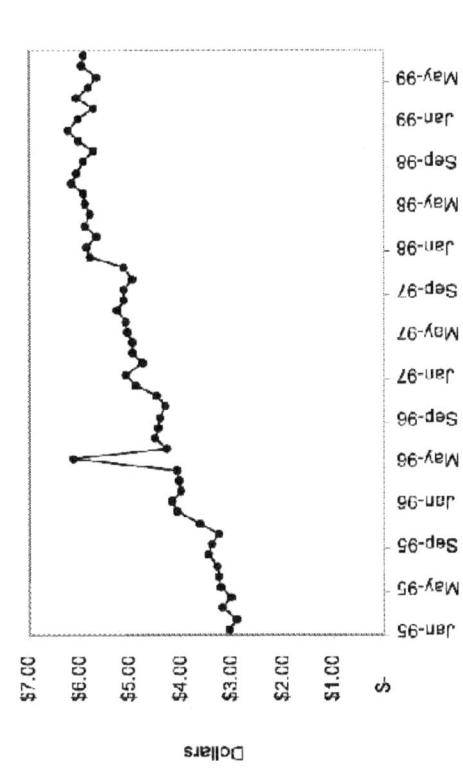

FIGURE 3.23 Average outpatient pharmacy spending per outpatient user by month on SSRIs.

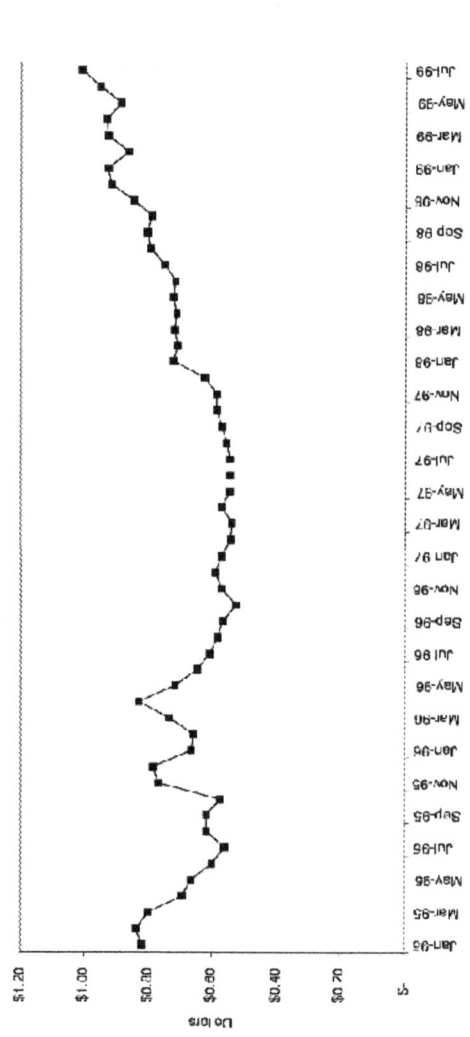

FIGURE 3.24 Average outpatient pharmacy spending per outpatient user by month on beta blockers.

The specific drugs chosen in each of the six closed or preferred drug classes examined are identified in Table 3.3. Percentage effects on class-level spending per VHA user are reported. The committee also reports the statistical significance level of the estimated effects and the overall explanatory power of the statistical model. Table 3.3 shows that for the five closed drug classes studied, closure was associated with a significant decrease in average per-user outpatient pharmacy spending in the class. This does not mean that there were absolute declines in spending (see Figure 3.17, and Figure 3.22), but, rather, that spending levels were lower than they would have been absent the changes in formulary policy. The one class studied for which a decrease was not seen was CCBs, a class with preferred status only. The estimate of the effect of CCB preferred status was not significantly different from zero at conventional levels, although it was quite precisely estimated ($p < .07$).

As shown, spending reductions associated with class closure for lisinopril and fosinopril (ACEIs), terazosin (alpha-blocker), lovastatin/simvastatin (HMG CoA RIs), lansoprazole (PPI), and famotidine (H_2R blocker) were 16.9 and 8.5%, 17.5%, 8.1%, 7.4%, and 41%, respectively, and the model explained 82, 83, 92, 95, and 65% of the variance in per-user spending, respectively. These reductions were statistically significant at the 99% confidence level. Finally, CCBs were designated as a preferred class, with felodipine as the preferred agent. This change was associated with a 7.9% increase in per-user spending on CCBs that was significant at the 93% confidence level. The model accounted for 66% of the variance in per user spending in the class.

IS THERE EVIDENCE THAT CHANGES IN FORMULARY POLICY HAVE RESULTED IN INCREASED UTILIZATION ELSEWHERE IN THE VHA SYSTEM?

Exploration of Changes in Hospital Discharges per VHA User

Figure 3.25 and Figure 3.26 show trends in the number of inpatient discharges for selected heart and ulcer-related diagnoses per outpatient VHA user by month.[8] Table 3.4 displays estimated effects of the formulary policy on rates of hospital discharges for illness related to cardiac care and treatment of ulcers.[9] These

---

[8] The following *International Classification of Diseases, Ninth Edition* (ICD-9) codes were used for the regressions focused on heart conditions (that is, ACEI related): 401.0, 402.0, 405.0, 410.0, 411.1, 413.0, 414.8, 414.9, and 428.0. The following ICD-9 codes were used for the regressions focused on gastrointestinal conditions (that is, PPI-related): 530.1, 531.0, 532.0, 533.0, and 535.0.

[9] Similar analyses for HMG CoA RIs and alpha blockers were not conducted because the conditions for which drugs in these classes are used most commonly would be less likely to result in hospital treatment if complications resulted.

analyses are aimed at identifying any shifts toward hospital treatment of heart disease and ulcers that might be associated with changes in the availability of the full line of products in the PPI and ACEI closed drug classes. The dependent variables in these models are the logarithm of the rates of discharges (disease-specific inpatient discharges/per veteran outpatient user) from the hospitals for a set of diagnoses for which ACEIs and PPIs are often used for treatment. The independent variables include demographic characteristics of each VISN's users, age, and gender. Also included are dummy variables for each VISN, a quadratic time trend, and an indicator variable for when the new formulary policy was in effect for each of the two classes. The full regression results are reported in Appendix C (Table C.2 and Table C.3).

TABLE 3.3 Outpatient Pharmacy Spending per Outpatient VHA User*

	Estimated Impact (%)	Significance
ACEI		
lisinopril	−16.9	$p<.01$
fosinopril	−8.5	$p<.01$
R^2	0.82	
Alpha Blockers		
terazosin, closed	−17.5	$p<.01$
terazosin, preferred	−0.1	NS
R^2	0.83	
HMG CoA RIs		
lovastatin, simvastatin (closed)	−8.1	$p<.01$
R^2	0.92	
PPIs		
Lansoprazole	−7.4	$p<.01$
R^2	0.95	
H_2R blockers		
Famotidine, closed	−41.1	$p<.01$
Reopened	−4.3	NS
R^2	0.65	
CCBs		
Felodipine, preferred	7.9	NS ($p<.07$)
R^2	0.66	

NOTE: NS = not significant.
* Complete regression results are available in Appendix C (Table C.2).

WHAT ARE THE POTENTIAL COSTS TO VA HEALTH CARE ASSOCIATED WITH THE NATIONAL FORMULARY FOR DRUGS?

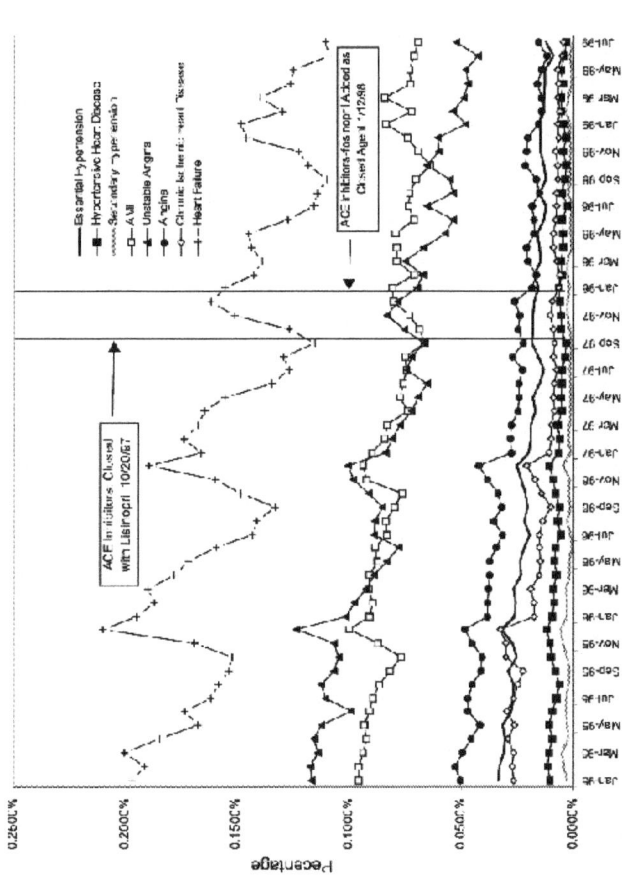

FIGURE 3.25 Number of inpatient discharges for selected diagnoses per VHA outpatient user.

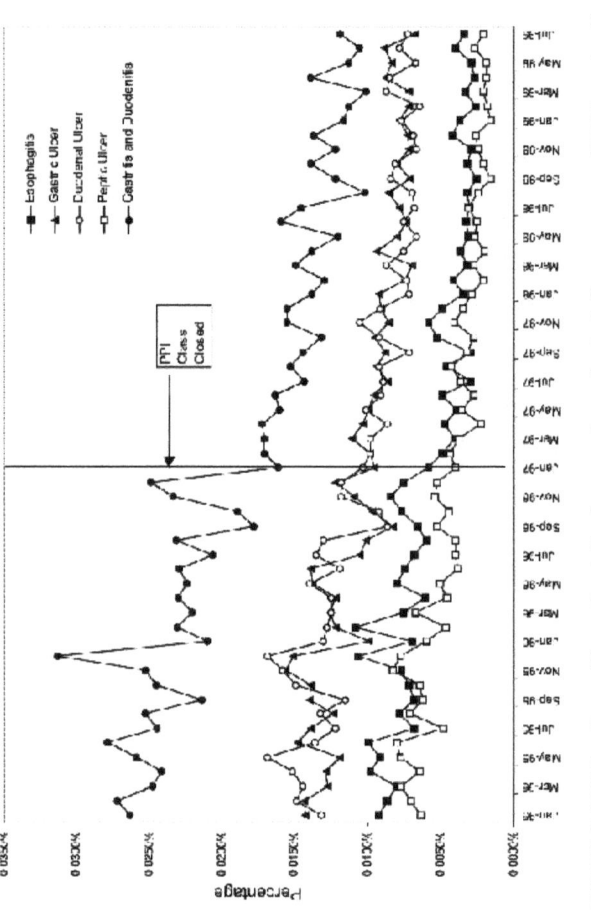

FIGURE 3.26 Number of inpatient discharges for selected diagnoses per VHA outpatient user.

TABLE 3.4 Estimated Impacts of National Formulary Class Closures on Disease-Specific Discharge Rates*

	Estimated Impact (%)	Significance
ACEIs	−1.3	NS
R^2	0.81	
PPIs	−4.9	NS
R^2	0.64	

NOTE: NS = not significant.
* The denominator of the discharge rate is the number of VHA outpatient users.

The first row of Table 3.4 displays the estimated effect on the rate of discharge per VHA outpatient user associated with closure of the ACEI class. The estimated effect implies that discharges for heart-disease-related care fell by 1.3% relative to what they would have been absent the change in formulary policy. However, this effect is not statistically significant at conventional levels ($p < .05$). The regression model accounted for 81% of the variation in discharges per user.

The second set of results on Table 3.4 reports the estimated effect of closing the PPI class on ulcer-related hospitalizations. Once again the dependent variable is the logarithm of ulcer-related discharges divided by the total number of veteran outpatient users in each VISN. The estimated effect implies a 4.9% reduction in the ulcer-related discharge rate. Again, this estimate was not significantly different from zero at conventional confidence levels. The regression model for ulcer-related discharges accounted for 64% of the variation in ulcer-related discharges per user.

The regression results suggest that there are no significant changes in hospital discharge rates related to heart disease and ulcers. However, these are very crude indicators of shifting utilization stemming from changes in the delivery system for treatment of ulcers and heart disease.

COSTS ASSOCIATED WITH IMPLEMENTING AND MANAGING THE NATIONAL FORMULARY

Evaluations of the cost effects of the VA National Formulary must consider both changes in pharmacy spending and costs imposed on the VHA associated with implementing and managing the National Formulary. To estimate these administrative costs, the committee requested total cost estimates of expenditures associated with National Formulary administration from the VA PBM. The PBM does not collect detailed information about these expenditures but estimated that roughly half of its budget was associated with National Formulary-related activities. The PBM estimated the following expenditures associated with the National Formulary: $400,000 each year for FY 1995 and FY 1996 (the PBMs total budget was $884,000 each of those years); and $900,000 each year from FY 1997 to FY 2000 (the PBMs total budget was $1,919,000 each year for FY 1997 to FY 1999 and $2,099,000 for FY 2000).[10] This estimate is limited to PBM expenditures and does not include a number of other costs, including time spent by VISN leaders and personnel in implementing and managing the National Formulary at the VISN level, time spent by the NAC in negotiating contracts for the National Formulary closed and preferred classes, procurement costs for the National Formulary closed classes, any extra staff that might have been added at the VISN or local facility level to handle increased pharmacy duties, and time spent at the local level administering nonformulary exceptions, therapeutic interchanges, and seeing patients again regarding prescription changes, among others. As a result, the committee could not provide a complete estimate of total administrative costs associated with implementing and managing the VA National Formulary.

Estimated National Formulary Savings

In this section, the IOM committee presents the estimated gross savings (that is, savings omitting costs associated with implementing and managing the National Formulary) attributable to VA National Formulary activities in six drug classes. This estimate should measure first-order effects such as the cost savings in each class attributable to formulary policy. In addition, any direct effects of formulary policy on all drug classes or secondary effects on the closed and preferred classes should also be measured. Finally, a complete estimate should also measure other effects of the VA National Formulary on prices for nonclosed or preferred classes stemming from the application of bargaining power created by the formulary system. For example, the threat of closing certain classes or using exclusive generic contracts in order to obtain more advantageous prices under BPAs or national contracts appears to have yielded price concessions in bargaining. The estimates presented below focus on the first-order effects of savings. Yet even the first-order estimates of savings are incomplete because complete data on prices and quantities purchased for the LHRH class of drugs were not available.

The IOM committee could not measure the effects of designating classes as closed or preferred on spending and utilization of related classes of drugs be

---

[10] To calculate the $900,000 estimate for each year from FY 1997 to FY 2000, the VA PBM reported that it "allocated the costs of the PBM clinical staff, the half full-time equivalent provided to support the MAP chair, travel related to [VA] National Formulary activities, and a portion of the data management, contracting, and supervisory staff to those activities directly related to [VA] National Formulary support" (e-mail correspondence with Michael Valentino, R.Ph., MHSA, associate chief consultant, PBM Strategic Healthcare Group, January 11, 2000). Additional details on PBM National Formulary expenditures were not available.

cause of lack of availability of data and time and resource constraints, although some evidence of cross-class effects for one class of antihypertensive drugs related to ACEIs (beta blockers) was investigated and is discussed later in this chapter. The committee also could not assess the effects of negotiations for drugs covered by BPAs and national contracts because of difficulties characterizing the precise features and timing of the implementation process for BPAs.

Several different approaches to estimating savings from formulary policy are described in the pharmacoeconomics literature. Many of these depend on being able to convert data into defined daily doses and to use detailed management information to predict purchasing patterns absent formulary changes. For example, some large private-sector health centers multiply total annual spending on a particular formulary agent by the percentage price decrease negotiated at the time of formulary selection and take this as a cost avoidance or savings for the year, unadjusted for possible coinciding factors affecting drug usage. Data limitations in this IOM study precluded such approaches. Instead the committee relied on a statistical method to estimate savings which is described below.

Table 3.5 summarizes the savings estimates for each of the six closed or preferred drug classes that were studied. The estimate for each class represents savings that accrued to the VHA beginning on the date the class was designated as closed or preferred and ending on either July 31, 1999 (the last date for which there were pharmacy spending data), or the date the class was reopened (in the case of H_2R blockers), whichever came first. The committee presents three estimates for each class: the nominal savings, the "real" savings, and the real discounted savings. The nominal savings are simply the sum of per-user dollars saved in each month multiplied by the number of outpatient VHA users. Projected per-user dollars are estimated by using coefficients from the regression models to predict national spending per user in each month. Using the regression model allowed the committee to hold constant the age, geographic, and gender composition of the population of veteran users in making projections, so the estimates reflect savings for the average population of VA outpatient users over the study period. The results from two models of per-user spending on each drug class are compared to estimate savings. The first model projects spending per user in each month for each class assuming that there was not a National Formulary in effect. The second model estimates spending per user in each month given the actual implementation of the National Formulary for each class. The estimated savings are the differences between the two estimates multiplied by the number of users in each month, summed over the duration of the policy.

The third column of Table 3.5 presents estimates of "real" savings, which represent nominal spending adjusted for changes in the general level of prices in the economy as measured by the Consumer Price Index. This adjustment is made so as not to include economy-wide price rises in the estimated spending over time. Real savings estimates reflect savings calculated retrospectively and adjusted for general inflation. In the fourth column of Table 3.5, the committee also

TABLE 3.5 Estimated Savings (in millions of dollars) from the VHA National Formulary for Closed and Preferred Classes

Class	Nominal Savings ($ millions)	Real Savings ($ millions)	Real Discounted Savings ($ millions)
Closed			
HMG CoA RIs	$14.4	$13.8	$13.5
PPIs	$4.9	$4.7	$4.6
ACEIs	$17.6	$16.9	$16.6
H_2R blockers	$47.1	$45.2	$44.2
Alpha Blockers	$1.8	$1.8	$1.7
Total	**$85.8**	**$82.4**	**$80.6**
Preferred			
CCBs	($13.2)	($12.8)	($12.7)

takes account of the time cost of money to the federal government as measured by the 30-year average of the short-term interest rate on federal securities (about 3% per annum in real terms). All real dollar estimates are presented as 1997 dollars. Because the committee is evaluating the effect of the National Formulary retrospectively, the focus below is on the real estimates of savings.

Table 3.5 shows very large differences in the level of savings across drug classes. In the case of H_2R blockers, a closed class initially, the nominal savings were estimated to be $47.1 million and the real savings were estimated to be $45.2 million. In contrast, the HMG CoA RI and ACEI classes realized moderate levels of savings following class closure. For HMG CoA RIs, the committee estimated $14.4 million in nominal savings and $13.8 million in real savings. Savings for ACEIs were estimated to be $17.6 million in nominal terms and $16.9 million in real terms. Closure of the PPI and alpha blocker classes yielded considerably smaller savings. Nominal savings for PPIs were estimated to be $4.9 million, while real savings were estimated at $4.7 million. Both estimated nominal savings and real savings for alpha blockers were approximately $1.8 million. Thus, the total savings associated with closing five of the six closed classes (that is, all but LHRHs) were estimated to be roughly $85.8 million in nominal terms and $82.4 in real terms.

The committee also examined one class (CCBs) that had a combination of committed-use contracts (for diltiazem and nifedipine) and a preferred status contract for one drug (felodipine) that accounted for about 25% of sales. As noted above, detailed information on the BPA for the largest selling drug in the category, diltiazem, was not available. Thus, the estimates are based on a somewhat incomplete model of the class. As reported in the regression analysis, the estimated effect on per-user spending in the CCB class of making felodipine the preferred drug was an increase, suggesting that the effect of National Formulary preferred status was to increase spending. However, the estimated coefficient was not significant at conventional levels although it was near significance ($p<.07$). Thus, any estimates of cost increases should be taken with caution. Nevertheless, if the estimated effect on spending for CCBs associated with making felodipine the preferred agent is accepted, CCB spending increased by an estimated $13.2 million in nominal terms and $12.8 million in real terms. Because of the existence of missing data on contracting in the CCB class, the committee presents estimated savings for the closed classes and this preferred class separately.

One possible outcome of class closure could be increased expenditures for other drug classes that include drugs treating the same conditions as those in the closed classes. To explore this hypothesis, the committee examined data on spending for beta-blockers to assess whether any changes were associated with closure of the ACEI class. A regression model for outpatient spending on beta-blockers per outpatient user, where the key variable of interest is the date of class closure for the ACEIs, was estimated for this purpose. An increase in per-user spending on beta-blockers followed the change in status of the ACEI class. However, it is difficult to view this association as causal. National quality-of-care standards for the use of beta-blockers were being implemented during the period of VA National Formulary implementation, creating a potential confounding between the National Formulary and changes in clinical practice. Nevertheless, this observation highlights the need to trace possible shifts in wider prescribing patterns that might occur coincident with changes in formulary policy and underscores the need to exercise caution in drawing conclusions about overall savings based on somewhat incomplete data.

The estimate of gross savings of approximately $82 million for the period beginning with National Formulary implementation through July 31, 1999, is a conservative lower-bound estimate of the true savings from instituting closed and preferred formulary status for a number of classes of prescription drugs for several reasons. First, the estimation method was designed to control for secular trends in VHA spending on prescription drugs. Some portion of these trends may be the result of activities associated with the National Formulary. Second, the data are incomplete. At the most basic level, all data on prices and spending for the LHRH class of drugs are missing. Within the classes analyzed, there were missing data for some specific products, although these were generally low-volume items. Third, the effects of instruments such as BPAs and other contracting vehicles that are made more effective by the threat of class closure are not included as part of the committee's estimates, partly as a matter of data availability on BPA agreements and partly because BPAs differ considerably in form from policies such as class closure. For these reasons, true gross savings in excess of $100 million are quite likely. The committee judged, however, that even the most generous assessment of the upper bound of its estimate would not reach the NAC estimate, which included savings from some contracting activities considered outside the scope of the VA National Formulary. Nor would the most pessimistic assessment of offsetting costs of formulary administration overwhelm the committee's estimated gross savings.

CONCLUSIONS

An important function of formularies in modern health care systems is to increase the bargaining power of a buyer of pharmaceutical products (for example, a health system or health plan). The enhanced bargaining power allows health care organizations to secure lower prices from manufacturers. The buying power stems from the ability to move market share among products. The VA National Formulary appears to have been quite effective in changing prescribing patterns and moving market share to chosen members of closed classes. This is evidenced by an average compliance level of 90% or more. As a result, the National Formulary has realized sizable price reductions from manufacturers of drugs in closed classes, ranging from 16 to 41% for the most commonly prescribed product forms.

The statistical analyses conducted showed that the National Formulary's closed classes are associated with reductions in average outpatient pharmacy spending per outpatient VHA user relative to what spending would have been absent the National Formulary. After controlling for secular trends in pharmaceutical utilization, time-invariant unmeasured differences between VISNs, and the changing demographic composition of VHA users, the statistical analyses yielded estimates that the National Formulary resulted in decreases in per-user outpatient pharmacy spending of between 7 and 41% for the closed classes.

A conservative, lower-bound estimate of gross savings achieved by the National Formulary on the closed and preferred classes (excluding LHRHs, for which data were unavailable) is approximately $82 million, as described above. To calculate net savings, an estimate of costs associated with implementing and managing the National Formulary is needed. A complete estimate of VHA systemwide expenditures associated with implementing and managing the formulary could not be calculated by the VA PBM. However, the magnitude of estimated expenditures by the PBM ($2.7 million in nominal terms over the period FY 1997 to FY 1999, or approximately 3% of estimated savings) suggests that systemwide management costs for the National Formulary are substantially lower than the estimated reductions in pharmacy spending associated with National Formulary adoption. In the fixed budget environment in which the VHA operates, any savings achieved by negotiating lower prices with pharmaceutical manufacturers can be used to expand health care services to veterans. Although the National Formulary has closed only a small number of drug classes, 6 of 254, these six classes represent a significant proportion of total VHA pharmaceutical expenditures and contain drugs that, on drug class review, are shown to have similar safety and effectiveness profiles. It is unclear whether expansions in the number of closed and preferred classes would continue to achieve similar levels of savings for the VHA. This issue is under consideration and evaluation by the GAO.

An exploratory analysis of cross-service sector impacts of the National Formulary was conducted. In examining inpatient discharge data for diagnoses potentially linked to two of the National Formulary closed classes (diagnoses of heart conditions for ACEIs and diagnoses of ulcer-related conditions for PPIs), the committee found no evidence of increases in hospital use per VHA user for conditions linked to these two National Formulary closed classes. Although this result is suggestive, it is important to recognize that these analyses were quite crude. Thus, the question of how the National Formulary might affect quality of care and other types of VHA health spending is far from settled.

Additional data are needed to provide a more complete evaluation of the effects of the National Formulary on VHA expenditures with respect to the effect on expenditures for the LHRH class and whether the National Formulary resulted in increased utilization in other drug classes or elsewhere in the VHA system. Efforts to construct a database to provide for a comprehensive assessment of the economic effects of the National Formulary revealed that the VHA does not currently have the capacity to provide a number of basic data elements for the purposes of evaluating programmatic innovations such as the National Formulary. The committee has noted several times that data problems and other constraints led to inclusion of fewer items in its analysis than in the NAC analysis of savings and to an underestimate of the savings due to the National Formulary. The VHA pharmacy expenditures for the time period analyzed (approximately July 1997 to July 1999), moreover, estimated from FY 1997, 1998, and 1999 VHA pharmacy expenditures (of $1,337,487,000, $1,548,424,000, and $1,844,742,000, respectively [GAO, 1999]), were slightly greater than $3 billion. The committee's more generous, upper-bound estimate of $100,000,000 in National Formulary savings over the 2 years in question is about 3% of total pharmacy expenditures, therefore, (or stated another way, about 15% of the cost of the six analyzed drug classes) a real, but perhaps not dramatic savings, nor one that likely approaches the potential if more preferred or closed classes were created. Undoubtedly, greater savings are realized currently by mandatory generic substitution (see that section of Chapter 2 and Figure 2.5 ; CBO, 1998).

4

What Are the Effects of the National Formulary and Related Policies on Quality of Care?

BACKGROUND INFORMATION

As health care costs have risen, organized health care delivery and financing systems have implemented cost containment measures, among them formularies and formulary systems. These measures attempt to balance control of costs of unnecessary services against appropriate expenditures for medically necessary care. The concerns Congress expressed about this balance reflect the public need for reassurance that quality of care has not been compromised by cost-conscious providers, or in fixed budget systems such as the VA. Convincing reassurance regarding quality effects of the VA National Formulary would require data relating formulary and formulary system elements to veterans' health outcomes. Since such data were typically not available, the committee relied on other kinds of information, surrogate or secondary measures, and a few outcome results determined by analyzing hospital discharge data or monitoring the effects of formulary therapeutic or disease management guidelines. Quality measurement in general and these data specifically are discussed below.

Assessment of quality depends on an understanding of what quality is and how it can be measured systematically. The IOM has defined quality of care as "the degree to which health services for individuals and populations increase the likelihood of desired health outcomes and are consistent with current professional knowledge" (Institute of Medicine, 1990b). Quality was discussed further in an IOM policy document emphasizing that the definition assumed contributions from diverse professionals and that even with the best of professional knowledge good outcomes were not ensured (Chassin and Galvin, 1998). Most recently, the IOM has emphasized the role of medical errors, such as adverse drug events, in affecting quality of care (Institute of Medicine, 1999). The IOM definition has been widely adopted. This definition and the contributions of professionals and medical errors to assessments of quality were accepted by the IOM committee in evaluating the VA National Formulary because they might affect the quality of care delivered to veterans by the VHA.

Classically, three elements of a health care system were said to be relevant to measuring quality of care: (1) structure, or the characteristics of the physical, organizational,and human components or resources of the system; (2) process, or the ways or procedures by which physical and human resources were used to deliver care; and (3) outcome, or the effects or results of care on the health status of patients (Donabedian, 1980). Another classification of health care quality categorized quality problems as underuse, overuse, and misuse of health care services (Chassin and Galvin, 1998). The subject of quality of care involving pharmaceutical services specifically was reviewed by Holdfield and Smith (1997). They discussed health care quality in general and also referred to the characterization of outcomes described by Kozma et al. (1993). These authors defined health quality in terms of clinical (effects on morbidity and mortality), humanistic (satisfaction and quality-of-life effects), and economic (costs of care balanced against benefits) outcomes. Because of data limitations, quality is assessed primarily by examining the structure of the VA National Formulary and formulary system in this chapter.

QUALITY ELEMENTS

1. **Structure:** the presence or absence of infrastructure that allows health care to be delivered, for example, formularies and pharmacists.
2. **Process:** the way in which health care is provided, for example, counseling.
3. **Outcome:** the result in terms of patient health status, for example, control or cure of illness, or rehabilitation.

Sources of Quality Data

Within the context of this background information on health and pharmaceutical quality of care, the IOM committee collected and analyzed data on the effect of the VA National Formulary on the quality of care for veterans. These data came from many sources, including peer-reviewed published reports, unpublished papers, conference abstracts, and conference presentations. VA sources included short IOM e-mail or telephone interview surveys of pharmacy and clinical personnel in all 22 VISNs and in many hospitals; collection of data from the VA PBM, MAP, and National Acquisition Center; personal communications from VA staff; official VA, VISN, and hospital policy and procedure documents; VA responses to questions from Congress and written questions from the IOM; VA manuals or handbooks; and the VA PBM Drug and Pharmaceutical Program Management website (www.dppm.med.va.gov). The committee asked the outcomes bureau of the VA and the VA survey team for any information that had been collected on clinical quality indicators related to the National Formulary or veterans' satisfaction with the National Formulary. Data on patient complaints were obtained from the patients' advocates at VA facilities. The Disabled American Veterans (DAV), Paralyzed Veterans of America (PVA), and Veterans of Foreign Wars (VFW) were also asked for data on formulary issues. Information on physician perceptions of the formulary system was also sought from the National Association of VA Physicians and Dentists and the Foundation for Veterans Healthcare. Additional information bearing on quality of care came from the National Committee on Quality Assurance, the Pharmaceutical Research and Manufacturers of America, the National Pharmaceutical Council, the American Association of Health Plans, the American Society of Health-System Pharmacists, the Academy of Managed Care Pharmacy, the National Institute for Health Care Management, Pfizer Inc., academic pharmacy experts, and the personal and institutional experiences of committee members.

QUALITY OF CARE IN THE VHA AND EFFECTS OF THE NATIONAL FORMULARY

The VA has recently reported an increased emphasis on measuring and improving varied aspects of quality of care in the VHA (Kizer, 1999). Health research and support activities aimed at understanding and improving VA quality of care have been initiated, and a number of quality of care and outcomes research centers and other activities, such as the VA Patient Safety Event Registry, are in operation at VA medical centers around the United States. These were recently reviewed and reported by Zimmerman and Daley (1997). However, the committee limited its focus to data that reflected effects of the National Formulary and formulary system. Such data proved scarce.

The committee has identified elements of the VA National Formulary that were relevant to quality effects and discusses them in this chapter. The data that were available for these elements were accumulated and analyzed. Often the committee was able only to describe elements and their possible relevance to quality rather than to analyze their effects in the VHA. As is true of other chapters in this report, some of the information and analysis in this chapter is also discussed elsewhere—for example, access to drugs in Chapter 2 and economic outcomes in Chapter 3.

In this chapter, the committee covers the implications of the VA National Formulary for quality of care, as indicated by the National Formulary's effects on structure, process, or outcomes of care, both clinical and humanistic. The committee looked predominantly at the structural elements of the formulary, including the local P&T committees, the VISN formulary committees, the VA PBM and MAP, and the quality and availability of existing drugs and drugs newly approved by the Food and Drug Administration (FDA). The committee also examined drug class reviews, therapeutic guidelines, the nonformulary process, therapeutic interchange policy, and drug utilization review (DUR).

The committee looked at the effect that the National Formulary and formulary systems have on process and outcomes criteria. Analysis of process is limited primarily to the effects on utilization of drugs. Outcomes are limited to the results of therapeutic interchanges and adverse drug events, where there are few or no data. The committee also examined changes in the distribution of hospital discharge diagnoses associated with implementation of the National Formulary or with important changes in drug utilization caused by closing classes or committed-use contracts, where some new data were gathered. Patient satisfaction and complaints about access to needed or wished-for drugs are outcome indicators of quality. The VA does not systematically gather and analyze these data; to do so might help communicate the VA's interest in these outcomes.

In addition to the lack of data on effects on quality of care from some elements of the National Formulary and formulary system, the committee noted other analytic problems. The use of outcomes research has limitations, including the length of time needed to conduct research; the difficulties in separating effects of health care from life-styles, environment, or other confounding variables; and the infrequency of some outcome events. Separation of National Formulary effects from other effects in a large, complex, and changing health care system such as the VA may not be possible. Furthermore, effects of the National Formulary and formulary system may not be easy to dissect from effects of the VISN or local formularies and formulary systems, as noted here and elsewhere in this report. This, however, is less of a concern since all the formularies were treated as part of the National Formulary. Nevertheless, the committee concluded that there was sufficient information to allow discussion and some inferences about formulary influence on the quality of health care to veterans.

PHARMACY, CLINICAL, AND FORMULARY PROGRAM ELEMENTS RELEVANT TO QUALITY OF CARE

Clinical Pharmacy

The development of clinical pharmacy services and the redefinition of the scope of pharmacy practice in the VA that occurred in the 1990s when the VHA was reorganized into 22 VISNs and redirected toward ambulatory and primary care has been described in a number of reports (Anonymous, 1988; Gray, 1992; Kizer, 1999; Ogden et al., 1997; Portner et al., 1996). These developments created an expanded pharmacy program and services. VA PBM activities involved the implementation of drug treatment guidelines, the National Formulary, and national contracts. Pharmacists assumed greater involvement in patient education activities and monitoring therapies. They increasingly joined clinical care teams in clinical settings and provided advice on pharmaceuticals and the formulary system to other health care professionals. Some special programs were initiated in which pharmacists monitored adherence to specific clinical guidelines in situations where national (Joint National Committee, 1993) and VA (http://www.dppm.med.va.gov/ newsite/treatment1.htm) drug treatment guideline compliance is poor (Siegel and Lopez, 1997). Through academic detailing, as described by others (Avorn and Soumerai, 1983), and other interventions involving education and cooperation with prescribing physicians, guideline compliance was improved. This significantly enhanced the quality and cost-effectiveness of care for hypertensive and diabetic veterans (J. Lopez, personal communication, VISN 21, 1999; Meier et al., 1999; Siegel et al., 1999). These structural enhancements in some cases are shown to enhance the quality of drug therapy for veterans and, in general, presumably would have a positive effect on quality of care. The committee did not audit the performance of these new roles, but clinical pharmacist advisers have had clear and positive effects on quality (for example, fewer adverse drug events, improvements in drug selection and dosing, and cost savings) in other systems when evaluated in research protocols (Baciewicz et al., 1994; Haig and Kiser, 1991; Hatoum et al., 1988; Leape et al., 1999).

Some changes in pharmacy practice in the VHA preceded and were to some extent independent of the National Formulary so that improvements in quality of care due to improved numbers, training, or activities of pharmacists in the VHA cannot always be related directly to effects of the National Formulary. Performance of VA clinical pharmacists was reported by Gray (1992) early in the 1990s to positively affect proper dosing, indications for drug treatment, laboratory monitoring, and nonformulary requesting. This investigator at the Long Beach VA also described the 1990 implementation of a computerized system for monitoring and reporting pharmacist-initiated clinical interventions. Pharmacists play an important role in the implementation of the National Formulary, and improvements in pharmacy services and expansion of their pre-National Formulary roles probably have affected the National Formulary positively. To the extent that better pharmacy services affect and participate in the implementation and management of the National Formulary and formulary system, they are relevant quality structural elements.

P&T COMMITTEES

The introduction to this report describes the history of P&T committees in hospitals and other settings such as MCOs. Later in Chapter 1, the establishment and some of the details of P&T committees in VA hospitals are reviewed. Today, private-sector P&T committees have evolved into hospitals' or other organized health systems' primary organizational tool to evaluate and select approved (or reimbursable) medications for inclusion on the formulary. An effective P&T committee has educational, communicative, and advisory roles (ASHP, 1964, 1992) and participates in ongoing review of formulary selections for effects on quality of drug treatment as recommended in guidelines of the NCQA (UM10). It is composed of a cross section of physicians, pharmacists, and nursing representatives, usually with 8–12 members. Most P&T committees meet monthly and have formal procedures for considering formulary additions. P&T committees, through their communications, serve as the primary link between the pharmacy and the medical staff. Traditionally, hospital P&T committees have been composed mostly of physicians (Rucker and Visconti, 1975). The primary goals of a P&T committee are to enhance the rational use of drug therapy and, at the same time, to minimize social and institutional costs.

As noted elsewhere in this report, VA policy requires VA hospitals to establish P&T committees that meet the standards of the JCAHO* and the ASHP. The P&T committees' functions are performed by the medical staff in cooperation with pharmacy and nursing services and management. Traditionally, a pharmacy service representative serves as the VA facility's P&T committee secretary and is responsible for the minutes of the committee meetings. Some VA P&T committees are said to consider staff requests for nonformulary drugs, ensure that mandatory contract sources are honored, develop and revise the facility formulary, monitor adverse drug events, ensure mandatory generic prescribing or substitution, and design and implement local therapeutic interchanges and approve pharmacist substitutions, among others (VA Manual, M-2, Part 1, Chapter 3, Clinical Programs, Pharmacy and Therapeutic Committee, Dec. 13, 1993). These VA committee functions are not dissimilar to those of P&T committees in other sectors of health care. The role of most VA P&T committees in formulary management is less clear, because in 16 of 22 VISNs that particular VISN's formulary is required in all facilities.

The IOM committee did not audit performance of the P&T committees at the 172 VA hospitals. These committees should be an important structural element in the quality of drug treatment and formulary effects at the local level. They preceded consideration of a National Formulary by decades, however, and they carry out functions in addition to the National Formulary. They would also appear to be the primary place where nonmanagement VA physicians can interact with the National Formulary, or at least the VISN and local formulary and formulary system, in an influential way, although this interaction may be weakened in VISNs with a policy that requires a single VISN-wide formulary. The committee could not determine if VA P&T committees are always chaired by physicians and made up mostly from the medical staff, although this is the generally accepted model. This has implications for local physician acceptance of the National Formulary and the effectiveness of formulary operations (Carroll, 1999).

The reorganization of the VA in 1995 divided the VHA into 22 VISNs. VISN formulary committees were established as an interface between the local and national units. The formulary committees have representatives from the facilities in their region, but they may differ in the ratio of physicians and pharmacists. Formulary committees average 15 members with a range of 6–28. The membership is primarily pharmacists (52%; range, 33–100%) and physicians (44%; range, 0–65%). Nurses are included in only six VISNs. In an occasional VISN, additional personnel are included, such as representatives from administrative units. One VISN formulary committee has no physicians, four have quite distinct minorities of physicians, and overall, pharmacists outnumber physicians.

---

* In 1993, the JCAHO ceased setting standards for P&T committees and began evaluating final outcomes rather than processes. The VA, however, still uses JCAHO P&T standards as medical guidance in hospitals.

This membership structure may weaken the role of VA P&T committees as mechanisms for medical staff management of quality drug treatment and as visible and important symbols of that role (see Table 4.1). A recent survey by the AMCP identified physician membership of PBM P&T committees at 63 % on average (Table 2.1).

Some VISN formulary committees may function as VISN P&T committees. Most of these VISN committees (16 out of 22) have a policy of a single network-wide formulary to control regional drug use. The role of the VISN formulary committees has not been standardized, nor do they have membership guidelines. This has resulted in some VISNs formulary committees' acting as an additional P&T committee and others evolving toward miniature PBMs. The latter committees could function more as formulary managers for VISN administrations than as medical staff drug treatment committees, and their composition with few or no physicians could reflect this role. National VA policies have allowed VISNs reasonable latitude in implementing and enforcing VHA policy. In general, written VISN policies were not found describing or specifying how individual VISNs implement national policies at the regional or local level. Implementation of most formulary policies appears to be somewhat informal, although VISNs are specific about nonformulary policy (as required by VHA Directive 97-047) and addition of drugs to the VISN formulary. National committed-use contract adherence in their regions, is also a responsibility of VISN formulary committees.

In focusing on budgetary matters, such as controlling items on VISN and the majority of local facility formularies, nonformulary policy, and contract adherence, VISN committees assume roles as little PBMs. In contrast to some P&T or formulary committees of traditional private-sector PBMs, the VISN committees, like traditional hospital P&T committees, do not include noninstitutional (that is, non-VA) members. VISN formulary committees tend to be made up of VA pharmacists who have a vested interest in the pharmacy budget. Since VISN budgets are allocated on a per capita basis and are fixed, pharmacy managers are responsible for control of their budgets to ensure that funds for other care are not jeopardized. There are no formal studies of VISN formulary committees' effects on veterans' care. The necessary, but not sufficient, conditions for producing higher-quality effects would be to maintain a quality listing of drugs, ensure access to drugs through a smoothly functioning nonformulary process, and provide competent management of the National Formulary at the regional level.

VISN formulary committees have evolved since their inception toward PBM functions. The committees vary in their membership. Inclusion of more physician representatives on some committees could improve acceptance by VA physicians with the implications this might have for effectiveness and quality of the National Formulary. The expertise of pharmacists will remain integral to the performance of these committees, however, and other aspects of the National Formulary system are probably more important to physician acceptance.

THE VA PBM COMPLEX

Private-sector pharmacy benefits managers have evolved from claims payers for employer plans, MCOs, and government-funded programs with a pharmacy benefit to more complex organizations that maintain formularies, have generic and therapeutic interchange policies, disease management, and other educational programs, and perform DUR. PBMs achieve cost-effective drug treatment through their cost-containment strategies, pharmacy networks and mail-order pharmacies, drug price negotiations aided by their formularies, and tiered copayments, as well as through careful review and guidance by the clinical staff. These and other activities of PBMs are discussed in Chapter 2 of this report (Friedmann and Hanchak, 1999; Gibaldi, 1995; Kreling et al., 1996; Navarro and Cahill, 1999; Schulman et al., 1996; Taniguchi, 1995; WyethAyerst, 1998). In eight of the largest U.S. PBMs, external representation in addition to internal staff on P&T or formulary committees is the rule. Private-sector PBM committee members can range from 1 outside physician with no vote to 17 outside physicians with full voting privileges. Usually from one to five pharmacists employed by the PBM round out the committee. Some PBMs have multiple local P&T committees and a central committee with local representation (Jones, 1998).

The VHA reorganization authorized and funded the creation of VISNs and VISN formularies, planning for the National Formulary, a VA Pharmacy Benefits Management Strategic Healthcare Group, a Medical Advisory Panel, and a VISN Formulary Leaders Committee. These are described briefly in Chapter 1 of this report. The VA PBM planning document (Pharmacy Benefits Managemerit: A Valuable Product Line, [1995]) describes VA PBM organization and functions. This document asserts that a VA PBM "has the advantage of having both clinical and pharmacological information by patient. The result is a PBM which truly can have a very positive effect on both the economics and quality of care we provide." For further comment on VA data, see Chapter 3 of this report. The MAP was described as a standing body of 10 practicing field-based physicians appointed to 2-year terms by the Undersecretary for Health on recommendation of the VA PBM. Currently it is comprised of 1 Department of Defense (DOD) and 11 VA physicians. According to the VA, the VA PBM, MAP, and VISN formulary leaders, acting together, are responsible for National Formulary addition and deletion decisions. These bodies are central structural elements related to the National Formulary's effects on quality of care, and the quality of their management and clinical decisions regarding the formulary and formulary systems

---

VA Pharmacy Benefits Management Strategic Healthcare Group: A pharmacy benefits manager created by the VA reorganization of 1994–1995 to administer the drug benefit of the VHA.

Medical Advisory Panel: A committee of practicing physicians appointed by the VA Undersecretary for Health that advises the PBM on medical drug issues for the VA National Formulary.

TABLE 4.1 Management of the Veterans Integrated Service Network (VISN) Formulary

VISN	VISN Formulary Relationship to Local Formulary	VISN Formulary Committee Membership			Addition of New Drugs to the VISN Formulary
		Pharmacist	Physician	Other	
1	Same	13	10	0	Local or VISN
2	Same	7	13	0	Prescriber or local
3	Same	9	7	0	Local[a]
4	Same	19	7	1	No information
5	Same	6	9	3	Local
6	Same	8	0	0	Local
7	Same	9	7	0	Local[a]
8	Minor restrictions	6	8	0	Local[a]
9	Can differ	7	4	0	Local[a,b]
10	Same	10	5	0	Local
11	Same	7	7	0	Local
12	Same	7	7	0	Evaluated at FDA-approval time
13	Same	6	5	0	Local

WHAT ARE THE EFFECTS OF THE NATIONAL FORMULARY AND RELATED POLICIES ON QUALITY OF CARE?

14	Same	4	5	0	Local[a,b,c]
15	Same	9	8	0	Local
16	Can differ	7	5	1	Local[a]
17	Minor restrictions	3	3	1	Local
18	Same	8	7	0	Local
19	Same	7	7	0	Local or some evaluated at FDA-approval time
20	Minor restrictions	3	8	2	Prescriber or local
21	Same	7	6	0	Prescriber or local
22	Minor restrictions	8	6	1	Prescriber or evaluation at FDA-approval time

NOTE: Local = local pharmacy and therapeutics (P&T) committee request for VISN formulary addition; prescriber = any prescriber can generate a request for VISN formulary addition independent of the P&T committee; VISN = VISN formulary committee can generate addition request to VISN formulary.

[a] VISN has a year wait on review.
[b] Additions considered in response to local physician-, P&T committee-, or VISN-generated requests.
[c] VISN does not generally add new drugs unless they are first added to the National Formulary.

is as important to the VA formulary as private-sector PBM management is to private formularies.

The VA PBM, MAP, and VISN formulary leaders are appointed by senior VA officials and do not include medical staff who could be seen as representatives of ordinary practicing VA physicians, outside expertise, or veteran consumers. The local facility P&T committee is, therefore, the focus of nonmanagement practicing physicians in a National Formulary and formulary system committee structure that is also devoid of formal patient input. Even at this level, it is not clear how much influence local physicians have on formulary listings or structure since in many cases such decisions appear to be made at the VISN level. Two surveys have suggested that a distinct minority of VA physicians feel some dissatisfaction with the VA formulary system. The ways the VHA finds to give representative physicians a sense of participation in the formularies, or the knowledge that their management of drug treatment is modified only by science-based controls, fairly implemented, and responsive to the clinical needs of veterans, may have implications for VA physician acceptance of, and satisfaction with, the National Formulary. Physician satisfaction and acceptance may influence how the National Formulary affects quality of care. The IOM committee assessed VA PBM performance by examining the quality of the formulary, additions of drugs, drug class reviews and therapeutic guidelines, the nonformulary process, therapeutic interchange policy, and other elements of the system that affect quality. These and other factors are discussed below and in other chapters (for example, Chapter 2) of this report.

Additions to, and Quality of, the National Formulary

The addition of existing and new FDA-approved drugs to the National Formulary and the overall quality of drugs on the present formulary are important factors in the availability of drugs and thus in quality of care. Because the availability of drugs is related to the restrictiveness of formularies, addition of new drugs to the National Formulary is taken up at some length in this report's Chapter 2. VA policy on considering the addition of new FDA-approved drugs requires a 1-year wait, except in cases of significant 1P (FDA priority) category drugs. In practice, the VA has added drugs primarily for HIV/AIDS treatment recently. In theory, veterans could still have access to new drugs if they were added to VISN or local formularies or if a smoothly working nonformulary process made them easily available. In practice (see Table 4.1), two VISNs do not add drugs unless they are first added to the national list, and these and four other VISNs also have a policy of a 1-year wait for new FDA approvals. Only three VISNs actively monitor FDA approvals, and they consider additions requested by their formulary committee, local P&T committees, or VA prescribers.

All local P&T committees can recommend existing drugs to the VISN formulary committee for inclusion in the VISN formulary. In four VISNs, an individual prescriber can request inclusion of a drug without local P&T committee approval. In one instance, a VISN (VISN 2) collected utilization data from all stations to explore whether nonformulary drugs being used locally were candidates for VISN review. The VISN review processes are similar. A form is available to make a request and provide supporting relevant information. This form is filled out either by the prescriber or by the local P&T committee and is sent to the VISN formulary committee, along with a drug review. This information and the VISN reaction are generally circulated to local facilities for a 30- to 60-day comment period. VISN decisions can be reversed if warranted by comments, but only one VISN (VISN 22) has an appeals process in place.

At the national level, drugs can be considered and added to the National Formulary after VISNs suggest a review. If multiple VISNs (usually five or more) add an existing drug or a new FDA approval, the drug will be reviewed at the national level for addition to the National Formulary. As discussed in Chapter 2, the National Formulary adds few drugs each year and considers relatively few new FDA approvals, adding primarily new HIV/AIDS drugs only. The committee is aware of complaints from veterans and from prescribers, as reviewed below.

There is no accepted standard for the number of items on a health system formulary, except that listings should reflect the judgment of the medical staff acting through a P&T committee (ASHP, 1992). As discussed in the chapter on restrictiveness, the VA National Formulary appears to be of reasonable size in comparison to other health system formularies, although it has fewer representatives in a number of drug classes than MCO or Medicaid formularies. The committee was aware of some past efforts to assess the quality of drugs on formularies (Rucker, 1982, 1982a). In these reports, the author listed drugs considered of questionable quality. Rucker has also criticized formularies for listing fixed combination drug products. More recently, GAO identified drugs considered inappropriate for the elderly (GAO, 1995). The P&T and medical experts on the IOM committee reviewed the VA national list against these lists of questionable drugs and questionable combination products, and concluded that the National Formulary contained few such products. Drugs included on the National Formulary appear to meet reasonable standards of numbers, variety, and quality based on committee members' professional judgment and experience. Timely consideration of new FDA-approved drugs is discussed in Chapter 2 of this report.

POLICIES AND PROCEDURES

Drug Class Reviews

Standards for drug class reviews have evolved since 1981 when ASHP published a comprehensive description of the elements of a drug class review (ASHP, 1981). The drug class review was originally a tool for the pharmacy administration to standardize therapies and reduce inventory. As formularies began to be used to manage drug benefits, drug class reviews came to provide comparative analyses of knowledge about a drug and drug class and the applicability of this knowledge to accepted medical practice. A drug class review is an important mechanism by which a formulary system evaluates and selects from among drugs and drug products those that are considered most useful in patient care. Choosing in this way has quality implications, but it also allows a formulary system to negotiate prices of selected drugs based on anticipation of volume use, as observed elsewhere in this report.

A review can be organized into four primary areas: (1) identification of the organization and reviewers; (2) objective of the review; (3) recommendations of the review; and (4) references. Reviews should also include absolute and relative data on pharmacokinetics, clinical trials and outcomes, safety and efficacy, dosing regimens and titration, routes of administration, multiple indications, and cost and pharmacoeconomic analyses. Detailed standards and guidelines for performing drug class reviews have been reported a number of times, for example, by a group purchasing organization, such as Premier, or in the literature (ASHP, 1981; Basskin, 1998; Langley and Sullivan, 1996; Lipsey, 1992; Majercik et al., 1985). VA drug class reviews generally conform to these primary and specific criteria, although they sometimes omit a specific item(s) or a specific section, for example, pharmacoeconomic analysis, which also occurs in the private hospital sector (Majercik et al., 1985). harmacoeconomic analyses are useful because, among other reasons, some lower-priced classes may require more resource intensive management or provide lower-quality results.

Conclusions drawn in VA reviews are based on current research and consultation with subject matter experts. Occasionally, other factors that may affect quality of care are assessed. For example, a VA drug class review of ACEIs recommended addition of two long-acting members of this class to the National Formulary because patient compliance is improved on once-a-day dosing, but it also provided for a shorter-acting agent (captopril) for frail patients in need of slow titration. Since decisions on the recommendations of drug class reviews are made jointly by the VA PBM, the MAP, and VISN formulary leaders, these recommendations are likely to be implemented in the National Formulary.

IOM committee members with experience and expertise as physician leaders of P&T committees and as responsible officials of MCOs and PBMs examined the conclusions and recommendations of nine VA drug class reviews (ACEIs, alpha blockers, prokinetics, LHRHs, CCBs, H_2R blockers, HMG CoA RIs, PPIs, and SSRIs). In all cases, the drugs recommended by the review were included on the National Formulary (July 1999 version). In two cases, CCBs and H2R blockers, the National Formulary listed more agents than the minimum recommended by the review. The committee concluded that VA reviews, both as stand-alone reviews and in comparison to reviews in private-sector organizations, were of high professional quality and reached recommendations based on scientific evidence and sound interpretation of clinical data. The experts on the VA committees look at the safety, efficacy, and cost of particular products. They can then make decisions that have a reasonable scientific and clinical basis and also may affect utilization, market share, and price negotiations. The National Formulary accurately reflects the results of good quality assessments of drugs and drug classes.

Clinical Guidelines and Drug Utilization Reviews

Therapeutic or clinical guidelines are a means to decide among, and educate clinical practitioners on, preferred management of diseases and clinical conditions. In 1990, the IOM examined clinical guidelines and identified eight attributes that are essential for guideline quality: validity, reliability, clinical applicability, clinical flexibility, clarity, multidisciplinary process, schedule review, and documentation (Institute of Medicine, 1990a). IOM committee members referred to these criteria in addition to their own expertise and institutional experience with guidelines in assessing the quality and effectiveness of VA therapeutic guidelines.

The VA PBM website has documented the process of developing guidelines, including the participants in the process. Guidelines are said to be updated regularly, although the exact periodicity is not specified. They are clearly written, and interested or key clinicians can review and comment on their appropriateness. Guideline treatment recommendations are consistent with current recommendations of outside organizations. For example, the guideline on congestive heart failure reflects recommendations of the American College of Cardiology, the American Heart Association, and the Department of Health and Human Services (see http://www.dppm.med.va.gov/newsite/DSMCHF.htm). The guidelines are also tailored to the older VA patient population. In the guideline for the pharmacological management of chronic obstructive pulmonary disease (COPD), special problems in theophylline use in older patients are discussed. The IOM committee reviewed all of the clinical guidelines found at the VA PBM drug and pharmaceutical product management website (www.dppm.med.va.gov). The committee concluded that the VA drug treatment guidelines are of high quality, are based on current scientific and clinical research data, and are reliable and equivalent to similar documents in the private sector.

The committee sought evidence that VA guidelines were known to, and used by, VA physicians caring for veterans. As noted earlier, the guidelines are available on the VA PBM website and are updated periodically. Based on interviews of VA physicians by IOM staff, they are also widely distributed via mail, e-mail, weekly meetings, and one-on-one counseling sessions. It is not known, however, to what extent VA physicians consult the guidelines in their daily practice. Responses of VA physicians to the IOM were varied. Most had reported looking at the guidelines, but not whether their clinical decisions had been affected. Some suggested that the guidelines were useful in the teaching of residents.

There was some evidence that implementation of guidelines was monitored and assessed. In general, an increase has been reported in the documentation of appropriate use of inhalers for COPD, in plans to manage cholesterol in patients with heart attacks, and in charting appropriate therapies in ischemic heart disease (beta-blockers) and diabetes (Kizer, 1999). It is hard to tell whether this reflects changes in charting or actual practice. Some specific programs to monitor and encourage compliance with guidelines have been implemented. At the national level, a DUR has recently been completed to evaluate the appropriate use of PPIs. Facilities that had the highest percentage of twice-daily dosing were identified for review. Recommendations for each individual patient were sent to the facilities in question.

At the VISN level, monitoring has varied. A program in VISN 21 to monitor antihypertensive drug treatment was described earlier. A DUR program to monitor appropriate use of troglitazone, a third-line agent for the treatment of diabetes eventually recalled by the FDA, was reported to IOM from VISN 22. Although proper indications for prescribing this drug were followed, monitoring of liver toxicity was spotty. A requirement for documentation of liver function test results on prescriptions improved compliance with monitoring for this adverse drug reaction. Some other VISNs have mounted similar DUR efforts, although most VISNs do not carry out formal DUR programs, presumably because of constrained resources. DUR programs are required at hospitals, but IOM did not survey VA hospitals' DUR programs. A few hospitals were queried and they followed JCAHO recommendations for establishing DURs. That is to say, they were looking at high-risk, high-use, and costly drugs as candidates for DURs. In some situations, the facilities would share their outcomes, either informally or formally, with other facilities in their VISN. Clinical guidelines and DURs are tools employed by the VA for improving quality of care, but programs that promote the use of guidelines and supplement them with DUR programs as appropriate would enhance the effectiveness of these tools.

The Nonformulary Process

When hospitals or organized health systems develop formularies, drugs in a class are evaluated, appraised, and selected that are at least equally, and preferably more, effective and safe and have at least the same, or preferably higher, probabilities of successfully treating most patients than other class members. Drugs that are essentially equivalent may be selected because, based on price, they are more cost-effective. Some patients in any population will have difficulty with the formulary drug(s) because of therapeutic failure, allergy, or other adverse reactions or contraindications. For this reason, any restricted formulary must have a mechanism to provide drugs that are not included or covered. A nonformulary process is a universally required component of a formulary system and is part of systems in MCOs and PBMs (AAHP, 1998; ACP, 1990; AHA, 1974; AMA, 1994; ASHP, 1983; Dillon, 1999). Prior to the introduction of the National Formulary, VA hospitals had restricted formularies and established procedures for obtaining nonformulary drugs. With the establishment of the National Formulary, the VA did not implement a standard national procedure, but rather outlined criteria in VHA Directive 97-047, and required VISNs to develop and implement a process in each region. VA criteria are consistent with the policies and criteria of most managed care organizations (Dillon, 1998). The VA is unlike many other organizations and Medicaid in that very rarely are drugs cluded, that is, unavailable even through a nonformulary process.

VHA Directive 97-047 requires the following: (a) A nonformulary request process must exist at each VA medical treatment facility; (b) This process should ensure that decisions are evidence based and timely; (c) Nonformulary drugs should be approved under the following circumstances—(1) contraindication(s) to the formulary agents, (2) adverse reaction to the formulary agents, (3) therapeutic failure of all formulary agents, (4) no formulary alternative exists, (5) the patient's previous response to a nonformulary agent and the risk associated with a change to a formulary agent, (6) other circumstances having compelling evidence-based clinical reasons; (d) Nonformulary approvals should require a reevaluation of the approval based upon clinical response; (e) Each VISN will identify key nonformulary approval components and establish a process to analyze and trend the information at the VISN and local level; (f) In therapeutic classes where national standardization contracts have been awarded, VISNs will report to the PBM quarterly the justification for nonformulary drug utilization. A template for the report will be provided to VISN formulary leaders by the PBM. As noted elsewhere, information from [e] and [f] is not available.

Since national policy does not dictate a specific nonformulary process, either a VISN or a local facility (depending on VISN policy) can design a procedure that is consistent with directive criteria. As a national average, 3.45% of all prescriptions dispensed by the VHA are for nonformulary drugs. However, this can vary from a fraction of 1% to about 30% by institution (based on closed-class nonadherence reports) depending on the local nonformulary process. These data depend on the national computerized system tracking drug dispensing and formulary adherence and are likely to be accurate. Comparisons of these percentages with percentages in hospitals and MCOs have been detailed in Chapter 2 of this report. In general, VA nonformulary dispensing volume is a comparatively lower percentage.

In a preliminary investigation, the IOM determined that there were many variants of approval processes in use (see Figure 4.1 for some common variants). The simplest and quickest process was a prescriber telephone call to the pharmacy or to the chief of staff to obtain a decision. More complicated and time-consuming processes involved completion of a form (of varying complexity) by the prescriber, which was submitted to the pharmacy for review, followed by a decision by the local P&T committee.

In response to a congressional inquiry, the VA PBM conducted a survey of all institutions in each of the 22 VISNs in December 1998. Survey results were reported to Congress in early 1999. The survey asked the physician chair of each P&T committee to rate the nonformulary system before and after implementation of the National Formulary. The process was rated "easy" (as opposed to "difficult") prior to the National Formulary by 84%. After implementation of the National Formulary, 97% of physician chairs gave the process an "easy" rating. The IOM committee noted that in many institutions the P&T committee is a step in the nonformulary approval process. The P&T chairperson cannot be considered a disinterested rater, and the rating itself is not an objective or quantitative one and is undoubtedly subject to varying interpretations. The time for approval

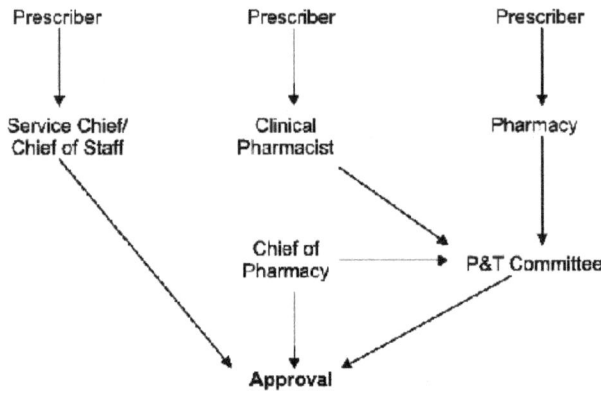

FIGURE 4.1 Variations of the VA nonformulary approval process.

was reported to decrease from 43 to 27 hours after the National Formulary became operational. The survey also reported that 88% of requests were approved. This compares with 70 to 90% approvals in other public-and private-sector formulary systems (Hoechst Marion Roussel, 1998; Jones, 1998; Kreling et al., 1996; Phillips and Larson, 1997; Schweitzer and Shiota, 1992; Sloan, 1989).

Many VA facilities have an informal nonformulary process, as noted in the minutes of the VA PBM Research Steering Committee meeting of March 1998. In a follow-up to its preliminary investigation, the IOM surveyed institutions in all 22 VISNs to explore qualitatively this informal system and its implications. Although institutions in all VISNs were queried, the total numbers (22) were too small to constitute a statistically valid sample. Nevertheless, the IOM survey discovered a range of interactions between physicians and pharmacy teams resulting in positive or negative nonformulary decisions that may not be documented (see Table 4.2). Historically, one large VA medical center reported that 7.7% (about 25 per month) of interactions between clinical pharmacists and physicians in clinical settings involved nonformulary requests (Gray, 1992). These were not tracked before the introduction of the National Formulary. Such interactions continue and are unlikely to be documented now. If this is prevalent, the nonformulary study reported to Congress may overestimate the percentage of requests approved.

Currently, in some facilities, if a prescriber sends a prescription for a non-formulary drug without a nonformulary request form, the pharmacist will call the physician to suggest formulary alternatives. In some institutions, the pharmacists will make similar calls even if a form is submitted. Although these are nonformulary requests, they are not always reflected in the approval numbers; that is, a change to a formulary item is not always counted in the approvals or denials for the month. In other institutions, physicians are called about denials and only approvals are tabulated. In still other institutions—for example, special units such as spinal cord injury centers—special negotiations by Paralyzed Veterans of America representatives, usually at the center or facility level, occasionally at the VISN or even undersecretary level, result in enhanced availability of sometimes hard-to-get items. These include supplies (which were listed in the VA National Formulary, at least in part, at the behest of the PVA). Of course, this kind of representation or sponsorship is not always available to most veterans (H. Bodenbender, PVA, personal communication, 1999).

The IOM committee appreciates the advantages of an informal system in flexibility and speed of response and the difficulty of recording informal discussions or advice. Spotty documentation of the process resulting from informal, or more formal but still unrecorded, interactions casts doubt on the accuracy of nonformulary request numbers and approval percentages, however. This may diminish confidence in the system. An informal and variable system also may result, in some instances, in processes that appear arbitrary or overly responsive to budgetary rather than medical conditions. In some facilities, the physician time necessary for multiple nonformulary requests, or the time spent if P&T committee review is required, might be perceived as a barrier and potentially detrimental to quality care. The nonformulary process appears to differ considerably across the VHA. It is often informal and unrecorded in national statistics.

TABLE 4.2 Results from IOM Exploratory Inquiry into the Nonformulary Approval Process

Nonformulary Process	Not Recorded[a] ($n = 22$)
Prescription is sent to the pharmacy without a form and is changed to a formulary item	22
Prescription is sent to the pharmacy without a form and is denied	6
Prescription is sent to the pharmacy without a form, and is denied, form is sent in but is denied.	0
Prescription is sent to the pharmacy without a form and is approved	5
Form is sent in, prescriber called, item changed to formulary item	9
Patient or drug representative initiates the nonformulary process	6
Prescriber and pharmacist talk about a nonformulary drug, but a formulary item is prescribed	19
Nonformulary item is discussed and approved, no form is generated	6
Nonformulary item is discussed and not approved, no form generated	4
A nonformulary item is discussed, and denied, a form is submitted and denied	1
Prescriber or facility is noncompliant	1

[a] Number of VISNs in which a facility might not record a nonformulary request in its monthly statistics.

Examination of nonformulary forms and some anecdotal reporting suggest that delays and burdens in obtaining nonformulary drugs also may vary and in some cases may be problematic. The current system has not provided reassurance about delay or access problems. The committee concluded that the National Formulary would be seen as fairer and more responsive if the nonformulary system were revised and simplified and improvements in accurate and consistent reporting were made. Among these, the VHA should consider pilot tests of non-formulary processes that include, for example, budget feedback to prescribers, request tracking and education through service chiefs analogous to academic detailing, or exploration of retrospective corrective discussions with prescribers who abuse the system.

Therapeutic Interchange, Policy, and Results

Therapeutic interchange policy and practice are reviewed in Chapter 2 of this report. In this chapter, the committee briefly discusses issues relevant to quality of care including policy direction, evidence for problems in VA interchanges, the relationship to a flexible nonformulary process, and prescriber control. Although the National Formulary and formulary system, like systems in most private-sector MCOs, PBMs, and hospitals (Doering et al., 1988; Hoechst Marion Roussel, 1998: Nash et al., 1993; Novartis, 1998, 1999; Reeder et al., 1997; Sloan et al., 1997; Wyeth-Ayerst, 1998) contemplate, therapeutic interchange in response to drug use criteria, formulary listings, or national standardized contracts, there is no national policy on the process of interchange. The VA PBM, MAP, and VISNs have left policy and procedure to local facilities, although directives leading to interchange often originate at the national or VISN level. Reports of therapeutic interchange at VA facilities describe various procedures and results. Overall they are reassuring (see references cited in Chapter 2), but they suffer from analyses of too-small numbers, often with too-short or otherwise less-than-adequate follow-up and other methodological shortcomings.

Interchanges generate a measurable level of dissatisfaction among VA physicians (Glassman et al., 1999; Yankelovich Partners, 1999) and complaints from patients (see below). Although current published reports in the medical literature, unpublished documents from VA facilities, and expressions of physician and patient dissatisfaction from surveys and patient advocate data, do not constitute compelling evidence of quality problems, they raise questions for exploration and suggest possible responses that might be taken by the VHA. Therapeutic failure of the formulary therapeutic alternate, medical complications, offsetting costs caused by extra visits and tests, and patient and physician complaints have all been discussed earlier (see Chapter 2). Elsewhere in this report it is suggested that desirable consistency in therapeutic interchange might include assurance of physician and patient education and advance notice, attention to drug treatment compliance, and provision for exceptions based on characteristics of at-risk patients, among others. The responsiveness and consistency of the local nonformulary process to problems that arise in interchange programs might also reassure patients and prescribers that quality considerations will be given priority.

VA P&T committee policy permits pharmacists to prescribe therapeutic alternates in a program of therapeutic interchange when authorized by the local P&T committee. The fact that the permission of prescribers may not be sought and often is not obtained at the time of dispensing an alternate emphasizes the desirability of ensuring prescriber (and patient) education and acceptance of the purposes of the National Formulary and formulary system to avoid unnecessary dissatisfaction and possible quality problems. Higher-quality investigations of interchange programs would engender greater confidence in VA study results. Furthermore, measures that promote physician understanding and acceptance of, and participation in, the formulary system and interchanges could diminish physician (and patient) dissatisfaction. Surely, if veterans receiving a drug on a long-term basis are subject to interchanges multiple times or too often because of changes in the formulary or committed-use contracting, there will be effects on acceptance and compliance, and there may well be changes in the effectiveness of treatment. In short, quality of care and possibly health outcomes will be affected. The VA has no policy on frequency, or limits on the number, of interchanges for veterans.

EFFECTS OF THE NATIONAL FORMULARY ON USE OF DRUGS BY THE VA

The committee evaluated the process of care by examining the number of prescriptions written for all drugs in closed and preferred classes from 1995 (prior to the National Formulary) until the second quarter of 1999. As expected, the selected drugs in closed classes were used significantly more than drugs not selected for the National Formulary. Figure 4.2 and Figure 4.3 (PPIs and LHRHs) illustrate how a formulary drug achieves more than 90% volume and use of the nonformulary agent drops to near zero. Inclusion in a closed class on the National Formulary, however, is not the only significant driving force for drug utilization. In drug classes where more than one agent is on the National Formulary, national contracts or drug usage criteria are also associated with prescribing changes.

This occurs in all classes. Figure 4.4 shows the effects of a national contract for ranitidine. Increases or decreases in utilization follow the negotiation or termination of a contract. Termination of the contract for famotidine was associated with a marked decrease in utilization of this agent. At the same time, ranitidine utilization changed in association with the contract for this drug. Nonadherence reports typically show about 4 to 6% nonformulary use in closed classes, although the range is much wider. In open or preferred classes, noncontract use varies over time. VISNs and local facilities also have the prerogative of negotiating favorable prices through blanket purchase agreements and/or initiating programs to influence prescribing toward the least costly alternate in a class. Figure 4.5 and Figure 4.6 illustrate VISN programs to encourage use of different

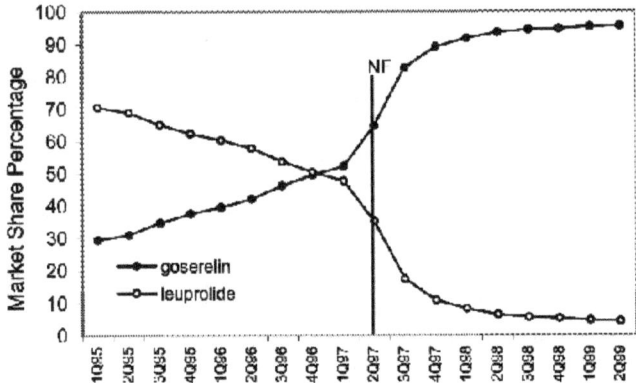

FIGURE 4.2 National formulary policies affect market share of the luetinizing hormone-releasing hormone against drugs.

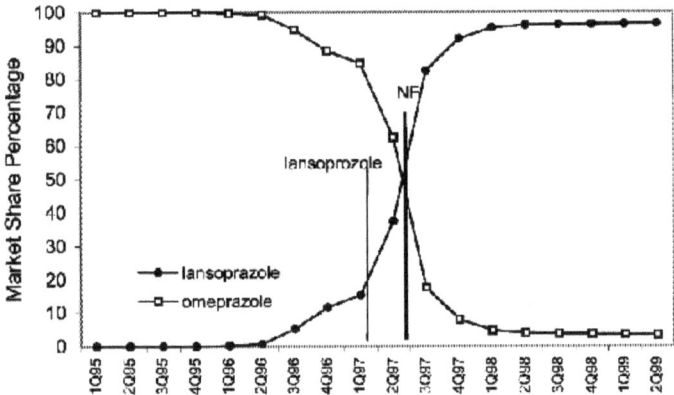

FIGURE 4.3 National formulary policies affect market share of the proton pump inhibitor drugs.

angiotensin II blockers for the treatment of high blood pressure, based on their assessments of cost and compliance factors. As illustrated, VISN 7 has shown a dramatic increase in the use of irbesartan with a decrease in the usage of losartan. Conversely, VISN 20 has shown an increase in the use of candesartan.

WHAT ARE THE EFFECTS OF THE NATIONAL FORMULARY AND RELATED POLICIES ON QUALITY OF CARE?

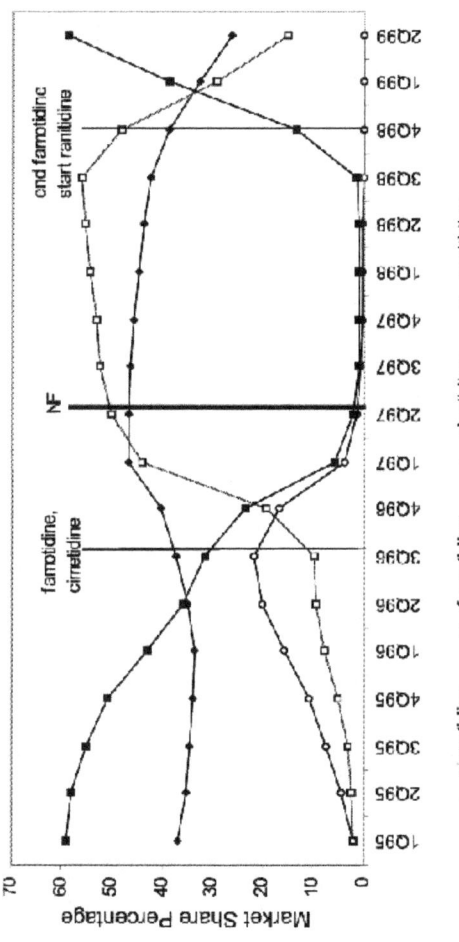

FIGURE 4.4 National formulary policies affect market share of the histamine$_2$ receptor (H$_2$R) blocker drugs.

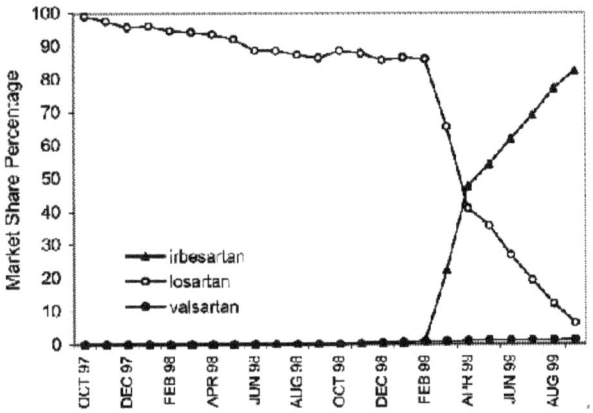

FIGURE 4.5 VISN policies affect the market share of the angiontensin$_2$ (A$_2$) antagonist drugs in VISN 7.

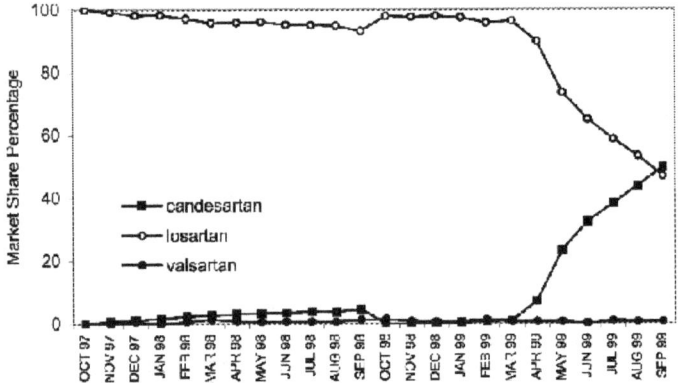

FIGURE 4.6 VISN policies affect angiontensin$_2$ (A$_2$) antagonist drug utilization for VISN 20.

If veterans travel to a different VISN where local or regional programs to encourage prescribing of particular members of a drug class are in force, they may experience quality problems unless interchange and nonformulary programs are responsive. These last two examples also demonstrate how local or VISN decisions may differ among themselves and from National Formulary decisions. The committee did not find any scientifically valid evidence that the changes in the number or variety of drugs by class closure were affecting the quality of drug treatment and the health outcomes of veterans, however. To analyze such effects, patient-specific tracking of drug utilization would be needed.

ADVERSE DRUG EVENTS

In the final sections of this chapter, the committee discusses outcomes as quality indicators. The World Health Organization defines an adverse drug reaction (ADR) as an effect that is "noxious and unintended, and which occurs at doses used in man for prophylaxis, diagnosis or therapy." An adverse drug event (ADE) encompasses medical error, that is, "an injury caused by medical management rather than the underlying condition of the patient" (Institute of Medicine, 1999). Included are unintended effects of drugs or errors in the process of dispensing. Adverse consequences range from rash, headache, and diarrhea to organ failure or death. The end result is that ADRs or ADEs may result in both increases in health costs and decreases in quality of life.

Although adverse drug events can occur at any age, the elderly are particularly at risk, due in part to their higher per capita consumption of drugs and in part to their decreased physiologic capacity for drug handling or to comorbidities. Many health care organizations have made decreasing the risk of ADEs a high priority and have developed strategies to achieve this (ASHP, 1996; Institute of Medicine, 1999). Strategies include using computerized prescription entry; using machine-readable (bar) coding in their medication use process; developing better systems for reporting and monitoring ADEs; using unit dose medication distribution and pharmacy-based intravenous medication admixture systems; assigning pharmacists to work in patient care areas in collaboration with prescribers; seeking systems to prevent ADEs; and using pharmacists to actively review medication orders prior to dispensing.

The VA has devoted resources to decreasing ADEs. Four sites (VA Palo Alto, VA Cincinnati, VA New England White River Junction, and VA Tampa) have been awarded contracts to establish "Patient Safety Centers of Inquiry." Two of these sites have a mission not only to collect information but also to implement systems to decrease errors. The New England center has been working with the Institute of Health Care Improvements to establish a breakthrough series to decrease ADEs. The programs are in their infancy and evaluations are not complete. The VA has completed switching to electronic prescribing, a system known to decrease errors. A program to implement machine-readable coding on all inpatient wards has been initiated and will presumably continue.

The main thrust of collecting and preventing ADEs in the VA is still at the local level. Few VISN formulary committees collect and discuss ADEs. VISN 2 and VISN 4 are part of the breakthrough series on ADEs. Another VISN (VISN 13) reports its ADEs during monthly teleconferences among facilities. Local facilities have employed different practices to decrease ADEs including programs such as the breakthrough series. ADEs are reported to local P&T committees for review and action. In addition, many facilities commonly include pharmacists on the inpatient and outpatient wards, a procedure found to have a positive outcome in both VA and the private sector (Gray, 1992; Haig and Kiser, 1991). These pharmacists provide a variety of interactions, including suggestion of drugs and doses, monitoring of drugs with narrow therapeutic ratios, conducting chart reviews, and education of physicians and patients on aspects of drug therapy.

In theory, the VA Patient Safety Event Registry, initiated in 1997, could collect VHA national data on medication errors. The Registry did, in fact, report 171 medication errors (with 22 deaths) after the first 19 months of operation, varying from wrong dose, dispensing error, and wrong medication to "other." The number of medication error reports was only 5.8% of the total events reported and varied 40-fold across VISNs. Some VISNs reported only one medication error during this period (Department of Veterans Affairs, 1999a). At present, the Registry does not appear to be a reliable source for identifying ADEs.

Although the VA National Formulary has introduced structural changes related to ADEs, other concurrent changes not resulting directly from the formulary (bar code recording, electronic prescribing, breakthrough series) confound a determination of formulary effects on ADEs. The committee did not find data on ADEs during therapeutic interchange, a specific element of the National Formulary. This is not surprising because reports to the FDA of ADEs associated with interchanges have also been infrequent from the health care system in general (FDA, 1997). The request for special reporting to the FDA presumably reflects this agency's interest in the consequences of therapeutic interchange. The FDA, however, has almost no data. Continued review of adverse event reporting has not resulted in reliable documentation of problems (P. Honig, FDA, personal communication, 2000). The system does not provide evidence of an association of poor health outcomes with interchanges; it only reports events, or anecdotes, with uncertain reliability.

Changes in Inpatient Hospital Discharges Associated with the National Formulary

In Chapter 3 of this report, the committee discusses gathering and analyzing new data on hospital discharges before and after the implementation of the National Formulary. These discharge data included discharges over 4 years for a group of diagnoses that might have been affected by changes in the availability of drugs used to treat them. These drugs were those known to be involved in restrictions by the National Formulary. The VA could not provide data on total pharmacy users, outpatient data for the relevant years, or patient-level drug data. These study years were also characterized by changes in hospitalization rates, movement to ambulatory care, and, undoubtedly, other confounding variables, including changes in medical practice and the clinical indications for the drugs involved. This analysis, therefore, is only suggestive that no major effects of the

TABLE 4.3 Most Frequent Formulary Complaints to Patient Advocates

3–4 Total Complaints	5–10 Total Complaints	>10 Total Complaints
bicalutamide (Casodex)	refecoxib (Vioxx)	omeprazole (Prilosec; 15)
Depens	loratadine (Claritin)	atorvastatin (Lipitor; 15)
Alendronate (Fosamax)*	troglitazone (Rezlin)	celecoxib (Celebrex; 27)
isosorbide (Imdur)	tramadol (Ultram)	sildenafil (Viagra; 60)
interferon	zolpiden (Ambien)	
amlodipine (Norvasc)	alprostadil (Muse)	
ranitidine (Zantac)		
tolterodine (Detrol)*		
tamsulosin (Flomax)		
fluticasone (Flovent)		
famotidine (Pepcid)		

* The committee notes that these complaints were generated by female veterans who comprise only 4% of the veteran population.

National Formulary and formulary system on health outcomes could be detected by this means (see Chapter 3 of this report).

PATIENT COMPLAINTS—ADVOCATE, VETERANS OF FOREIGN WARS, AND SURVEY DATA

Patient complaints may suggest program areas where changes or improvements could be considered. Patient satisfaction is a generally accepted element of quality of care. Patient dissatisfaction discovered through significant levels of complaints to advocates or through surveys could be an important indicator of the need for a system response. The IOM contacted VA patient advocates at each facility for formulary-related complaints. Patient advocates did not code for formulary complaints prior to establishment of the VA National Formulary. Thus, data were available only from July 1997. Of course, some veteran dissatisfaction may not be expressed in complaints to patient advocates. Furthermore, not all visits to patient advocates are documented. The number of formulary-related complaints may be higher than reported, therefore.

Enough information was available to make some observations, however. Approximately 92% of all VA facilities representing all 22 VISNs responded to the committee's request for information. Nationally, only 2,385 of 570,937 complaints (0.4%) were attributed to the National Formulary. No VISN had significantly more complaints. The committee was able to identify the medications in question for 462 complaints. Not surprisingly, medications that are subject to direct-to-consumer marketing generated a number of complaints, as did lack of access to specific drugs that were considered desirable such as sildenafil (Viagra) (see Table 4.3). Since the collection of these data, the VA has developed clinical guidelines for the treatment of erectile dysfunction and criteria for the use of sildenafil. Most complaints were from veterans unable to get a desired drug because it was not on the National Formulary or on VISN, or local formularies. In some other instances a local decision had been made not to stock a National Formulary drug or the local medical staff had decided to restrict it for medical reasons (H. M., Farrow, personal communication, VISN 16, 1999). Patient advocates interviewed agreed that the inability to obtain medications was not a major veteran complaint. Advocates near VISN regional borders received complaints about the availability of medications because of differences in VISN formularies. Overall, however, patient advocates heard few complaints concerning the National Formulary. The committee also contacted veteran groups for their formulary data to verify that formulary-related issues were not a major complaint among veterans. In 1997, the VFW established a toll-free complaint line as an additional advocate source for veterans. Nearly 20,000 complaints have been counted in 98 categories. Complaints concerning the formulary amounted to less than 0.2% of the total.

A large VA multicenter study of a therapeutic interchange program between HMG CoA RIs (switching fluvastatin to simvastatin) was carried out in 1999. In the course of this project, 3,153 surveys were mailed to patients, and 1,800 (57.1%) were returned. Although there were problems with the survey design and some confusion and incomplete responses from veterans, this study provided evidence of satisfaction with a National Formulary program based on adequate numbers and a reasonable response rate. An attempt was made to sort responses by whether veterans learned of the interchange by letter or were told by their pharmacist or physician. Among the former, 21–24% of veterans were neutral, that is, neither satisfied nor dissatisfied, and 6–8% were dissatisfied or very dissatisfied with how they learned of the exchange. Among the latter, similar results, 21% and 6–11%, respectively, were obtained. In 91–92% of responses, veterans believed the replacement medication was as effective as the original. About one-quarter to one-third of veterans reported that they received either no or inadequate information on the replacement medicine, however (W. N. Jones, personal communication, VISN 18, 1999).

Based on these data, the committee speculated that many veterans are aware (or are made aware through interchange notices) that there are budgetary restraints in the VHA and that some restrictions or cost-saving reactions are necessary. Most veterans seem to be tolerant of cost controls, although they could not be said to be enthusiastic, and some either complain or express their dissatisfaction when asked. As noted elsewhere in this report, there are potential improvements in VA programs that might address some concerns of these veterans. Overall, the committee did not find data on significant numbers of veterans expressing dissatisfaction with the National Formulary.

PHYSICIAN COMPLAINTS AND SURVEY DATA

Studies of physician satisfaction with formulary systems from the private sector and from the VHA specifically are reviewed in detail elsewhere. Insofar as physician dissatisfaction is a quality indicator, these studies are relevant here, although they have sampling, numbers, and other design problems that weaken any conclusion that can be drawn from them. The data appear to identify a minority of VA physicians who have concerns about quality effects of the VA National Formulary and formulary system and are dissatisfied with the National Formulary (see Chapter 2 of this report). Most observers agree that physician compliance is essential to the success of a formulary and formulary system, and to that extent, dissatisfied, noncompliant physicians may impair the quality of the National Formulary. General surveys in the medical literature suggest that physicians do not automatically approve of formulary systems, especially those that practice therapeutic interchange. Navarro and Cahill (1999) have pointed out the natural antipathy that results when a professional (or indeed anyone) is faced with restrictions that prevent customary freedom and enforce cost-conscious behavior. These physicians need to feel a part of such formulary systems and to subscribe to formulary objectives.

The IOM committee is of the opinion, based on physician comments recorded in the Yankelovich Partners (1999) survey and others, that VA physicians by and large understand that the VHA has a fixed appropriation. They understand that overruns in one budgetary component obligate cutbacks in others. The discussions in this chapter raised the possibility that quality might be enhanced and physician acceptance of the National Formulary improved with some adjustments to the system. These included empowering physicians through more membership on influential committees involved with the National Formulary. Improvements in consistency and responsiveness of the nonformulary process should be implemented. Physician nonformulary performance could be examined retrospectively or through education. In a similar vein, one VA facility has given physician services target drug budgets for the year, and it reports expenditures and progress toward the target each month to each service. Although there is no penalty for exceeding the target, physicians are expected to support appeals for financing budget overruns. In principle, the involvement of practicing physicians in drug program management seems likely to help them understand the goals of the National Formulary.

SUMMARY STATEMENT

In this chapter, as its title indicates, the committee has explored the effects of the National Formulary and related policies on quality of care. Such an exploration inevitably questions whether there are quality effects sufficient and certain enough to support a decision to either abandon, continue, or strengthen the VA National Formulary. A completely firm and final answer to this question would require scientifically sound evidence of formulary influences on quality of care that affect process of care and health outcomes of veterans. However, there are no epidemiological or other well-designed studies of the VHA that conclusively provide such evidence one way or the other, that is, of either improvements or impairments in outcomes. The VA has apparently not completed any such studies or reported any such research. Some early and incomplete steps in this direction have been taken, including some information in this report on hospital discharge distributions associated with the National Formulary. There are anecdotal reports of quality problems or successes, few veteran complaints, and some worrisome indicators of physician concerns. The absence of persuasive reports of substantial worsening of health outcomes in the medical literature attributable to a closed or partially closed formulary either for the VA or for millions of covered lives in MCOs or PBMs is not proof of no effect, although it is somewhat reassuring.

The committee fell back on, and relied primarily on a review of structural elements of the National Formulary related to quality. This review was also somewhat reassuring, including communications with, and reports of, an active and apparently skilled pharmacy service, observation of an active and thoughtful MAP, evidence of quality drug class reviews and a careful and rather parsimonious class closure process, reviews of therapeutic guidelines, an assessment that the formulary was of adequate size and quality, and an analysis of the formulary's effects on drug prices, with the implication that prudent drug purchasing freed funds for increased services to veterans.

Based on this information and analysis, the committee concluded that there is no reason to discontinue the National Formulary and every reason to try to improve it. In this latter regard, concerns are expressed in this chapter about the nonformulary process; the composition of committees; physician and patient satisfaction, therapeutic interchange policies, notice of interchanges, and education; follow-up and monitoring of clinical guidelines; and addition of newly FDA-approved drugs among others. The committee also strongly urges the VA to focus its considerable health services research capacity on National Formulary and drug treatment issues, in a way that hitherto has not been the case, as the responsibility of a national program to illuminate these issues. The absence of good data on quality effects is a concern, as is the need for better data to enable prudent management of the National Formulary. In the meantime, the committee supports the continuation of the National Formulary and formulary system. This includes the careful closure of classes where good therapeutic alternates exist and clinical and economic data are supportive, and an emphasis on quality of care for veterans as the highest priority.

5

How Does the VA National Formulary Compare with Private Insurance Formularies for Drugs and Devices and with Other Government Formularies?

INTRODUCTION

The majority of Americans are covered by private-sector pharmacy benefits with formularies and formulary systems. These benefits must be flexible and responsive to public needs and preferences if they are to compete in the private marketplace. The VA has explicitly attempted to model its recent reorganization and pharmacy benefits after many aspects of those in the private sector (Kizer, 1996, 1999; Ogden et al., 1997). The committee found that comparisons of the VA National Formulary and formulary systems with private-sector plans are the most informative. There are clear and substantive differences between the VHA and MCOs (as described elsewhere in this report), which suggest the need for caution in making comparisons. Nevertheless, the VA and private-sector plans have similar formulary control objectives, as noted in Chapter 2 of this report. The committee also concluded that specific details of MCO formularies and state statutory controls on MCO performance would be helpful in understanding MCO formularies and formulary systems in comparison to the VA National Formulary.

That information is reviewed in this chapter. The information to characterize these formularies was gathered from the open, peer-reviewed literature, company websites, and the annual surveys supported by Hoechst Marion Roussel, Novartis, and Wyeth-Ayerst. The IOM committee did not find any surveys of MCO and PBM formularies that were similar to the survey of pharmacists about hospital P&T committee activities done by Mannebach et al. (1999). To address this deficiency, a special survey responding to questions concerning important controls or elements of restrictiveness that the committee identified was carried out by the Academy of Managed Care Pharmacy, as noted earlier (see Appendix B and Table 2.1). This survey covered two small MCOs and six PBMs serving 176 million covered lives. The committee also relied on information from the personal and institutional experiences of committee members in the managed care and pharmacy benefits management industry (E. Dichter; J. Jones; O. Wolke; and A. Zimmerman, personal communications, 2000).

MCOs or PBMs may know what effect prior authorization, therapeutic interchange or generic substitution, or copayments and other cost controls that are commonly used have on choice of drugs for their patients. The committee found no national quantitative quality or cost data in the peer-reviewed literature, however, and therefore could not compare these restrictions to the VA National Formulary effects on utilization (examples of which are displayed * in the figures in Chapter 3 and Chapter 4 of this report and discussed in both chapters). Clearly, these controls are intended to restrict choice and direct prescribing. It is well known that copayment size is inversely related to utilization of health care services (Brook et al., 1983), including prescription drugs (Leibowitz et al., 1985; Smith, 1993), and may possibly affect health outcomes (Johnson et al., 1997).

Most MCOs/HMOs offer prescription drug benefits (98.1%, although only about 90 to 92% of enrollees buy these benefits). They usually have formularies (92.9%, but 97.8% of all HMO enrollees are covered by plans that have formularies), and 92% of HMOs contract with PBMs to handle part or all of their pharmacy programs. This most often involves claims processing (Hoechst Marion Roussel, 1998), but PBMs carry out formulary management for 46% of MCOs and 63.2% of employer plans according to Novartis (1998). Most formularies are closed (26.9%) or partially closed (45.4%) (Novartis, 1999). Similar results—35% closed, 24% partially closed—were reported by Luce et al. (1996). Kreling and Mucha (1992) reported 60% restricted or restricted with exceptions. These figures document the increase in restrictive formularies in managed care (72.2%); most hospital formularies have been restrictive for some time.

Only 17.5% of MCOs provide brand name drugs without a penalty when generics are available, which occasionally (17%) amounts to the entire cost of the brand drug, but usually (66.4% [or 44.4%; Novartis, 1998]) to the difference in cost (Hoechst Marion Roussel, 1998). Employer plans are more generous, but 20% require dispensing generics when available; otherwise the enrollee must pay either the entire prescription cost or, more often, the difference in cost between the brand and the generic drug (Wyeth-Ayerst, 1998). MCO and PBM coverage of members of major drug classes is usually more extensive than the VA National Formulary, but financial penalties for nonformulary drugs, non-preferred drugs, or brand name drugs when generics are available are more and more common. This cost control was applied by 86.4% of HMO pharmacy benefit programs estimated in 1999, but less frequently by PBMs (Lipton et al., 1999). MCO copayments on formulary genetic prescriptions average $6.17, and on formulary brands $9.65. Nonformulary genetic copayments average $7.32, and nonformulary brands $13.77. About 80 to 90% of MCOs require prior authorization for some drugs (Novartis, 1998, 1999).

IMPLEMENTATION OF DRUG MANAGEMENT STRATEGIES IN MANAGED CARE

MCO drug management strategies include formularies and formulary systems, generic substitution, therapeutic interchange, tiered copayments, DUR, and prior approval, among others. These, as in the case of the VA, are intended to direct prescribers and patients to lower-cost, but similarly safe and effective drugs and to help in price negotiations to obtain such lower-cost drugs. As described later, some of these strategies are applicable to Medicaid managed care recipients within certain limits. Others, such as tiered copayments, are not. MCO formularies also restrict access by prior approval or lists of excluded drugs, ranging from a few to more than 200 different agents. Earlier in this chapter, MCO formulary systems were discussed. Here, some specific formularies are examined.

The committee reviewed MCO or PBM formularies in whole or in part from six Mountain State MCOs (R. Valuck, personal communication, 1999), five major Massachusetts MCOs (Massachusetts Outpatient Formulary Guide, 1999), Geisinger Health Plan (PennState Geisinger Health Plan, Formulary, 1999), PCS Health Systems (1999), Humana (http://www.humana.com, under member services), United (www.uhc.com, under pharmacy programs), and Aetna/U.S.Health Care (www.aetnaushc.com, under members and consumers) and from the experiences of committee members. About 70 million covered lives and hundreds of formularies are represented by MCO or PBM officials serving on the IOM committee. Because managed care formularies undergo constant revision, these formularies will undoubtedly be different by the time this report is published.

MCOs usually list more drugs than the VA National Formulary, but they also exclude more drugs, have more drugs on required prior authorization, and occasionally have quantity or volume limits. They may also list only one agent in a class, which may be different or the same as that listed in the VA National Formulary (although, according to the AMCP survey [see Table 2.1], the surveyed PBMs and MCOs usually do not limit closed classes to only one agent). For example, in Massachusetts, Fallon Community Health Plan listed lansoprazole, Neighborhood Health Plan, omeprazole; and BlueCrossBlueShield, Harvard Pilgrim Health Care, and Tufts Health Plan, both lansoprazole and omeprazole in the very popular and costly PPI class (Massachusetts Formulary Guide, 1999). At the same time, some of these plans listed five or six ACEIs or HMG CoA RIs compared to two or three in these classes in the VA National Formulary. Tufts Health Plan publishes its list of noncovered drugs as part of its Prescription Alternative Program (www.tufts-healthplan.com, under member information). The list of noncovered drugs includes both the restricted product and the health plan's suggested alternative (s). For example, the HMG CoA RIs cerivastatin (Baycol), lovastatin (Mevacor), and simvastatin (Zocor) are on the noncovered list. The suggested alternatives are atorvastatin (Lipitor), pravastatin

(Pravachol), and fluvastatin (Lescol). A modest number of other drugs have quantity limits or require prior authorization.

Humana's on-line drug formulary notes 12 products and some injectables requiring prior approval. These products include the ache drug isotretinoin (Accutane), alendronate sodium (Fosamax) for osteoporosis, antifungals terbinafine tabs (Lamisil) and itraconazole (Sporanox), finasteride (Proscar) for prostatic hypertrophy, troglitazone (Rezulin) for diabetes, and NSAIDs celecoxib (Celebrex) and rofecoxib (Vioxx). United Health Care's on-line list of preferred drugs includes 19 products that require prior approval and 69 that have some type of quantity limit. The prior approval list includes antihypertensives losartan (Cozaar) and losartan/hctz (Hyzaar), etanercept (Enbrel) for arthritis, antifungals fluconazole (Diflucan), terbinafine (lamasil), and itraconazole (Sporanox); and the antidepressant bupropion (Wellbutrin SR). Drugs subject to some sort of prescribing limit include: interferon beta 1B (Betaseron); alprostadil (Caverject) for erectile dysfunction; SSRIs paroxetine (Paxil), citalopram (Celexa), fluoxetine (Prozac), and sertraline (Zoloft); fluticasone propionate (Flonase) for allergy; alendronate sodium (Fosamax); drugs for migraine sumatriptan succinate (Imitrex), rizatriptan benzoate (Maxalt), and zolmitriptan (Zomig); and HMG CoA RIs simvastatin (Zocor) and atorvastatin (Lipitor).

Aetna US Health Care lists 46 drug products that require precertification and more than 120 that are excluded from the formulary. Of the newer antidepressants, Aetna excludes payment for fluvoxamine (Luvox) and citalopram (Celexa) and lists paroxetine (Paxil), fluoxetine (Prozac) and sertraline (Zoloft) as alternatives. For HMG CoA RIs, Aetna excludes cerivastatin (Baycol), atorvastatin (Lipitor), pravastatin (Pravachol), lovastatin (Mevacor) and includes simvastatin (Zocor) and fluvastatin (Lescol) as alternatives. A number of drugs such as rofecoxib (Vioxx) and celecoxib (Celebrex) require step therapy under the Aetna formulary plan.

A comprehensive analysis of MCO formularies is not available. The restrictiveness data assembled for this report from the AMCP survey and from publicly available sources are the most extensive and up-to-date currently available. MCOs may have different formularies, prior approval, and copayment provisions for different clients such as employers, individuals, Medicare, and Medicaid programs. Some insurers have numerous health plans, each with a unique drug benefit structure. For example, the Aetna US Healthcare on-line formulary notes exceptions for California (injectable drugs require precertification) and Indiana (no precertification program) residents. The Humana on-line formulary lists unique formularies for Tampa, Florida, South Florida, and Illinois. Other large MCOs are similarly variable. VA formularies are also variable, as noted elsewhere in this report. This variability among formularies in different health care sectors and the variability in controls or elements of restrictiveness prevented the committee from reaching a definitive conclusion about comparative restrictiveness. In some respects the VA National Formulary is more, and in some respects less, restrictive than comparison formularies.

IMPACT OF STATE LEGISLATION ON MCO PRACTICE

Reacting to the studies cited in this report, to professional and trade groups, and to consumers, legislators in many states have become actively involved in the issues of managed care and the use of formularies. To date, 33 states (see Figure 5.1) have passed legislation authorizing the use of formularies. The majority of these states have also required public disclosure of the formulary and nonformulary process. California Law SB625 requires the filing of the nonformulary procedure and that the process be expeditious (http://www.leginfo.ca.gov/pub/97–98/bill/sen/sb_0601–0650/sb_625_bill_19980622_chaptered.html). Maine Law 63-2550.4 requires nonformulary request approvals within 24 hours or provision of a 72-hour supply of the prescribed drug. Fifteen states require access to nonformulary drugs if, (1) they are medically necessary, (2) they are prescribed by a physician, and (3) the preferred drug is ineffective or reasonably expected to cause an adverse or harmful reaction (see www.ganet.state.ga.us/cgi-bi...code/g/33/20A/9 for Georgia's law).

Tennessee Bill SA0684 amends SB0637 and prohibits managed care organizations from either switching or discontinuing an enrollee's prescription drug unless the patient's provider determines that this change would not harm or prolong the patient's treatment (www.legislature.state.tn.us/Bills/100gahtm/l00_amnd/sa0684.htm). California Bill AB974 requires that health plans continue coverage of a drug that is appropriately prescribed and medically necessary (www.leginfo.ca.gov/pub/97–98/bill/asm/ab_0951–1000/ab_974/bill/19980622_chaptered.html). States have also addressed off-label usage. When scientific results reported in the

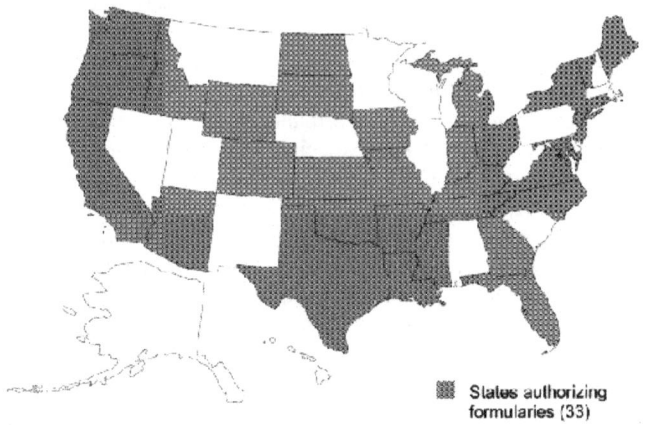

FIGURE 5.1 States specifically authorizing formularies.

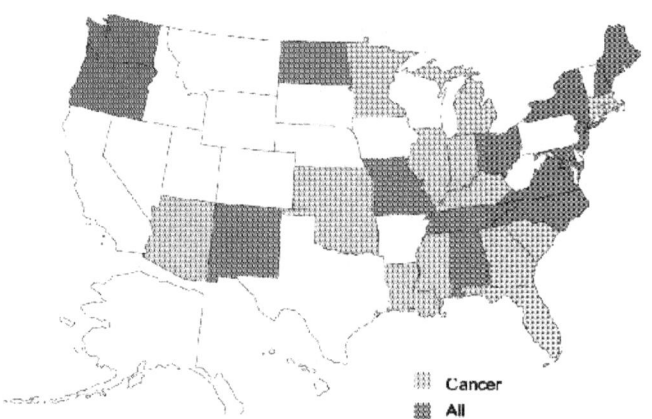

FIGURE 5.2 States enacting off-label usage legislation.

medical literature support the off-label use of a drug for a medical condition, MCOs in 15 states must provide coverage. An additional 15 states specifically require off-label coverage for the treatment of cancer (Figure 5.2).

In 1999, 12 states (Connecticut, Florida, Iowa, Maryland, New Hampshire, North Carolina, North Dakota, Oklahoma, Rhode Island, South Dakota, Texas, and Virginia) passed legislation, in some cases further restricting MCOs. Connecticut legislation prohibits a managed care plan from increasing cost sharing or copayment conditions or eliminating or decreasing covered prescriptions during the contract year (www.cga.state.ct.us/ps99/fc/pdf/1999sb-00125-r000430-fc.pdf). Similar legislation was passed in Texas and was effective as of September 1999 (http://tlo2.tlc.state.tx.us/tlo/76r/billtext/SB01030F.htm). Other provisions enacted include establishing quality-of-care and performance measurement systems (Maryland) or requiring formulary approval by a special committee (Virginia) (Centeon, 1999). Most of the provisions of these state laws are not relevant to the VA National Formulary, which is characterized by complete disclosure (www.dppm.med.va.gov), off-label coverage, low or no copayments, and relatively stable drug coverage. Nevertheless, the basic thrust of many of these provisions is to ensure that access to drugs is not restricted unless there is a reasonable decision on medical necessity, a concern for all formularies including the VA National Formulary.

PUBLIC-SECTOR PROGRAMS

The VHA is a government health care program. For this reason, two relevant public-sector programs with formularies and formulary systems were reviewed in addition to MCO programs. The VA and Congress had specified such a comparison and specifically suggested the Medicaid program. The Medicaid program also is the largest government pharmacy benefit. It has been functioning with formularies for several decades. Its effects have been studied extensively, and it is described annually in some detail in surveys supported by the National Pharmaceutical Council (NPC). The committee appreciates that Medicaid serves a population with entirely different demographics (principally women and children), has different eligibility standards (primarily economic rather than national service), and is subject to quite different federal and state law and regulatory program requirements. Information on Medicaid was gathered from an extensive consultant's report (Brown, 1999), committee experience, the NPC surveys, and the open, peer-reviewed medical literature.

The committee also decided to review the Department of Defense (DOD) formulary and formulary system. The DOD health system and pharmacy benefit budgets are similar in size to the VHA and VA Pharmacy budgets, and there is considerable interest in coordinating DOD and VA formularies and pharmacy benefits or in making changes that would bring the DOD pharmacy benefit design closer to that of the VA (see P.L. 105-85, P.L. 106-65, and P.L. 106-117). Although the DOD health system serves a larger total population with somewhat younger active duty personnel and more women, there are similarities because of the large numbers of retired military personnel using DOD health care. DOD and VA programs are already cooperating in purchasing for example, but as described below, the formularies are quite different. Data for the committee's comparison of the DOD system came primarily from GAO audits and personal communications (GAO, 1998) and from the publicly available DOD website.

Medicaid

The Medicaid outpatient pharmacy benefit is administered through state Medical Assistance programs under Title XIX of the Social Security Act (SSA) and applicable state laws. The program provides drugs to recipients through the U.S. retail pharmacy market, which dispensed about 2.97 billion prescriptions in 1999. It spent slightly less than $12 billion in this marketplace in FY 1997 (Baugh et al., 1999; www.nacds.org/news/releases/nr_082999_projections.html; www.hcfa.gov/medicaid/mstats.htm). In comparison, the total VHA pharmacy budget for FY 1997 was $1.3 billion (GAO, 1999).

Medicaid Fee for Service

In this section, the committee discusses Medicaid fee for service. Medicaid managed care is taken up later in this chapter. The Medicaid program was enacted in 1965 to provide health care services to the poor and is jointly funded by the federal government and the individual states. Originally a fee-for-service program, it is now increasingly managed care (discussed later in this chapter). Federal law and regulation require states to provide Medicaid benefits to specific categorically needy groups in order to receive federal matching funds. These groups include those eligible for Aid to Families with Dependent Children (AFDC) prior to July 16, 1996; the aged, blind, and disabled receiving Supplemental Security Income (SSI); and children, pregnant women, and elderly who meet certain income criteria. The Personal Responsibilities and Work Opportunity Reconciliation Act of 1996 (P.L. 104–193) repealed the AFDC program and replaced it with Temporary Assistance for Needy Families (TANF). Most persons covered by TANF are eligible to receive Medicaid benefits, but it is not an automatic entitlement. States may also extend Medicaid benefits to other groups that do not meet the basic federal eligibility guidelines, for example, the medically needy.

Although the Medicaid program covers a wide range of eligible groups, the Medicaid population is not representative of the U.S. population. The majority of Medicaid recipients are poor women and children. Of the 41.5 million Medicaid eligibles in FY 1997, 58% were women; 45% were less than 14, 55% less than 21, and 77% less than 45 years of age (www.hcfa.gov/medicaid/mstats.htm). This compares with a VA population that averages 53 years of age and is 95% male (see VA Annual Reports). In general, 26% of Medicaid eligibles are SSI aged, blind, or disabled and more than 68% are adults or children meeting income standards, for example, TANF or AFDC eligibles. The aged Medicaid eligibles, however, obligate a disproportionate share of Medicaid expenditures, primarily due to long-term (nursing home) care, which alone consumes about 25% of the total Medicaid budget. These Medicaid recipients resemble the VA population more closely.

Only 55% of Medicaid recipients remain continuously eligible for the full year. The rest enroll and disenroll throughout the year. Over 34.8 million (83%) Medicaid eligibles received one or more health care services during 1997 (www.hcfa.gov/medicaid/mstats.htm). Although VHA eligibles are to some extent stratified by income, as veterans they remain eligible for life. Only 3.3 million of a total of about 26 million veterans are enrolled in the VA health care system, and they tend to be older, disadvantaged, and minorities (VA *Annual Report,* 1998; Fonseca et al., 1996).

Title XIX of the SSA specifies the types of services that must be provided to Medicaid recipients if states are to qualify for federal matching funds. These include inpatient and outpatient hospital care; physician services; vaccines for children; prenatal care; x-ray and laboratory services; and nursing home care for recipients over 12 years of age. Title XIX also lists a variety of optional services eligible for federal matching funds. These include diagnostic and screening services; optometrist services; eyeglasses; intermediate-care facilities for the mentally retarded; rehabilitation and physical therapy services; transportation to and from medical services; and outpatient prescription drugs. Most of these services are provided by the VHA, including some highly specialized care for spinal cord injury and blindness, among others.

The basic Medicaid program is described as a fee-for-service system, but states have wide latitude in determining payment methods and rates. Federal law requires that payment be sufficient to enlist enough providers to reasonably deliver the care required by recipients. In addition, providers must accept Medicaid payment as full payment for their services. States may require small deductibles, coinsurance, or copayments for certain recipients, but cost sharing cannot be imposed on pregnant women, children, or nursing home patients, or required for emergency or family planning services. States may apply for waivers allowing them to enroll recipients in prepaid managed health care plans. These waivers, called Section 1915 and Section 1115 waivers, allow states to experiment with different health care delivery systems.

Medicaid programs operate within broad federal guidelines. As a result, state programs have developed in various ways over time. Some states have enrolled all Medicaid recipients in managed care; and others have not enrolled any. Some states have imposed strict drug utilization and payment guidelines, while some have only nominal drug cost and use control procedures. Some states have expanded eligibility to include a broader range of needy individuals. In addition, 17 states have implemented expanded drug coverage programs for elderly and/or disabled individuals who would not normally qualify for Medicaid coverage. Nine of these programs were implemented more than 10 years ago.

Total Medicaid vendor payments amounted to more than $123.5 billion in FY 1997. This figure does not include payment by Medicaid of aged recipients' Medicare Part B premiums (see Glossary) or Medicaid managed care premiums, or payments to "disproportionate share" hospitals (those with large numbers of poor patients). Almost 25% of vendor payments in 1997 were associated with nursing home care, and 20% went to hospitals. Pharmaceuticals accounted for 9.7% of vendor payments. Almost two-thirds of Medicaid recipients, about 21 million individuals, used the pharmacy benefit in 1997 (www.hcfa.gov/medicaid/mstats/ htm). Since Medicaid is an entitlement, its budget is open ended. If prescription drug costs increase, they will be paid without affecting other care budgets. In the VHA, a fixed appropriation requires savings in one or more parts of the budget to offset overruns in other parts. This may make VA providers and managers more sensitive to budget overruns and to the need for controls that demonstrably achieve their intended purposes.

Medicaid Prescription Drug Benefit

Every Medicaid program provides coverage for prescription drugs. Federal law and regulations set the basic requirements for this coverage. Each state has leeway in designing drug benefits within these federal requirements. Federal law regarding prescription drug coverage has changed over the past decade. In addition to Title XIX of the SSA, the current Medicaid prescription drug benefit is governed by provisions enacted in the Omnibus Budget Reconciliation Acts of 1990 and 1993 (OBRA 1990, 1993). Prior to the passage of OBRA 1990, states faced fewer limits on the implementation of drug management strategies, such as formularies, prescription limits, generic substitution, prior approval systems, refill limits, and copayments (NPC, 1989). To address rising drug expenditures in the late 1980s, Congress proposed that a national P&T committee create a national formulary and designate therapeutic interchanges. Pharmaceutical companies responded to this proposal by offering to pay rebates on drug purchases to state Medicaid programs in exchange for a statutory prohibition on restrictive state formularies. Under a compromise enacted in OBRA 1990, Congress prohibited restrictive state Medicaid formularies, allowed prior approval under certain conditions, required Medicaid programs to reimburse all new drugs for at least 6 months after FDA approval, and required manufacturer rebates based on the lesser of a discount of about 15% below AWP or the best price offered to other purchasers.

After OBRA 1990 and the elimination of restrictive formularies, many states reported increases in drug expenditures, and Congress began considering a repeal of the prohibition on restrictive formularies. In addition, other drug purchasers complained that the best price language of the Medicaid rebate agreement led to an increase in the prices they paid as manufacturers tried to reduce their rebate liability (CBO, 1996). Provisions in OBRA 1993 responded to these concerns, repealing the prohibition on restrictive formularies in OBRA 1990 as well as the requirement to cover all drugs for 6 months after FDA approval.

OBRA 1993 and 1990 mandated that manufacturers sign rebate agreements to qualify their products for reimbursement. Standardization of state formularies and prior approval systems is required. Medicaid now covers products of manufacturers that have signed rebate agreements (as essentially all do) and may only exclude products in accordance with specific federal regulation described below. An excluded product must be made available through prior approval, but certain statutorily designated classes of drugs may be excluded from reimbursement and the prior approval requirement at the discretion of the states.

The best-price language of the rebate agreements continues to require that the best price a manufacturer gives to any other purchaser, including any cash or volume discount or rebate, is automatically given to every Medicaid program. A minimum rebate amount is now set at 15.1% below AWP (42 USC Section 1396r–8 (c)(1)(C)). Prices charged under the Federal Supply Schedule, depot prices, and single-award contract prices are excluded from the best-price calculations. Also specifically excluded are covered (that is, brand name) drug prices charged to the Indian Health Service, the Department of Veterans Affairs, the Department of Defense, and the Public Health Service, according to the Veterans Health Care Act of 1992 (42 USC Section 1396r-8(c)(1)(C)).

The current Medicaid prescription drug benefit also allows prior approval of any drug as long as the prior approval system provides a response within 24 hours and a 72-hour emergency supply of the drug under review. Requirements for formularies are more complex. States may create a formulary if it is developed by a committee consisting of physicians, pharmacists, and other appropriate individuals appointed by the governor of the state, and it includes the drugs of any manufacturer that has entered into a rebate agreement unless the product is excluded in accordance with other regulatory requirements.

These latter requirements specify that a covered outpatient drug may be excluded only if it does not have a significant, clinically meaningful therapeutic advantage in terms of safety, effectiveness, or clinical outcome over other drugs included in the formulary and there is a written explanation available to the public of the basis for the exclusion (42 USC Section 1396r–8(d)(4)(C)). In any event, excluded drugs must be made available under a prior approval program unless they are members of a specifically listed class. These are (a) agents when used for anorexia, weight loss, or weight gain; (b) agents when used to promote fertility; (c) agents when used for cosmetic purposes or hair growth; (d) agents when used for the symptomatic relief of cough and colds; (e) agents when used to promote smoking cessation; (f) prescription vitamins and mineral products, except prenatal vitamins and fluoride preparations; (g) nonprescription drugs; (h) covered outpatient drugs for which the manufacturer seeks to require as a condition of sale that associated tests or monitoring services be purchased exclusively from the manufacturer or its designee; (i) barbiturates; (j) benzodiazepines.

These federal statutory and regulatory requirements have left prior approval as one of the last flexible drug management strategies available to state Medicaid programs. After meeting the requirement for a 24-hour response and a 72-hour emergency supply, states have significant leeway in designing and implementing prior approval. States may adopt their own clinical or nonclinical criteria for approving a request. States may restrict a particular drug to patients of a certain age, to those with a specific and verified diagnosis, or even to those who have been treated with other drugs prior to the request. Prior approval and formulary programs vary depending on factors such as the specific drugs or classes restricted, the criteria for approval, and the system for granting exclusions to the regulations. No two Medicaid drug benefit programs are exactly alike, but no state has the flexibility in designing formularies and formulary systems, including exceptions processes, enjoyed by the VA.

Medicaid Controls Prior Approval and Formulary Systems

Formularies, prior approval systems, copayments, exclusions, and prescription limits or quantity controls are the most common restrictions found in Medicaid programs. Table 5.1 outlines the basic control elements of each state's Medicaid fee-for-service drug benefit. Seven states (California, Colorado, Illinois, Michigan, Montana, Ohio, and South Dakota) report a closed formulary, although all states restrict some medications or therapeutic classes. Every state restricts some or all of the OBRA 1990 excludable drugs (see Table 5.1), most commonly amphetamines, barbiturates, antihistamines, drugs used for cosmetic purposes, and benzodiazepines. Although not required, some states allow coverage of these products with prior approval. States also require prior approval for drugs other than those listed in OBRA 1990, although these requirements change periodically. These restricted drugs and drug classes include the antipsychotic drug clozapine (Clozaril), growth hormones (for example, Protropin),

TABLE 5.1 Medicaid Fee-for-Service Drug Benefit[a]

	Formulary Design	Prior Approval System in Place?	Limits			Number of Prescriptions per Month	Patient Cost Sharing
			Quantity[b]	Refill			
Alabama	Open	✓	✓	5 per Rx		None	$0.50–$3.00
Alaska	None			None		None	$2.00
Arkansas	None	✓	✓	5 refills within 6 months		3	$0.50–$3.00
California	Closed	✓	✓	None		6[c]	$1.00 (optional)
Colorado	Closed	✓		None		None	$0.50, generic $2.00, brand
Connecticut	Open	No PA	✓	6 month limit		None	None
Delaware	Open	No PA	✓	None		None	None
Florida	Open		✓	Up to 1 year		6 (8 for institutionalized)[d]	None
Georgia	Open		✓	None		5 (6 for children)[e]	$0.50
Hawaii	Open		✓	None		None	None
Idaho	Open		✓	None		None	None
Illinois	Closed		✓	11 per Rx		None	None
Indiana	Open	No PA	None	None		None	$0.50–$3.00
Iowa	Open		None	None		None	$1.00
Kansas	Open		✓	Up to 1 year		None	$2.00
Kentucky	Open		✓	5 refills in 6 months		None	None
Louisiana	Open	No PA	✓	5 refills in 6 months		Impotence drugs limited to 6 per month	$0.50–$3.00

State	Formulary		Refill Policy	Limit	Copay
Maryland	Open	√	2 per Rx	None	$1.00
Massachusetts	Open	√	5 refills in 6 months	None	$0.50
Michigan	Closed	√	None	None	$1.00
Minnesota	Open	√	Limit of 1 year or 11 refills	None	
Mississippi	Open	√	5 maximum	5	$1.00
Missouri	Open	√	None	None	$0.50–$2.00
Montana	Closed	√	25% grace period over 3 months	None	$1.00, generic $2.00, brand
Nebraska	Open	√	None	None	$1.00
Nevada	Open	√	None	3	None
New Hampshire	Open	No PA √	None	None	$0.50, generic $1.00, brand
New Jersey	Open	√	None	5 in 6 months	None
New Mexico	Open	√	3 per 90-day period	None	None
New York	Open	No PA √	Limit of 6 months or 5 refills	None	$0.50, generic $2.00, brand
North Carolina	Open	√	None	6	$1.00
North Dakota	Open	√	Up to 12 months	None	None
Ohio	Closed	√	11 within 12 months for noncontrolled drugs[f]	None	None
Oklahoma	Open	√	1 year maximum	3 unlimited for patients under 21	$1.00–$2.00

Oregon	Open	✓	None	None	None
Rhode Island	Open	✓	5 per Rx [g]	None	None
South Carolina	Open	✓	None	3, unlimited for patients under 21	$1.50
South Dakota	Closed		None	None	$2.00
Texas	Open	✓	5 refills, total cannot exceed 6-month supply	3, unlimited for patients under 21	None
Utah	Open	✓	5 per Rx	None	$1.00
Vermont	Open	✓	5 per Rx	None	$2.00
Virginia	Open	✓	None	None	$1.00
Washington	Open	✓	2 per 30-day period, with exceptions[h]	None	None
West Virginia	Open	✓	5 per Rx	10	$0.50–$2.00
Wisconsin	Open	✓	11 per 12 months	None	$1.00

HOW DOES THE VA NATIONAL FORMULARY COMPARE WITH PRIVATE INSURANCE FORMULARIES FOR DRUGS AND DEVICES AND WITH OTHER GOVERNMENT FORMULARIES?

	Open	No PA		up to 1 year	3	$1.00
Wyoming						
Total	41 of 48 have open formularies	41 of 48 have a PA system	45 of 48 have a quantity limit	28 of 48 have a refill limit	14 of 48 have prescription limits	31 of 48 require patient cost sharing
Veterans Administration Formulary System	Partially closed	√	√	√		√

NOTE: PA = prior approval.

[a] The information in this table is not a comprehensive listing of drug benefit designs. It is based on each state's response to an annual survey conducted by the NPC and the level of detail provided by each state varies from extensive to minimal. Many states listed only a subset of their restricted drugs. Nevertheless, the NPC report is the most comprehensive source of information available.

[b] Most states limit the quantity dispensed to 30- or 34-day supplies except for maintenance drugs, which generally have 100-day supply limits.

[c] Exceptions for family planning, AIDS, or cancer drugs.

[d] Antiulcer, antianxiety, and sedative hypnotic drugs limited to 1 per therapeutic class per month, 1 refill per prescription.

[e] H_2Rs and other antiulcer drugs limited to 2 Rxs per lifetime; nonsedating antihistamines Toradol and Dolobid are limited to 1 Rx per year.

[f] Limit of 5 refills for schedule II, IV, and V drugs, no refills allowed for schedule II drugs.

[g] Five refills are limited to certain products (e.g., antihypertensives, diuretics, anticonvulsants, and antidepressants). No refills for certain products, including central nervous system stimulants and schedule II and III products.

[h] Antibiotics, antiasthmatics, schedule II and III drugs, antineoplastics, topicals, and any propoxyphene drug may have 4 refills.

[i] Arizona and Tennessee are excluded because they run statewide Medicaid managed care plans.

SOURCE: National Pharmaceutical Council (1998).

nonsedating antihistamines, isotretinoin (Accutane) for acne, branded NSAIDs, the Alzheimer's drugs tacrine hydrochloride (Cognex) and donepezil hydrochloride (Aricept), and antiulcer medications. Restrictions also include biotechnology products such as somatropin rh-GH (Serostim), aldesleukin, or interleukin-2 (Proleukin), filgrastim G-CSF (Neupogen), and erythropoietin alpha (Epogen, Procrit) used in the treatment of cancer and chronic kidney disease, and interferon beta-1 (Betaseron) for multiple sclerosis. Only seven states reported having no prior approval process (Connecticut, Delaware, Indiana, Louisiana, New Hampshire, North Carolina, and Wyoming).

Implementation of formularies and prior approval systems varies widely. California requires prior approval for any drug or indication not listed in its MediCal list of contract drugs, essentially a nonformulary exceptions process. Maryland requires approval for drugs prescribed for 34 days or more with usual and customary charges above $100 or for any drugs with usual and customary charges above $400. Florida limits the use of antiulcer, antianxiety, and sedative or hypnotic drugs to one prescription per month and one refill per prescription. Georgia limits antiulcer medications to two prescriptions per lifetime, and the nonsedating antihistamines ketorolac tromethamine (Toradol) and diflunisal (Dolobid) to one prescription per year. Limitations on time, amount, or dollar value are rarely employed by the VA. Veterans can get up to a 90-day supply per prescription, but not more. These prescriptions can be refilled, however. A few drugs, such as sildenafil citrate (Viagra), may be limited to a specified number of doses per unit time. Volume or time restrictions may result in restrictions on patient access to needed, medically indicated drugs as noted in studies reviewed later in this chapter.

Uses of prior approval requests vary from state to state. For example, Florida has a special request form for approval of growth hormones for adults and a general request form for other nonformulary products. Both are one-page forms, although the growth hormone form requires more detailed clinical information. New York's program for clozapine (since discontinued) required patients to have a diagnosis of schizophrenia, be at least 16 years of age, and be refractory to treatment by other antipsychotic medications (New York Office of Mental Health, 1991). If the request for clozapine was approved, an 8-digit prior approval number had to be provided to the participating pharmacy to permit reimbursement. Considerable additional data were required for continuing clozapine, which appear to have represented significant time burdens for prescribing physicians.

Copayments and prescription limits are additional forms of drug use and cost controls. Sixteen states impose some copayments, and 12 have limits on the number of reimbursable prescriptions per month. Copayments vary from $0.50 to $3.00 and are waived for certain patient groups (children, pregnant women, nursing home or long-term-care residents) or drug categories (family planning). Pennsylvania has a $1.00 copayment, but it does not apply to patients receiving drugs in classes such as anticonvulsants, antidiabetic agents, antineoplastics, antiparkinsonian agents, and psychotherapeutics. Five states limit reimbursement to three prescriptions per month, two have a limit of five prescriptions per month, and three have a limit of six per month.

An interesting example of a difference between the VA and the Medicaid program was recently provided by the introduction of sildenafil for erectile dysfunction. This new and expensive medication generated concerns in both the VA and Medicaid about potentially significant inflation in drug costs. In the case of Medicaid, the Health Care Financing Administration (HCFA) concluded that, "Viagra does not fall within any of the allowable exclusions or restrictions listed in section 1927(d)(2) and section 1927(d)(3) of the Act. Therefore, the law requires that a State's Medicaid program cover Viagra when medical necessity dictates such coverage for the drug's medially accepted indication" (www.hcfa.gov/medicaid/drpolicy.htm). Of course, states can and do restrict the use of Viagra to specific indications via prior approval, limit the number of refills and/or quantity of pills, and monitor and discipline prescribers found to be prescribing the medication inappropriately (www.hcfa.gov/medicaid/drpolicy.htm). Only after a much longer interval was sildenafil removed from the list of excluded drugs and approved for use by the VA, and this was a VA option not a statutory requirement.

Although most states use some combination of prior approval, exclusions, prescription limits, and copayments, the effects of these controls are unclear. The impact of any particular prescription drug control measure is dependent on its design and management. If the clinical criteria associated with a prior approval program are strict and requests are carefully managed and scrutinized, then the program may be effective in limiting uses of a particular product that exceed uses approved by the program. If a prior approval system is burdensome, it may impose a resource cost that deters physicians from submitting requests. On the other hand, a minimally burdensome system with clear clinical guidelines may simply encourage physicians to meet all the criteria before submitting a request.

Whether or not the effects on drug utilization of these administrative level drug management strategies are sustained is open to debate. No long-term studies have addressed whether they are maintained beyond the first year or two after implementation. Prescribing patterns may eventually return to previous levels once physicians become familiar with the specific regulations, learn how to navigate the system, and become less fearful of oversight of their prescribing practices. In any case, as discussed later in this chapter, the cost effects on other parts of the Medicaid program pharmacy benefit or on nonpharmacy program components may be of concern and are often unrecognized or unmeasured. Some of these cost effects have resulted from restrictions in the optional outpatient pharmacy benefits and their formularies (which are the primary subject of this chapter) that divert recipients to the mandatory inpatient hospital or long, term care benefits and the drugs provided in these settings which depend more on the policies of these facilities (Soumerai et al., 1991).

Comparison to the VA

The committee noted that although there are some standardizing factors such as the requirement for a timely response and emergency supply of drug, the differences among states in exceptions, prior approvals, and other drug-specific restrictions have led to a Medicaid formulary or drug access entitlement that varies considerably for some products (see Table 5.1). The VA National Formulary provides a basic, uniform entitlement that is expanded by differing VISN and local formularies. The VA exceptions process is perhaps even more variable than Medicaid's, although in the absence of good data on either the VA or Medicaid, this is uncertain. Exclusion of OBRA classes and some kinds of limits on the amount and frequency of dispensing by Medicaid are more restrictive than VA controls. With the exception of sildenafil (Viagra) and new prescriptions for troglitazone (since recalled by the FDA), the VA has not excluded drugs except insofar as nonformulary requests are disapproved. The VA National Formulary provides fewer choices in some drug classes, particularly the closed classes, although Medicaid prior approval in some of these classes may hinder unfettered access to drug members. Copayments in the VA were authorized by P.L. 101-508. They are small ($2.00) and limited to more affluent veterans and to non-service-connected treatment. Copayments linked to income may increase in the future as allowed by recent legislation, however (P.L. 106-117, Section 201). Copayments may be meaningful barriers to access, particularly in poor populations in either the VA or Medicaid.

Since the VA nonformulary process requires approval before a nonformulary drug can be dispensed, it is similar to the Medicaid prior approval process which requires approval before the program will pay for a prescribed drug that is subject to prior approval requirements. Programs in states without prior approval requirements are clearly less restrictive in this respect than the VA. However, other states have more prevalent or more burdensome requirements. It is not certain, therefore, that Medicaid prior approval processes are always less restrictive than the VA nonformulary process. The committee assumed that the 88% VA National Formulary nonformulary approval percentage is based on incomplete reporting and is an overestimate, as the IOM survey of VISNs' nonformulary exceptions processes implies. Several authors suggested that the states' approval processes, in general, resulted in higher approval rates than are current in the VA, with variations in the burden imposed (Jones, 1999; Kreling et al., 1996; Schweitzer and Shiota, 1992; Sloan, 1989; see Chapter 2 of this report).

Effects of Medicaid Formularies and Formulary Systems

Medicaid administrative-level cost containment studies focus on the use of formularies and, specifically, the effect of limiting reimbursement through formulary exclusions. Their findings are generally consistent (see Table 5.2). The review of the formulary literature by Jang (1988) found the assumption that restrictive formularies result in a reduction in drug expenditures unsubstantiated and suggested that formularies shifted costs to other parts of the health system.

Jang concluded that restrictive formularies lead to dynamic changes in the total Medicaid program of a complex and often costly nature. Schweitzer and Shiota (1992) also found the evidence of cost reduction by restrictive formularies inconclusive.

Unfortunately, there is a lack of high-quality formulary studies. This severely limits understanding of the impacts of formulary systems (Soumerai et al., 1993). Common problems with the current formulary literature include short follow-up periods and a lack of control groups. Follow-up periods must be long enough to distinguish between short-term and long-term effects. An adequate comparison group is necessary to control for underlying trends in drug and non-drug utilization (Soumerai et al., 1993). Of the 12 administrative-level studies evaluated by Soumerai et al., only three met their criteria for adequate controls. It is often difficult for researchers to obtain data appropriate for conducting well-controlled studies (for example, time series, comparison series data sets). Nevertheless, as noted in Chapter 4, there is a need for more well-controlled studies on the drug and nondrug effects of formulary restrictions.

Soumerai et al. (1990) used New Jersey Medicaid data to assess the effect of withdrawing reimbursement for drug efficacy study implementation (DESI) drugs. Drugs referred to as DESI drugs, all approved before the 1962 Kefauver-Harris Amendments to the Food, Drug and Cosmetic Act, were those found to have questionable efficacy. As a result, they were determined to be nonreimbursable by government payers. These researchers conducted interrupted time-series analyses of data on almost 400,000 Medicaid recipients over 42 months (July 1980 to December 1983) to determine how the withdrawal of reimbursement affected their use of DESI and substitute medications.

Withdrawal of reimbursement led to an immediate reduction of 21.7 DESI prescriptions per 1,000 recipients per month, an almost total elimination of prescriptions for these drugs. This decrease was more than offset by an increase of 33.7 prescriptions per 1,000 recipients per month in the use of substitute medications. There was no change in total drug use or expenditures during the study period. These authors concluded that reimbursement restrictions result in desirable and unimproved therapeutic substitutions and, for marginally effective therapies, may not reduce costs. Education may be necessary in order to achieve desirable therapeutic and economic practices (Soumerai et al., 1990).

The findings of an earlier study (Smith and McKercher, 1984) eliminating reimbursement for DESI drugs are consistent with the results of the study conducted by Soumerai et al. This 6-month case study (3 months before and 3 months after the change in reimbursement policy) followed Michigan Medicaid recipients who received one of the study drugs the month before the formulary restriction was implemented. Of 137 patients whose pharmacy records were reviewed, 46% discontinued therapy, 30% paid out of pocket, and 23% substituted a covered drug. Although this uncontrolled exploratory study found some changes in utilization and costs, the small sample, short follow-up period, and lack of a control group limit the reliability of the results.

TABLE 5.2 Summary Table of Medicaid Studies

Authors	Study Population	Study	Result or Conclusion
Soumerai et al., 1990	New Jersey Medicaid	Withdrawal of reimbursement for DESI drugs	Fewer prescriptions of DESI drugs and proportionately more prescriptions of substitute medications. Same total cost
Smith and McKercher, 1984	Michigan Medicaid	Withdrawal of reimbursement for DESI drugs	46% discontinued therapy, 30% paid out of pocket, 23% substituted another drug
Kreling et al., 1989a, 1989b	Wisconsin Medicaid	Withdrawal of the analgesic propoxyphene napsylate from the Wisconsin formulary	Inconsistent changes. Formulary restrictions do not always result in savings and may have unpredictable economic and quality-of-care impacts
Cromwell et al., 1999	Florida Medicaid	Limit of one antiulcer prescription drug at a time, limiting all antiulcer prescriptions to one refill, and covering high-dose antiulcer treatment for maximum of 60 days	Number of doses reimbursed decreased by 33% but started to increase 1 year later. Peptic ulcer hospitalization was unchanged.
Moore and Newman, 1993	47 states between 1985 and 1989	Retrospective study of the effect of Medicaid formularies on utilization and expenditures	Formularies reduced drug expenditures, but service substitutions resulted in no aggregate Medicaid savings
Kozma et al., 1990	South Carolina Medicaid	Expanding Medicaid formulary coverage by removing restrictions	An 81% increase in the number of drugs used. A broader approach was recommended

Study	Setting	Intervention	Findings
Walser et al., 1996	States with or without restrictive formularies prior to OBRA 1990	Availability of the top 200 prescription drugs in 1989 after OBRA elimination of restrictive formularies	Increased coverage was of uncertain effect. Formularies are complex policy instruments
Dranove, 1989	Illinois Medicaid	Studied the effects of lifting formulary restrictions on new anti-infective drugs on office and outpatient hospital visits and costs for eight disease categories	A significant increase in drug costs for 3 of 8 categories and in physician visits in one category Concluded that neither an open or a closed formulary is best
Kotzan et al., 1993	Georgia Medicaid	Implementation of prior approval for NSAIDs	Decrease in single-source NSAID use and costs
Smalley et al., 1995	Tennessee Medicaid	Implementation of prior approval for NSAIDs	Increased generic NSAIDs. Decreased total NSAID use and costs
Bloom and Jacobs 1985	West Virginia Medicaid	Implementation of cimetidine prior approval	Reduced use of cimetidine and overall ulcer medications. Increased physician and hospital costs and surgical procedures
Soumerai et al., 1987, 1991, 1994	New Hampshire Medicaid	Effect of a limit of 3 prescription per month. Replaced by $1.00 copayment after 11 months	Reduced prescriptions, reduced access to effective drugs, increased nursing home admissions, increased use of mental health services
Martin and McMillan, 1996	Georgia Medicaid	Reduction in prescription limit from 6 to 5 per month	Fewer Medicaid prescriptions and more out-of-pocket expenses. Potential exposure to adverse health consequences

NOTE: DESI = drug efficacy study implementation.

Kreling et al. (1989a, 1989b) studied the effect of removing propoxyphene napsylate (an analgesic) from the Wisconsin Medicaid formulary. Propoxyphene napsylate products were placed on the negative drug list because they were determined to be no more efficacious than aspirin or acetaminophen. Wisconsin officials recommended that physicians replace propoxyphene napsylate prescriptions with propoxyphene hydrochloride. These investigators used a pretestposttest study design over 6 months to examine changes in expenditures and the number of prescriptions. There was no comparison state, a short follow-up period, and no control for prior trends in analgesic prescribing patterns. The effect of the formulary was inconsistent across drug categories and treatment settings. For example, NSAID prescriptions rose, and the number of schedule III and OTC analgesic prescriptions fell for noninstitutionalized patients. Adjusted program expenditures fell slightly for institutionalized patients who were more likely to be switched to the recommended substitute product. The authors concluded that formulary restrictions do not always result in savings. They can have a variety of unpredictable economic and quality-of-care impacts.

Cromwell et al. (1999) conducted a before-and-after study without a comparison state on the cost, utilization, and hospitalization effects of reimbursement restrictions on antiulcer medications. In early 1992, the Florida Medicaid program imposed a policy of reimbursing only one antiulcer prescription drug at a time, limiting all antiulcer prescriptions to one refill, and covering high-dose treatment for acute disorders for a maximum of 60 days. The study used quarterly Medicaid drug claims data, nonfederal short-stay hospital discharge data, and monthly Medicaid eligibility data for 1989 through 1993. The number of doses reimbursed by Medicaid decreased by 33% after the policy was implemented but began to increase about 1 year later. Peptic ulcer disease-related Medicaid and non-Medicaid hospitalization rates did not change over the course of the study.

As with many of the other studies, it is difficult to interpret the results of this study. Medicaid drug use could not be linked directly to hospital data because the drug use data were aggregated by drug and the hospital data were organized by patient. The lack of a comparison state makes it impossible to determine whether the trends found are the result of the policy or just general trends in prescribing behavior. The impact of the policy on potential substitute medications, especially antibiotics used to eliminate a recently discovered bacterial cause of peptic ulcer disease, was not evaluated. It is possible that the trend in medication use was the result of a change in medical practice, not the result of the policy.

A study by Moore and Newman (1993) analyzed the effect of Medicaid formularies on utilization and expenditures for 47 states between 1985 and 1989. Per capita instead of per recipient measures were used because data on the number of eligible Medicaid recipients by state by year were not available. The relevant variables were measured on a yearly basis; monthly or quarterly measurements may have provided more reliable results. The investigators attempted to address these potential biases by including a number of control variables. They found that restrictive formularies were associated with a 13.4% reduction in drug expenditures but, presumably because of service substitution, 8% more physician visits and 28.7% increased per capita expenditures for physician services. Formularies were also associated with a 39% increase in inpatient hospital mental health expenditures. The authors ran two additional regressions for 1988 and 1989 that included state-level information on prescription limits, refill limits, and unit limits per prescription. Inclusion of these variables eliminated the significant association between restrictive formularies and reduced per capita drug expenditures, and resulted in an association of restrictive formularies and increased per capita Medicaid expenditures. Overall, Moore and Newman concluded that formularies reduce drug expenditures, but that service substitution results in no aggregate Medicaid savings. This type of retrospective research design is fraught with internal validity problems related to differences between states and over time in Medicaid program, state, and service-specific regulatory characteristics. This report was 1 of the 12 reviewed by Soumerai et al. (1993). Methodological problems preclude a reliable interpretation of the findings according to that analysis.

A few studies address the effects of expanding Medicaid coverage for pharmaceuticals. Kozma et al. (1990) studied the utilization and expenditure effects of expanding drug coverage by eliminating formulary restrictions in the South Carolina Medicaid program. Their 2-year study (1983–1984) of more than 12,000 Medicaid recipients found an 81% increase in the number of drugs used after the expansion of coverage. New drugs accounted for 8% of total drug claims, although the percentage of total claims accounted for by new drugs varied substantially among drug classes. For example, new drugs represented only 3.3% of total central nervous system prescriptions, but 17 and 69% of miscellaneous anti-infective and blood formation agents, respectively. The authors also found an increase in the number of prescriptions, physician visits per person per period, and expenditures in every sector except inpatient hospital (which experienced decreased admissions). This study lacked an adequate preintervention period to evaluate prior trends, however, making it difficult to know the true cause of any of the findings. The proportion of variance explained by the formulary change was small (see Soumerai, 1993). The authors concluded that medical care is composed of a series of interrelated services and that a broader approach to cost containment is warranted (Kozma et al., 1990).

Walser et al. (1996) analyzed the projected clinical impact of increased access to drugs following the elimination of restrictive formularies that resulted from the enactment of OBRA 1990. They compared the availability of the top 200 prescription drugs (defined by sales volume) in states with and without restrictive formularies in 1989, the year before restrictive formularies were banned. After OBRA 1990, there was no change in the mean number of drugs (196) covered in states that had not had restrictive formularies, and there was a 10% increase—from 169.3 to 186.2—in covered drugs in states that had. The use of prior approval increased from an average of 1.4 to 3.8 drugs in states that had, and from 0.7 to 1.4 drugs in states that had not had, restrictive formularies.

The investigators surveyed assessments by panels of physicians of the therapeutic importance of expanded availability of a selected subset of 18 of the top 200 drugs. The surveyed physician panels agreed that expanded access to four of the 18 drugs resulted in a net therapeutic benefit. They agreed that expanded access to four other drugs provided no additional therapeutic benefit. The remaining products provided questionable therapeutic benefit or produced no agreement among the panels. Medicaid programs around the country reported increases in drug expenditures after the elimination of restrictive formularies. These authors warned that formularies are complex policy instruments that may lead to intended and unintended consequences (Walser et al., 1996).

Dranove (1989) used Illinois Medicaid data to study the effect of lifting formulary restrictions on a group of new anti-infective drugs on office and outpatient hospital physician visits and costs for eight disease categories (all infections). He found significant increases in drug costs for three of the eight disease categories (genital tract infection, severe acne, and chronic lung disease). There was also an increase in the number of physician visits for patients with respiratory infections. Interestingly, physicians tended to prescribe the newer and more expensive drugs only after trying the older and cheaper ones. The study did not address the possibility that new drugs may provide patients with improved health more quickly, offsetting their increased cost. Dranove concluded that neither an open nor a closed formulary is best. The study did not control for previous trends in drug utilization and cost and had no comparison state.

Effects of Medicaid Prior Approval Systems

Two recent studies have focused specifically on the effect of prior approval for NSAIDs (Kotzan et al., 1993; Smalley et al., 1995). Both studies reported savings from increased use of generic NSAIDs as a replacement for proprietary, single-source drugs. Kotzan et al. analyzed 19 months of utilization and cost data (12 months before and 7 months after beginning prior approval) for 80,000 continuously enrolled patients in the Georgia Medicaid system. They found an immediate decrease in the number of single-source NSAID prescriptions and an increase in the use of multiple-source drugs. The increase in multiple-source prescriptions replaced slightly more than half of the single-source prescriptions. This absolute reduction in prescribing accounted for a total cost savings for NSAID therapy of $3 million. There was no increase in the use or cost of physician or hospital services during the 7 months after the program began. The results of the study are limited by the lack of a comparison group and the short postintervention period.

The findings of Smalley et al. (1995) were similar. They studied the effect of the Tennessee prior approval program for NSAIDs, initiated in October 1989, on the use and cost of pharmacotherapy, outpatient, and inpatient services. There was no comparison state to control for general trends in the use of study drugs. They found that expenditures fell by 53%, resulting in a savings of approximately $12.8 million, due to increased use of generic NSAIDs and an overall reduction of 26% in the total number of days of NSAID use. Regular users of single-source NSAIDs experienced a 28% decrease in the number of days of NSAIDs use and an associated 64% decrease in NSAID cost. There was no change in the use of other health care services associated with the prior approval program. Both measures began to rise within 3 months after the prior approval program began and continued to increase throughout the 2-year follow-up period. The authors concluded that prior approval for NSAIDs may reduce NSAID costs. The savings may be a function of the large number of generic substitutes, similar efficacy and safety profiles of most NSAIDs, and the large variations in cost among the various drugs.

The claim that NSAIDs have similar safety profiles was questioned in a subsequent letter to the editor (Lehman, 1995). The writer noted that two of the generic preparations in the study by Smalley et al. (1995)—fenoprofen and phenylbutazone—"have higher rates of severe organ toxicity than other NSAIDs." In a reply to the letter, the authors acknowledged that use of one of the two drugs noted (fenoprofen) doubled after the implementation of the prior approval program. Concern that prior approval restricts access to new and effective therapies and may result in the substitution of less safe alternatives has been expressed by academic investigators (Soumerai and Lipton, 1995) and the public at large (Pear, 1993; The Pink Sheet, 1993; PMA Newsletter, 1993b).

Bloom and Jacobs (1985) studied the effect of restricting the availability of cimetidine (Tagamet) on Medicaid expenditures. They found that prior approval led to a 79% reduction in per-patient per-month Medicaid pharmaceutical expenditures for peptic ulcer disease and an 85% reduction in cimetidine use. However, the average per-patient per-month expenditures for physician and in-patient hospital services increased 3 and 24%, respectively, during the same period, and total expenditures rose in every health service category except out-patient pharmaceuticals. There was also a significant increase in the number of surgical procedures for patients with newly diagnosed peptic ulcer disease. Although the study had a number of methodological flaws (for example, it lacked a comparison group and had a short follow-up period), the results support the conclusion that denying access to medically needed, effective drugs is shortsighted policy. At the time of the study, cimetidine was the only member on the market of a drug class (H_2R blockers) that is highly effective for peptic ulcer disease.

Effects of Medicaid Prescription Limits

Several studies have focused on the effect of prescription limits, or quantity controls, on utilization and expenditures in Medicaid (Martin and McMillan, 1996; Soumerai et al., 1987, 1991). In general, these studies have found that prescription limits lead to an immediate reduction in pharmaceutical utilization, but not necessarily to a reduction in overall Medicaid spending, and they may adversely affect clinical outcomes. A study by Soumerai et al. (1987) was the first in a series of studies on the consequences of a three-prescription-per-month limit for New Hampshire Medicaid recipients in 1981. This policy was replaced

11 months later by a $1.00 copayment for all prescriptions. The investigators used a time-series, comparison-series analysis of patient-level changes in the number of prescriptions dispensed (controlling for prescription size) and expenditures. New Jersey was used as the comparison state. The time series covered 48 months: 20 months before the prescription limit, 11 months during the limit, and 17 months after the limit was replaced by the $1.00 copayment. The study cohorts consisted of Medicaid recipients who were continuously enrolled for 10 or more months during each of the 4 study years. More than 10,000 patients in New Hampshire and 74,000 patients in New Jersey fit the study criteria.

These investigators found that the prescription limit reduced prescriptions from 1.1 to 0.7 per patient per month. Analysis of a cohort of primarily disabled or elderly, female, multiple-drug recipients ($n = 860$) found that their utilization fell from 5.2 to 2.8 prescriptions per patient per month. Although the report noted that the greatest reduction in use was for ineffective drugs, there were large reductions also for essential medications such as insulin (28%) and furosemide (30%). When New Hampshire replaced the prescription limit with a copayment, prescriptions increased to just below the prelimit level (Soumerai et al. 1987).

A second study by Soumerai et al. (1991) extended their 1987 findings. This study focused on the effect of the prescription limit on admissions to nursing homes and hospitals for a group of high-risk patients. The study ($n = 411$) and comparison ($n = 1,375$) cohorts consisted of elderly, multiple-drug users (more than three medications per month) taking at least one medication for certain chronic diseases during the baseline year. The authors reported that the prescription limit reduced drug use by 35%, but it was associated with a significant risk of being admitted to a nursing home (relative risk 1.8; 95% confidence interval, 1.2–2.6) compared to similar Medicaid recipients in New Jersey. Although the use of the study medications returned to near baseline after the prescription limit was replaced with a copayment, the patients admitted to nursing homes remained there. The authors concluded that limiting reimbursement for effective drugs puts patients at increased risk of institutionalization and may increase Medicaid costs (Soumerai et al., 1991).

A third report by Soumerai et al. (1994) studied the effect of the New Hampshire prescription limit on the use of psychotropic agents and acute mental health services for schizophrenics. They found that the use of antipsychotic drugs, anxiolytic and hypnotic agents, and antidepressants and lithium fell 15, 37, and 49%, respectively. Per-patient per-month visits to community mental health centers increased, as did the use of emergency mental health services. The reduction in drug expenditures was more than offset by an increase in cost for other mental health services, estimated at $1,530 per patient or about 17 times the saving in drug costs. Health care utilization returned to baseline levels after the policy was discontinued.

The findings of a study by Martin and McMillan (1996) on a prescription limit regulation in Georgia are consistent with previous findings of Soumerai et al. (1987, 1991, 1994). In November 1991, the Georgia Department of Medical

Assistance reduced the number of monthly reimbursable prescriptions from six to five. These two investigators conducted interrupted time-series analyses on 12 months (6 months before and 6 months after the reduction) of patient-level data for 743 high prescription drug users. There was no comparison cohort. Overall, Martin and McMillan found a 6.6% reduction in total prescriptions, a 9.9% reduction in prescriptions reimbursed by Medicaid, and a 9.7% increase in prescriptions paid out of pocket. Each of these changes was abrupt and continuous except for the out of pocket, which was temporary. Miscellaneous, palliative, and pulmonary drugs experienced a significant, abrupt, and sustained decrease in the number of prescriptions filled. It is likely that the policy reduced the use of cardiovascular drugs, but the effect was not immediate. Chemotherapy, central nervous system, gastrointestinal, and hormone prescriptions did not change. These authors concluded that prescription limits alter prescription regimens, potentially predisposing elderly Medicaid recipients to clinical consequences. The lack of a comparison cohort and the short follow-up period limit interpretation of these results.

The impression left by many of these studies, despite their methodological flaws, is that denying patients access to medically needed drugs is neither good medicine nor good economics. These denials occur when formularies exclude or deny reimbursement for drugs or classes of drugs or limit prescriptions without providing exceptions or therapeutic alternates or when drugs that represent therapeutic advances are not available. Although costs for these drugs or drug classes may decrease, costs for substitute drugs or substitute care modalities or settings may escalate and patient outcomes deteriorate. The evolution of Medicaid formulary management over the past two decades reflects this realization. As a result, legislation has been enacted in many states to address some of these issues in managed care, as reviewed earlier. Other studies are more difficult to assess, show mixed results, or may indicate some effects of controls. With few exceptions, these reports should be interpreted with caution. The committee also observed that most of the formulary systems and controls studied in these reports differ from the VA National Formulary and their restrictions are generally not those used by the VA, for example, prescription limits, or prior approval of the only member of a class. These studies, therefore, are not very helpful in evaluating the restrictiveness of the current VA formulary system.

Medicaid Managed Care: Background

Medicaid managed care is not new, but it has expanded dramatically in the past 10 years. In 1991, less than 10% of all Medicaid recipients were enrolled in Medicaid managed care plans. Currently, more that half are enrolled (21,167,485 recipients in 585 plans as of June 30, 1998; www.hcfa.gov/medicaid/ plansum8.htm). All of the states except Alaska and Wyoming are enrolling Medicaid recipients in managed care plans (National Academy for State Health Policy, 1999). Two states, Tennessee and Arizona, administer their entire Medicaid programs through managed care plans. Provisions in the Balanced Budget Act of

1997 made it easier for states to enroll Medicaid recipients in managed care, so it is likely that the trend will continue (NPC, 1998).

Most Medicaid managed care plans are authorized by HCFA through approval of Section 1915b Freedom of Choice waivers or Section 1115 Research and Demonstration waivers. Section 1915 waivers allow states to forgo some requirements of Medicaid law, such as freedom of choice, comparability, and statewide access. They permit states to increase access to managed care plans, but they do not allow an expansion of benefits or coverage of populations that would not meet the eligibility requirements of Title XIX of the SSA. In addition, they are generally limited to a small geographic area, such as a county, and are approved for 2-year periods. Section 1115 waivers allow states broader exclusions from Medicaid law and are approved for 5-year periods. These waivers permit states to implement statewide programs to test new health care delivery and financing systems, expand coverage to different populations, and expand benefit packages. States are required to demonstrate that the waiver will not increase Medicaid spending; that is, the program must be budget neutral. HCFA has approved 19 Section 1115 waivers for Medicaid managed care.

The Balanced Budget Act of 1997 further eased the way for states to enroll Medicaid recipients in managed care by adding a new section (Section 1932) to Title XIX of the SSA, which allows states to enroll recipients in managed care without a waiver if they comply with the new section. With some exceptions, states must offer a choice between at least two managed care organizations or primary care case managers, or at least one plan and one primary care case manager. Lesser restrictions apply in rural areas. States may also "lock in" recipients for 12 months instead of 1 month unless the recipient can show just cause for disenrollment. The act also removed the requirement that contracted health plans have no more than 75% of enrollees from Medicaid. Plans have enrolled mostly women and children eligible through AFDC or TANF, not the more vulnerable and costly SSI aged and disabled population. The Medicaid managed care programs that have begun to enroll the SSI populations have started with small pilot programs limited to a specific geographic area (National Academy for State Health Policy, 1999). As with state Medicaid formularies, it is not easy to characterize the complex and variable benefits provided by the average managed care organization that will affect Medicaid recipients.

Drug Benefit in Medicaid Managed Care

There is no standard prescription drug benefit package in Medicaid managed care. It is possible that each of the hundreds of different Medicaid managed care programs has a unique drug benefit plan. The benefit provided to Medicaid managed care enrollees is based on the specific contract(s) negotiated between the state and the plans and, when relevant, on Section 1915 and Section 1115 waivers approved by HCFA. Some states have carved out the drug benefit from their managed care benefit package and continue to provide drug benefits through the fee-for-service system.

In general, the drug benefit found in any particular Medicaid managed care plan is similar to the fee-for-service benefit found in that state. The Center for Health Policy Research at George Washington University asked states whether their managed care contracts or requests for proposals (RFPs) included language regarding drug formularies (Center for Health Policy Research, 1998). The level of specificity in the contracts was found to vary widely. For example, the Michigan RFP noted only that health plans may use a drug formulary, whereas the Florida Medicaid managed care contract specified that the plan should not have a pharmacy benefit more restrictive than Medicaid fee for service. The plan could use a preferred formulary as long as adherence was voluntary. New Jersey permits health plans to have a formulary but requires them to provide all medically necessary legend and nonlegend drugs covered by the Medicaid program and to ensure the availability of quality pharmaceutical services for all enrollees. The contract mandates that health plans include in their formularies new drugs that will have a significant impact on patient care and permits exclusion without prior approval only of drugs and drug categories listed in OBRA 1990.

The Pennsylvania RFP is another example of the limits placed on Medicaid managed care plan drug benefit design (Commonwealth of Pennsylvania, HC-SW PH RFP #10-97, 1997). This RFP requires that formularies be developed by P&T committees; include drugs in the therapeutic categories currently covered in the fee-for-service program; provide access to all new drugs within 10 days of FDA approval (either through inclusion on the formulary or by prior approval); exclude coverage of all DESI drugs; and exclude any drug marketed by a company that does not participate in the fee-for-service rebate agreement. The document also requires prior approval systems to abide by the OBRA 1990 requirements of a 24-hour response time and access to a 72-hour emergency supply of any reviewed product. The RFP prohibits therapeutic substitution without explicit consent from the attending physician. Similarly, the South Carolina contract requires that service limits such as a drug formulary may not be implemented unless there is a mechanism to cover drugs outside the formulary that are determined to be medically necessary in the treatment of a particular Medicaid managed care enrollee.

The Center for Health Policy Research survey responses and the sample RFPs and contracts indicate that although there is variation in the contract language from state to state, the drug benefit in Medicaid managed care plans is generally limited by the conditions outlined in OBRA 1990 and 1993. Perhaps most importantly, the contracts described in this report provide that drugs not listed on the managed care formulary must be made available through a prior approval program. Furthermore, these prior approval programs are generally required to adhere to the statutory requirements for Medicaid fee-for-service prior approval programs listed in OBRA 1993, that is, 24-hour response time and access to a 72-hour emergency supply (Center for Health Policy Research, 1998). OTC coverage was provided by 25 states through their managed care contracts.

A more detailed study of Medicaid managed care plans conducted by the National Academy for State Health Policy (1998) found similar variations in the drug benefit across states and types of enrollees. Of the 45 Medicaid systems reporting information, including Washington, D.C., 34 provided prescription drug coverage. The remaining 11 states carved out their Medicaid pharmacy benefit from the Medicaid managed care system, and subsequently 2 more states (Massachusetts and New York) have done so. States that carve out the drug benefit are able to retain participation in the Medicaid rebate program and guaranteed best-price discounts that otherwise would be lost for the managed care portion of their Medicaid pharmacy benefit.

Presumably, state legislation on disclosure of formularies and nonformulary processes, continuation of needed drugs, and off-label coverage, reviewed earlier in this report, would apply to Medicaid managed care but would have relatively minor effect since Medicaid fee-for-service and therefore managed care programs do not usually present barriers that these laws are designed to address.

DEPARTMENT OF DEFENSE

Health Care System and Pharmacy Benefit

The Department of Defense's primary medical mission is to maintain the health of 1.6 million active duty personnel and to provide health care during military operations. The secondary mission is to offer health care to 6.6 million non-active duty beneficiaries, including dependents of active duty personnel and military retirees, their dependents, and survivors. Most care is provided in about 587 military hospitals and clinics (military treatment facilities, MTFs) operated worldwide by the uniformed services. This system is supplemented by care that is paid for mostly by DOD but provided by civilian physicians under the TRICARE program. The TRICARE health care system provides services to both active duty and retired military personnel and their families. TRICARE is DOD's managed care replacement for CHAMPUS (Civilian Health and Medical Program of the Uniformed Services), which was phased out between 1995 and 1998. TRICARE offers military and retired military beneficiaries three health care options: TRICARE Extra, Standard, or Prime which are preferred provider, standard fee-for-service, and health maintenance organization benefits, respectively (C. Kirby, GAO, personal communication, 2000).

DOD health care services were provided at a cost of $14.7 billion in FY 1998. The DOD pharmacy benefit cost $1.3 billion (9%) in FY 1998 and is available through the 587 military treatment facility outpatient pharmacies, TRICARE contractor network or nonnetwork retail pharmacies, and a national contractor mail order program. MTF pharmacies filled about 55 million prescriptions and consumed about three-fourths of the pharmacy budget in FY 1997. Many retired personnel obtain their health care in the private sector but use the DOD pharmacy benefit to fill their private physician prescriptions at no or reduced cost, a practice not condoned by the VHA for veterans (C. Kirby, GAO, personal communication, 2000). Like the VA and the private sector, DOD pharmacy costs are increasing more rapidly than overall health care costs.

The structure and management of the DOD pharmacy benefit will undergo considerable change under the terms of the National Defense Authorization Act (NDAA) for Fiscal Year 2000 (P.L. 106-65, Section 701, enacted October 5, 1999). The following description applies to the current status of the DOD pharmacy benefit. Relevant potential changes and their implications are noted as appropriate. MTF drugs are free to eligible personnel, but varying copayments, which can reach 50% of prescription cost (and a $300 deductible) for nonnetwork retail drugs, are imposed in other settings, retail pharmacies, and the mail order program. MTF drugs are distributed through a prime vendor at prices negotiated by the Defense Supply Center Philadelphia *(sic)*. These prices vary from the Federal Supply Schedule (FSS) discount for covered drugs of 24% below average manufacturer price (AMP) to as much as 70% lower than AMP. TRICARE contractor network pharmacies provide discounted drugs (although at lesser discounts than the FSS), but nonnetwork pharmacies are reimbursed at retail prices. According to GAO (1998), the data collected to monitor and operate the DOD pharmacy benefit are uncoordinated and inadequate. Therefore, it is difficult to be sure of program costs, drug utilization statistics, appropriateness, or safety. The pharmacy benefit also varies significantly across the United States (GAO, 1998).

DOD Formulary and Formulary System

MTF pharmacies devise and monitor their own closed formularies. According to the Policy for Basic Core Formulary and Committed Use Requirements Contracts (HA Policy 98-034, 27 April 1998), all MTF full-service pharmacies are required to stock and list on their formularies all the items on a Basic Core Formulary (BCF). When there are joint VA and DOD committed- use contract drugs, they represent the mandatory source and use for MTFs just as for VA facilities, and they may be the only members in formulary closed drug classes. The BCF, as of the last quarter of 1999, is a limited formulary with 159 listings (some differ only with respect to dosage or routes of administration forms) in 41 categories (www.pec.ha.osd.mil/BCF/BCFqckr.htm). This formulary requires a single mandatory source for amoxicillin, albuterol inhalers, extended-release diltiazem and verapamil, oral captopril, lisinopril, nortriptyline, cimetidine, and ranitidine. HMG CoA RIs and PPIs are closed classes and limited to cerivastatin and simvastatin, and omeprazole, respectively. At least one SSRI is required. Two ACEIs; two H2R blockers; two alpha blockers; three CCBs; a limited, mostly generic, group of antibiotics; and only first-generation cephalosporins are listed. Under the terms of the NDAA, DOD is required to establish by October 1, 2000, a Uniform Formulary ensuring the availability of drugs in the complete range of therapeutic classes. The details of the new formulary are currently under development, but it will apply to the MTF, retail, and mail order pharmacies.

BCF policy requires a quarterly update by the DOD P&T committee, and changes may be requested by MTF P&T committees. The DOD P&T committee meets at the DOD Pharmacoeconomic Center in Texas and consists of armed forces physicians and pharmacists, representatives from the VA, the Defense Supply Center Philadelphia, TRICARE contractors and the mail order program contractor, and the DOD pharmacoeconomic center. According to the NDAA, this P&T committee must be supplemented by a Uniform Formulary Beneficiary Advisory Panel that will include DOD beneficiary representatives and provide comments to the Secretary of Defense on the new Uniform Formulary.

Currently, nonformulary exceptions to MTF formularies require submission of a request and approval of the MTF commander. Mail order exceptions are handled according to the contractor's exceptions and prior approval procedures. The NDAA requires the Secretary of Defense to establish nonformulary procedures, including an appeals process. Since there are no formulary system restrictions, except for copayments and deductibles, at TRICARE network or non-network retail pharmacies, eligible personnel (that is, non-Medicare, non-active duty) can short-circuit formularies and the nonformulary exceptions or prior approval processes by filling prescriptions at these pharmacies at increased cost to themselves and DOD. Presumably, TRICARE network pharmacies will provide drugs according to the new Uniform Formulary in FY 2001, however.

The DOD mail order program provides drugs to patients with chronic health conditions at Defense Supply Center Philadelphia negotiated prices using Merck-Medco as the contractor. All categories of military personnel (except Medicare retirees, although the NDAA has ordered a study of a more comprehensive pharmacy benefit for these retirees) are eligible for the program and, except for active duty personnel, are subject to copayments of $4.00 to $8.00 for each 90-day supply. Until the Uniform Formulary is implemented, the mail order program has a limited formulary of preferred and nonpreferred drugs that was devised by the DOD P&T committee. The formulary lists covered drugs, excluded drugs, and drugs under review. As at MTFs and network pharmacies, generic substitution is mandatory. The mail order formulary, as of the last quarter of 1999, had about 80 preferred, contract, injectable, and OTC listings and about 30 nonpreferred or noncontract listings. Less than 10 individual drugs were excluded, as were 10 drug classes, such as immunizations, smoking deterrents, and anabolic steroids, among others. Drugs for cosmetic, weight reduction, or investigational use were also excluded.

The committee concluded that the present DOD BCF, mail order formulary, and multiple MTF formularies are not comparable counterparts to the VA National Formulary and formulary system. The DOD formularies cover a limited number of products, and nonformulary exceptions do not appear to be based on the kinds of clinical criteria and review process required by the VHA. The committee has little information on MTF formularies except that they are free to add drugs in many categories or drug classes to the BCF and undoubtedly do. They are also free to restrict access to new or expensive drugs and are reported to do so (GAO, 1998). Presumably, this creates a highly variable pharmacy benefit. Little information was available about the nonformulary exceptions process, except that a request approved by the MTF commander is required. Presumably this, too, might create highly variable access to drugs. Since active duty

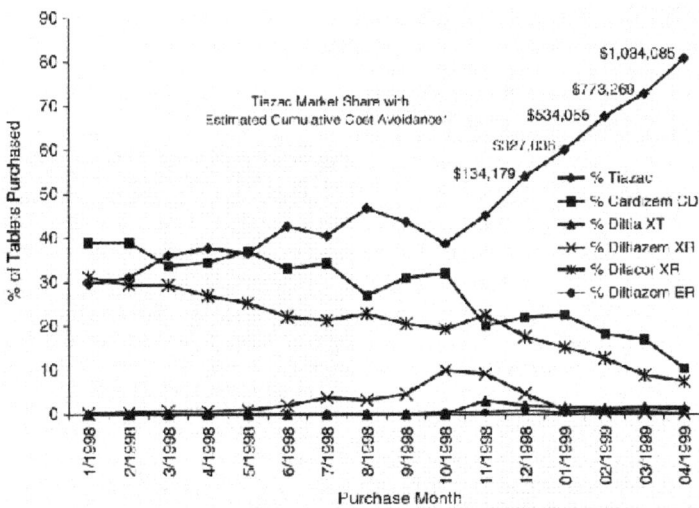

FIGURE 5.3 Effect of contract on relative market shares of CCBs. SOURCE: Department of Defense P&T committee minutes (Aug 1999).

and Medicare-eligible retired personnel are not eligible for TRICARE contractor retail pharmacy drugs, they must deal with this fragmented and restrictive system as best they can. The committee has no information on the level of satisfaction or health implications of this.

The BCF formulary itself is highly restrictive in comparison to the VA National Formulary, which has about eight times as many listings. The effects of this formulary system on quality of care are not known as far as the committee could determine. Some data on cost implications have been collected, for example, Figure 5.3 from the minutes of the DOD P&T committee. Existing DOD databases do not allow detailed cost analyses according to GAO (1998), although the NDAA mandates implementation of the Pharmacy Data Transaction Service to address this problem. Furthermore, as noted earlier in this chapter, restrictions on access to medically indicated drugs by the BCF or some MTFs may divert utilization and costs to other settings, that is, retail pharmacies, other MTFs, or in the case of Medicare-eligible retirees, to the VA (although they would have to see VA physicians to obtain VA pharmacy benefits), where these treatments or alternatives are available. The committee concluded that the DOD BCF and other formulary and formulary systems are in earlier stages of development than the VA National Formulary and do not provide useful comparisons. How they will compare after full implementation of improvements under the NDAA is unknown and presumably will depend on the details of changes.

GENERAL COMMENTS ON COMPARISONS

In examining private-and public-sector formularies and formulary systems in comparison to the VA National Formulary and formulary systems, the committee concluded that some formularies are more open. For example, Medicaid programs are required to offer all drugs on the Federal Supply Schedule. Some formularies are more restricted. For example, they require prior approval for many drugs and entirely exclude some drugs or drug classes. Drugs or drug classes are not excluded in the VA systems. All are variable, and some perhaps much more so (DOD) than the VA. Access barriers are sometimes more frequent, and sometimes less, and they vary in how burdensome they are in both the private and the public sectors. Some controls that may present real impediments to obtaining needed drugs, especially for low-income patients, such as relatively costly copayments and deductibles, are not features of the VA formulary system. Other controls, such as generic substitution and therapeutic interchange are in common use in many systems. The committee could not reach blanket conclusions on the relative restrictiveness of these highly variable comparison formularies and formulary systems. If a formulary appropriately controls drug costs, it may be more important to the VA since cost overruns and cost shifting have entirely different implications in a fixed budget system like the VA (or to some extent managed care) than they do in an open-ended entitlement like Medicaid. As has been concluded so often in this report, the key issue does not appear to be the details of a formulary, providing it is of reasonable size, inclusiveness, and quality. The important element for quality and restrictiveness is timely availability of a safe and effective, medically necessary drug, if not listed, through an exceptions process. A good formulary supports this element and, through its capacity to make quality choices, enhances price negotiations and prudent purchasing.

6

The VA National Formulary and Veterans Health Care

INTRODUCTION

In this report, a committee of the Institute of Medicine (IOM) describes and analyzes the role of the Department of Veterans Affairs' (VA) National Formulary in veterans health care. In requesting this study, the Congress and the Department of Veterans Affairs (VA) asked that four aspects of the National Formulary be evaluated: its restrictiveness, its effects on both cost and quality, and how it compares with other formularies. After an introductory chapter that provides background and context, these evaluations are reported in Chapter 2, Chapter 3, Chapter 4 and Chapter 5, each of which covers one of these aspects. This final chapter is a narrative summary of the preceding chapters. The specific conclusions and recommendations of the committee are found in the Executive Summary of this report.

In 1998, House Report 105-610 noted that serious concerns had been raised about the impact of the VA National Formulary and directed the VA to contract with the IOM to conduct an independent analysis of its effects on quality of care and potential costs and to compare it with other public and private insurance formularies. The IOM and the VA entered into a contract to address the congressional concerns, effective April 12, 1999. Implementation of this contract was begun with the appointment of staff and a committee of independent experts to carry out the necessary work. This committee consisted of representatives of two veterans service organizations; health professionals knowledgeable in clinical pharmacology, pharmacy and therapeutics activities, and clinical medicine and geriatrics; and pharmacists and others with experience in managed care and pharmacy benefits management. The committee delivered an interim report on January 28, 2000, and this final report was scheduled for delivery not later than July 11, 2000.

BACKGROUND AND CONTEXT

The history of formularies dates back hundreds or even thousands of years in other parts of the world, and to the American Revolution in this country. Formularies began as simple lists of remedies and their formulas. In the United States, they developed along with changes in health care delivery and the science of pharmacology. Primarily used in hospitals, they gradually came to include purified and standardized drugs identified by generic nomenclature. More recently, they have focused on the cost-effectiveness as well as the quality of drugs that are included and controlled. Beginning in the 1950s, professional societies, government programs, and accreditation agencies began to define formularies and to require them in health facilities. The facilities and organizations using formularies evolved with changes in health care financing and delivery to include managed care plans, pharmacy benefit management organizations, all kinds of health care settings, and government programs such as Medicaid, the Department of Defense, and the Veterans Health Administration (VHA). Veterans health facilities have used formularies to control inventory and the cost-effectiveness and quality of drug treatment for veterans for the last 40 or 50 years.

Fundamentally, formularies are lists of drugs that may be more or less inclusive. They can be differentiated by the formulary system, that is, the restrictions, controls, or modifications that are employed in their management to achieve objectives for the pharmacy benefits of a health care system. At the simplest level, formularies may be open—that is, they list many drugs and place few limits on access or coverage; they may be closed, in which case, they list a limited number of drugs and place more limits on access or coverage; or they may be partially closed.

Aside from listing or not listing a drug in the formulary itself, the limits or controls that characterize a formulary and formulary system include generic prescribing, generic substitution, therapeutic interchange, use of step protocols, restrictions by certain specialties or clinical settings or conditions, nonformulary exceptions and prior approval or authorization processes, prescription copayments that vary in amounts and differ for generics and brands covered or not covered in the formulary, specific exclusions of drugs or drug classes, or closure of drug classes and designation of drugs or drug classes as preferred, among others. These are defined and discussed in the body of this report. Limits on prescription size, numbers, dollar values, or frequencies are restrictions or controls parallel to direct formulary management that are also discussed in this report, primarily in Chapter 2. Committees made up of practicing physicians, pharmacists, and some other professionals in a health system (pharmacy and therapeutics [P&T] committees), drug class reviews, and treatment guidelines are also important to decision making and management of formularies and formulary systems.

THE VETERANS HEALTH ADMINISTRATION

The VHA consists of 146 medical centers, including 172 hospitals, more than 600 ambulatory care and community-based clinics, 132 nursing homes, 40 domiciliaries, and a number of other programs. In 1995, a reorganization of the VA affected the status of all VA facilities and the relationships of the VA formularies and formulary systems, the control of drug use, and pharmacy operations. This reorganization created 22 Veterans Integrated Service Networks (VISNs), that is, essentially 22 managed care organizations with their own capitation-based budgets. Each VISN, on average, encompasses 7 to 10 hospitals, 25 to 30 ambulatory clinics, 4 to 7 nursing homes, 1 or 2 domiciliaries, and various other assets. The VHA is a unique health care system (and different from private-sector managed care) in terms of its size, cost, and budgeting; diversity of settings; geographic scope; role in the use and training of young physicians; and its permanently eligible patient population.

In November 1995, a VISN-level formulary was required in order to provide a uniform drug benefit in each network or region and to prepare for a national formulary. At about the same time, a VA Pharmacy Benefits Management Strategic Health Care Group (VA PBM), a central Medical Advisory Panel (MAP), VISN formulary committees, and a VISN Formulary Leaders Committee were created. VISN formularies were then merged into the VA National Formulary which was issued in May 1997. In October 1997, VHA Directive 97-047 required each VISN to develop a nonformulary exceptions process and specified criteria for granting exceptions. In December 1997, supplies were added to the National Formulary. Additional minor changes have been made periodically.

The VA National Formulary is controlled by the VA PBM, the MAP, and the VISN formulary leaders. These bodies issue drug class reviews and treatment guidelines, and make decisions on drug additions to and deletions from the formulary and the designation of closed and preferred classes. VISN formularies differ among themselves and from the National Formulary, but local formularies are usually the same as the VISN formulary. Specific restrictions by specialty, setting, or condition may differ among the formularies depending on local practice patterns, antibiotic resistance profiles, and the like. At present, there are four closed classes, that is, therapeutic classes in which a selection has been made among member drugs. Those selected must be listed and used systemwide. Those not selected cannot be listed on a formulary at any level and can be used only by nonformulary exception. Two classes are preferred; that is, a selection has been made among drugs in the class, and the drugs selected are preferred and subject to national contracts that provide for favorable prices. Other drugs can be listed on VISN or local formularies, however.

As described further in the cost sections of this report, drug prices depend on competition—the ability to choose among competitors, to purchase in volume, and to enforce compliance with market share agreements. By choosing among drugs in a class, the National Formulary and formulary system enable prudent purchasing of drugs. For the VA, the National Acquisition Center

(NAC), which administers the Federal Supply Schedule (FSS), uses National Formulary selections in closed or preferred classes as leverage to make market share or volume commitments and to negotiate prices that often are substantially lower than the already favorable prices for brand drugs on the FSS. National Formulary cost savings achieved through these selections and prices are supplemented by mandatory generic prescribing and substitution, negotiation of favorable prices among genetic manufacturers, and a substantial number of blanket purchase agreements that take advantage of various market conditions from time to time to get good prices on a range of products at the regional (or occasionally national) level.

RESTRICTIVENESS

Restrictiveness is a multifactorial attribute of a formulary and formulary system. It is a measure of the stringency of the controls on veterans' access to prescribed medicines at the appropriate times. If formulary structure or formulary system controls deny or significantly delay access to drugs that, in the reasonable judgment of medical experts, are clinically indicated, then the VA National Formulary meets the definition of overly restrictive. National Formulary elements of restrictiveness include formulary size, number of classes closed and number of drugs in closed classes, timeliness of addition of newly approved drugs, appropriateness and responsiveness of the nonformulary exceptions process, sensitivity of therapeutic interchange policies to patient risks, coverage of over-the-counter (OTC) drugs, and generic substitution. Other limits incorporated into restrictive designs include exclusions of drugs or drug classes, volume or quantity limits, high copayments, and prior approvals. Restrictiveness can be judged by comparison among public and private formularies and formulary systems, by comparison to reasonableness standards in the literature or in the informed judgment of the IOM committee, by comparison to objective standards where these exist, and by effects on satisfaction of patients and prescribers.

The VA National Formulary (July 1999 version) contains about 1,200 items, of which about 170 are OTC and 133 are medical-surgical supplies. Although there is no standard that specifies a particular formulary size for a given health care system, most managed care formularies contain less than 1,000 items. Also, before 1997, some VISNs were functioning, apparently satisfactorily, with formularies about 70% the size of the current National Formulary. The VA closed classes account for about 13 to 16% of VHA drug costs. Drugs in closed classes have important therapeutic effects. The conditions they treat are prevalent. Many prescriptions are written for these drugs. These classes are in the top five contributors to drug costs in managed care, and they are frequently closed in managed care and hospital formularies.

VA choices of classes to close and of drugs within closed or preferred classes are based on good-quality drug class reviews. There is no convincing evidence that choice is overly restricted in VA closed and preferred classes. Unlike Medicaid, managed care, or PBM plans, the National Formulary rarely designates drugs or drug classes that are excluded from coverage. Sildenafil citrate (Viagra), which was excluded, is now available although with limitations. The effects of class closure and committed-use contracts on utilization of drugs in the VA are impressive. Preferred or formulary agent market shares in some classes are driven to 95% or more. The committee found no scientific evidence that this detracted from, or posed risks to, veterans' care.

Drugs newly approved by the Food and Drug Administration (FDA) are considered for addition to the VA National Formulary only after a 1-year delay, except in special cases of important new (FDA priority) 1P category drugs. The VA considers this a safety precaution, allowing evidence of adverse drug effects or studies on comparative safety, efficacy, and cost-effectiveness to accumulate during that interval. In practice, few comparative studies are published in the first year after market entry of a new drug. Most FDA recalls in the 1990s involved drugs that were not being actively marketed, occurred well after the first year on the market (and in one case, troglitazone, was available in some of the VISNs in the VHA), were not 1P drugs in the first place, or were, in fact, on the National Formulary (cisapride). Although most VISNs can add new drugs without delay, the blanket national policy of delay may occasionally protect veterans from exposure to a drug that will be recalled but has not always protected veterans from a problem drug. Given the higher cost of new drugs, costs will probably be avoided. However, veterans will not have the advantage of new treatments. Also, the VA policy is more restrictive than Medicaid and managed care policies on new drugs. The committee recommended that this policy be abandoned in favor of examining new drugs on their merits as they appear.

By the end of 1999, a net of 20 mostly existing drugs (that is, drugs already on the market) had been added to the National Formulary. VISN formularies, in the aggregate, had added 260 different, mostly existing drugs. In addition, VISN formularies differed from the National Formulary from the outset, sometimes by more than 100 items. VISN and local policies and procedures on drug additions, nonformulary exceptions, and therapeutic interchange—all important attributes of formulary systems—are different from the National Formulary and vary among themselves, as discussed further below. These differences and inconsistencies across the VHA potentially expose veterans to variable access to drugs and restrictions on drug treatment. The tension between national standardization and uniformity and local autonomy and preferences is difficult to balance, depending on time and place. Recalibration in favor of a more consistent, uniform national approach for these key attributes is desirable.

A nonformulary exceptions process should involve procedures for obtaining nonformulary drugs that are simple, fair, and reasonable and do not involve needless delays and complicated technicalities. In 1999, the VHA reported that 3.45% of total prescriptions, and 4 to 6% of prescriptions in closed classes, were filled with nonformulary drugs. Apparently, compliance with the National Formulary is excellent. According to a standard in the literature, hospital formularies were deemed restrictive if less than 5% of the pharmacy budget was spent on nonformulary drugs, and in managed care, a survey reported 10% of prescriptions filled with nonformulary drugs.

The VA nonformulary exceptions process is often informal and variable across VISNs and facilities. Not all VISNs have standard forms. The procedures for assessing and acting on a request appear to require different amounts of time and impose different administrative burdens in different VISNs. Because some requests are unrecorded, program statistics are not reliable. The National Formulary would appear fairer and more responsive if the nonformulary system were revised and simplified, and reporting was accurate and consistent.

In closed or preferred classes, anticipated or promised volume of drug use supports better negotiated prices. There is, therefore, an expectation that VHA prescribers will discontinue prescribing nonformulary or noncontract drugs so that veterans are not started on them. Alternatively, veterans on nonformulary or noncontract drugs may be converted to the formulary therapeutic alternates. The VA PBM, MAP, and VISNs have left policy and procedure on such therapeutic interchanges to local facilities, although directives leading to them often originate at the national or VISN level. These interchanges are often made without the authorization of individual prescribers at the time of dispensing.

Therapeutic interchange is an accepted practice driven by price differentials and market share commitments in about half of managed care plans. Very often MCO interchanges involve the same drug classes as VA interchanges. They almost always are carried out with the permission of the prescriber at the time of dispensing. Therapeutic interchange is common in hospitals, generally also in the same drug classes. Since hospital medical staffs agree in advance to interchanges, individual prescriber permission at the time of dispensing is usually not sought. Therapeutic interchange is not practiced in Medicaid fee-for-service. It is uncertain how frequent it is in Medicaid managed care or Department of Defense (DOD) programs.

Although evaluations of VA therapeutic interchanges in the medical literature are generally reassuring, these studies frequently have methodological deficiencies; they can generate discontent, and occasional problems are reported. VA interchanges respond to national contract (and sometimes blanket purchase agreement) volume commitments and negotiated price differentials. They are left to local facilities without national VHA guidelines or written policies at the VISN level, however. Some veterans report not having received adequate, or any, information on the replacement drug, and some physicians have registered complaints. There should be consistency throughout the VHA in ensuring interchange program quality, patient and prescriber acceptance, adequate advance notice and education, and protection against risks to certain vulnerable patients. A responsive nonformulary process would also help provide this assurance.

Since VA contracts with drug manufacturers are renewable annually, they and the prices they set may change, obligating new interchanges. At some point, the VHA will have to evaluate how frequently veterans taking a drug chronically should be subjected to interchange or determine the total number of interchanges that is reasonable for an individual patient.

The IOM committee compared the coverage of OTC drugs and the use of generic substitution in the VA National Formulary with coverage and use in other formularies and formulary systems. Few health maintenance organizations (HMOs) offer OTC coverage as a specific pharmacy benefit, and the number of OTC drugs or drug classes covered in managed care is limited mostly to insulin and diabetic supplies with lesser coverage of antihistamines, histamine$_2$ receptor (H$_2$R) blockers, nonsteroidal anti-inflammatory drugs (NSAIDs), and cough and cold remedies. Medicaid OTC coverage is also less generous than that of the National Formulary. In comparison to other public and private-sector formularies the VA is less restrictive in this respect.

Generic substitution is an accepted medical practice. In hospitals, it is usually automatic. About half of the states require dispensing of the generic drug, if there is one, in their Medicaid programs. Managed care organizations also commonly mandate or encourage generic substitution. The VHA requires genetic substitution, and is more successful than the private sector in promoting the use of generics. This practice relies on FDA determination of the equivalence of a generic to the branded "innovator" product. It is unexceptional and has no implications for restrictiveness.

The committee examined information on veterans' complaints about the National Formulary and surveys of physician opinions of the formulary and formulary system. Complaints and dissatisfaction may be indicators of the restrictiveness of the formulary and may point to areas that have to be addressed. Veterans complained primarily about access to nonformulary drugs, in particular sildenafil citrate (Viagra). These complaints about the National Formulary comprised 0.4% (2,385 out of 570,937) of the total complaints recorded by official patients' advocates in VA facilities.

A number of surveys of physician attitudes about the National Formulary or other formularies have been reported. Of these, the most helpful was performed by the RAND Corporation for the VA. This survey had problems limiting the conclusions that could be drawn from it, but it did find that a minority of physicians complained about not being able to prescribe needed drugs. Other surveys suffered from more substantial problems of a similar nature, that is, very low response rates, survey design, and support by interested parties that made any conclusions highly suspect. The committee appreciates the normal human tendency to want unfettered access to available benefits without (even reasonable) economic or other restrictions. Nevertheless, complaints of patients and prescribers should be evaluated seriously, and their acceptance of the formulary should be a priority objective. Physician support, especially, is essential to the success of a formulary, and refusal of doctors to cooperate may greatly reduce anticipated savings.

COSTS

The VHA is one of the larger purchasers of drugs in the United States. Prices for most brand drugs are set in the Federal Supply Schedule, which is administered by the National Acquisition Center. The NAC also negotiates and administers contracts for drugs for the VHA. The NAC, using the leverage of a large purchaser and the selection among agents by the National Formulary, reports substantial savings resulting from implementation of the formulary. As of February 2000, these savings (that is, the difference between NAC estimates of actual expenditures on drugs and what would have been spent in the absence of the National Formulary and other contracting activities) were said to amount to at least $572,521,352. This included savings due to closed or preferred classes, selected blanket purchase agreements (BPAs), generic drug purchases under contract, bulk purchases of pharmacy-related supplies, and savings from patent expirations on brand drugs, among others, from FY 1996 through FY 2000. Using a limited scope (that is, only savings accruing from favorable prices negotiated for six closed or preferred National Formulary drug classes) and a more limited time period (that is, from the date of designation as a closed or preferred class to class opening or the end of available data [July 1999]), the IOM arrived at a conservative, lower estimate, approximating $100 million in the aggregate.

In economic terms, the objective of the VA National Formulary is to make the demand for specific prescription drugs more responsive to price than might otherwise have been the case. Formularies increase a buyer's bargaining power, enabling buyers to be more aggressive in price negotiation. By excluding certain products or by shifting demand significantly between competing products, the buyer presents a seller with a more elastic, or price-responsive, demand, thereby inducing a lower price. The greater the ability to direct the volume of prescriptions between competing products, the more elastic the demand and the greater the bargaining power of the buyer.

Because only drugs selected through drug class reviews by the National Formulary in a closed class are available throughout the VHA unless a nonformulary exception is approved, class closure exerts strong effects on prescribing behavior. Prescribing of preferred drugs in preferred classes is encouraged by drug usage criteria, information about the preferred drugs, and other administrative directives. Alternatives to preferred agents can be provided by VISN or local facility formularies, however. BPAs can also affect drug choices at the VISN, local, or, occasionally, national level. Other factors affecting drug use in the VHA include the shift to outpatient services (and outpatient pharmacy), greater numbers of veterans using the VHA (and the VHA pharmacy benefit), and the introduction of a number of effective, popular, but expensive new drugs.

To assess the effect of the VA National Formulary on VHA drug expenditures, ideally person-level data should be used to compare per-person expenditures for 1 to 2 years before and after formulary implementation. Such data would allow examination of changes in drug spending, in overall health care spending, and in shifts among VHA budgets associated with the National Formulary. Instead, VA data limitations required the IOM to employ aggregate drug use data per VISN per month for FY 1994 through FY 1999 for 14 classes of drugs, 6 of which were, or had been, closed or preferred (angiotensin-converting enzyme inhibitors [ACEIs], hydroxymethylglutaryl coenzyme A reductase inhibitors

[HMG CoA RIs], alpha blockers, H_2R blockers, proton pump inhibitors [PPIs], and calcium channel blockers [CCBs]), and 8 of which were open. Price data by VISN by month, with some gaps, were obtained from the VA, and these prices were multiplied by drug use by VISN by month to get expenditures. Expenditures were controlled for changes in the VHA user population and age and gender distribution. To explore for cost shifting or other secondary effects, aggregate data on VA inpatient discharges for conditions treatable with drugs affected by class closure were also examined for any association with implementation of the National Formulary.

Several different approaches to estimating savings from formulary policy are described in the pharmacoeconomics literature. Many of these depend on being able to convert data into defined daily doses and to use detailed management information to predict purchasing patterns absent formulary changes. For example, some large private-sector health centers multiply total annual spending on a particular formulary agent by the percentage price decrease negotiated at the time of formulary selection and take this as a cost avoidance or savings for the year, unadjusted for possible coinciding factors affecting drug usage. The data limitations in this study precluded such approaches.

The IOM committee compared pre-National Formulary prices for the most commonly prescribed product in each affected class with post-National Formulary prices calculated as the average VISN prices over the 3 months after the class was closed. Price reductions varied from 16 to 41%. Market shares of selected drugs in these classes changed substantially in most cases, reaching 97% in one case. Price, utilization, and market share changes were generally not found or were consistent with existing trends in the open classes for which data were obtained. Trends in outpatient pharmacy spending varied considerably. In three closed classes (ACEIs, H_2R blockers, alpha blockers), implementation of the National Formulary was associated with a decreased spending level per user relative to previous trends. In two classes (PPIs, HMG CoA RIs), the spending increase was consistent with increasing numbers of prescriptions per outpatient user. In the sixth class (CCBs), spending did not change significantly. Regression analyses were performed to control for key variables, and coefficients of interest were reported to assess the spending effect for each closed or preferred class relative to what would have occurred absent the VA National Formulary.

Effects were reported as reductions in spending, nominal spending change, change adjusted to real present discounted value, and nominal spending adjusted for changes in the general level of prices in the economy as measured by the Consumer Price Index, that is, "real" savings. For ACEIs, reductions were 16.9% (lisinopril) and 8.5% (fosinopril); nominal savings, $17.6 million; and real savings, $16.9 million. For alpha blockers, reductions were 17.5%; and both nominal and real savings, about $1.8 million. For HMG CoA RIs, reductions were 8.1%; nominal savings, $14.4 million; and real savings, $13.8 million. For PPIs, reductions were 7.4%; nominal savings, $4.9 million; and real savings, $4.7 million. For H_2R blockers, reductions were 41%; nominal savings, $47.1 million; and real savings, $45.2 million. For CCBs, there was an increase of 7.9%, nominal extra spending of $13.2 million, and real extra spending of $12.8 million. There was additional (BPA) contracting for drugs in this class for which data were not available, and these changes were not statistically significant. Because of this uncertainty, the effects in the CCB class should be interpreted with caution.

As noted earlier, the committee explored the possibility of changes in inpatient use associated with VA National Formulary activities. Trends in the number of discharges for selected heart- and ulcer-related diagnoses were plotted to explore possible associations with National Formulary policies on drugs for treatment of these conditions. The regression analyses showed an estimated decrease in heart disease-related discharges of 1.3% relative to the numbers expected in the absence of the National Formulary, and a decrease of 4.9% in ulcer-related discharges. Although neither of these changes was significant, they are very crude indicators of shifting utilization that might be caused by changes in the delivery system.

The committee also attempted to estimate the costs of developing and operating the National Formulary using data from the VA PBM. About half of the VA PBM budget was said to be associated with the formulary, that is, $400,000 for FY 1995 and FY 1996, and $900,000 for each year thereafter. Costs not captured in this estimate would include time spent by VISN leaders and personnel in implementing and managing the National Formulary at that level, time spent by the NAC on National Formulary contract work, procurement costs for the formulary's closed classes, and time spent administering National Formulary exceptions and therapeutic interchanges at the local level, among others. The committee had no information that would allow an assessment of these costs or an overall estimate of VA National Formulary operational expenditures.

The committee estimated the aggregate gross savings associated with five of the six examined classes to be $85.8 million in nominal terms and $82 million in real dollars. As noted, incomplete information—that is, the effect on expenditures of a BPA for diltiazem, the highest-volume drug in the class—prevented a complete estimate of cost trends for CCBs, the sixth class studied. The seventh closed or preferred class, luteinizing hormone-releasing hormones (LHRHs), could not be studied due to the unavailability of data. Overall, the committee found that the National Formulary's closed classes were associated with notable reductions in average outpatient pharmacy spending per outpatient VHA user. After controlling for secular trends in drug utilization not related to the formulary, time invariant unmeasured differences between VISNs, and the changing VA population, the committee estimated decreases in per-user pharmacy spending of between 7% and 41% for these classes. Given the fact that effects of BPAs and other activities of the VA PBM were not measured in the IOM assessment, it is likely that aggregate gross savings may have exceeded the previously cited figures. True gross savings approximating $100 million are quite likely to have been realized over the first 2 years of operation of the VA National Formulary. This figure is about 3% of total pharmacy or 15% of the six analyzed drug class expenditures over those 2 years.

The cost savings directly attributable to the VA National Formulary enable the VHA to provide additional services of other kinds to veterans. Continuation of the formulary is justified on the basis of these savings, especially since, as discussed below, there are no scientifically valid reports of adverse quality effects from the National Formulary. The committee has observed some deficiencies in the data needed to assess various effects of the National Formulary or to ensure knowledgeable formulary management. Improvements in cost data would help the VHA to assess per-person expenditures and cost shifts among various VHA budgets.

QUALITY

The committee has evaluated VA National Formulary and formulary system effects on quality of care using structural elements. Effects of the formulary and formulary system, using process and outcome criteria, have also been discussed. Process criteria include effects on utilization: whether veterans have access to the fight drug at the right time. Outcome criteria refer to whether clinical or human outcomes are affected. They would be the most persuasive indicators, as noted in the IOM definition of quality. By this definition, quality of care is the degree to which health services for individuals and populations increase the likelihood of desired health outcomes and are consistent with current professional knowledge. In fact, there are few data on anything other than structural characteristics of the VA National Formulary. The committee, therefore, concentrated on these characteristics.

The committee looked predominantly at clinical pharmacy services, local facility pharmacy and therapeutics committees, VISN formulary committees, the VA PBM and MAP, the quality and availability of existing and new FDA-approved drugs on the National Formulary, drug class reviews and therapeutic guidelines, the nonformulary process, therapeutic interchange policy, and drug utilization review (DUR). The development of clinical pharmacy services and the redefinition of the scope of pharmacy practice in the VA that occurred in the 1990s are important structural elements. However, these changes began well before the VISN formulary and the National Formulary and are important in overall quality of drug therapy and management of the pharmacy benefit. They are also important to the quality-of-care effects of the National Formulary, but they cannot be said to be a specific structural element of the National Formulary itself.

Local facility pharmacy and therapeutics committees (P&T) predated VISN formularies and National Formulary by several decades. They have other than National Formulary functions. They also are important to the quality-of-care effects of formularies at the local level. They consider staff prescriber nonformulary requests, ensure proper contract drug use and generic prescribing, implement therapeutic interchanges, and monitor adverse drug events, among others. Their role in the design of local formularies is unclear since most of these are the same as the VISN formulary, but they can originate requests to add drugs to a VISN formulary or to the National Formulary.

VISN formulary committees usually have 15 members (range 6–28), and average 52% pharmacists (range 33– 100%) and 44% physicians (range 0– 65%). Some VISN formulary committees appear to focus on VISN and National Formulary management and budgetary matters, that is, to function as little PBMs. As such, they will affect quality of care, but there are no formal studies of this. Other formulary committees may be more like traditional pharmacy and therapeutics committees and may affect quality of care as these committees do. Formulary committees appear to be highly variable in membership, and the presence of no or very few physicians on some of them may have implications for physician acceptance of the VISN or National Formulary.

The VHA reorganization that authorized 22 VISNs also led to the creation of a Pharmacy Benefits Management Strategic Healthcare Group located in Washington, D.C., and Chicago; a Medical Advisory Panel made up of 1 DOD and 11 VA field physicians; and a VISN Formulary Leaders Committee, as described earlier. These bodies are central structural elements related to the National Formulary's effects on quality of care. The quality of their management and clinical decisions regarding the formulary and formulary systems is as important to the VA formulary as are similar management and decisions of private-sector PBMs to private formularies. The IOM committee assessed VA PBM performance by examining the quality of the formulary, additions of drugs, drug class reviews and therapeutic guidelines, the nonformulary process, therapeutic interchange policy, and other elements of the system that affect quality. The committee observed good quality discussions and decision making at a MAP/VA PBM meeting in August 1999.

Addition of existing and newly FDA-approved drugs to the National Formulary and the overall quality of drugs on the formulary are important factors in the availability of drugs and thus in the quality of care. The committee recommended more timely consideration of additions and a better balance between a uniform national entitlement and local preferences. The size of the National Formulary was found to be reasonable. The committee evaluated the quality of the drugs listed against available lists of questionable drugs, questionable combination products, and drugs considered inappropriate for the elderly by the General Accounting Office (GAO). The national list was found to contain few such products. Drugs included on the National Formulary appear to meet reasonable standards of numbers, variety, and quality based on IOM committee members' professional judgment and experience.

A drug class review is an important mechanism by which a formulary system evaluates and selects from among drugs and drug products those that are considered most useful in patient care. Choosing in this way has quality implications, but it also enables a formulary system to negotiate favorable prices for selected drugs based on anticipation or commitments of high-volume use, as observed elsewhere. Detailed standards and guidelines for performing drug class reviews have been published several times. The committee also has professional and institutional experience with drug class reviews at academic medical centers, managed care organizations, and PBMs. Using these standards and its experience, the committee examined the conclusions and recommendations of nine VA drug class reviews. In all cases the drugs recommended by the reviews were included on the National Formulary. Both intrinsically and in comparison to reviews in private-sector organizations, the reviews were of high professional quality and reached recommendations based on scientific evidence and sound interpretation of clinical data.

VA clinical guidelines are clearly written, and their recommendations are consistent with current recommendations of other organizations, such as the American College of Cardiology, the American Heart Association, and the Department of Health and Human Services. The guidelines are also tailored to the older VA patient population. These guidelines are based on current scientific and clinical research data and are equivalent to similar documents in the private sector. Evidence on the use of these guidelines is scanty, but some facilities or VISNs are monitoring their effect on clinical practices and following up with appropriate interventions.

The IOM committee surveyed pharmacy or medical personnel in all 22 VISNs and discovered a wide range of circumstances in which nonformulary prescriptions, requests, and decisions might not be recorded or appear in monthly statistics. As a result, reports of the percentage of requests submitted or approved are probably not reflective of the actual situation in the VISNs. The access of veterans to nonformulary drugs, other effects of the nonformulary process, and their implications for quality are therefore hard to assess or compare with other systems. Although the committee appreciates the advantages of some degree of informality, the VA system should be made more consistent and likely to be portrayed accurately in program statistics.

Current published reports of VA therapeutic interchanges, unpublished documents from VA facilities, and expressions of physician and patient dissatisfaction from surveys and patient advocate data have not made a compelling case for quality problems. They do reinforce that therapeutic interchanges are often viewed as problematic, and they raise questions for exploration and suggest possible responses that might be taken by the VHA. Some of these questions have been discussed earlier. If veterans receiving a drug on a long-term basis are subject to interchanges multiple times or too often because of changes in the formulary or committed-use contracting, there will be effects on treatment acceptance and compliance, and there may well be changes in the effectiveness of treatment. In short, quality-of-care and health outcomes may be affected. The VHA has to address the consistency and policy gaps in therapeutic interchange to ensure that quality is not affected.

The use of drugs, as part of the process of care, was examined by the committee. Class closure, committed-use contracts, preferred drug designations, drug usage criteria, and separate negotiations for drug prices, such as blanket purchase agreements, all may affect the utilization of drugs in certain classes. Dramatic changes in utilization may follow class closure, National Formulary selection, and contracting for drugs. These changes are indicated in Chapter 3 (Cost) and Chapter 4 (Quality) of this report. If some of these changes are not systemwide, as is often the case due to BPAs, for example, veterans traveling from VISN to VISN may experience different preferred drugs. They will then have to depend on the uncertainties of the nonformulary process to ensure access to their current drug treatment. The committee did not find any scientifically valid evidence that changes in the number or variety of drugs by class closure were affecting the quality of drug treatment and health outcomes of veterans. To analyze such effects, person-specific tracking of drug utilization would be needed, as noted in Chapter 3.

Changes in the prevalence or types of adverse drug events associated with implementation of the National Formulary and formulary system would be important evidence of health outcomes affected by the formulary. The VHA has taken steps, such as electronic prescribing and machine-readable coding of prescriptions, to reduce adverse events. Other programs, such as the VA Patient Safety Event Registry, do not reliably collect adverse event data or are in early stages. These programs are not a part of the National Formulary. Statistics on adverse events during therapeutic interchange are not available in the VHA or nationally in other health care systems.

The IOM committee, as part of its analysis of cost effects of the National Formulary, collected hospital discharge data before and after formulary implementation in 1997. As reported earlier, no association was observed between changes in the distribution of discharge diagnoses for specific conditions and changes in National Formulary policies on drugs to treat these conditions. This analysis suggests only that there are no quality effects of sufficient magnitude to be demonstrated by this imprecise measurement tool.

Patient satisfaction is a generally accepted element of quality of care. Patient dissatisfaction discovered through significant levels of complaints to advocates or through surveys could be an important indicator of the need for a system response. Data from surveys are not conclusive, but physician acceptance of the formulary is important to its success and has to be addressed.

Based on what is known about its effects on quality of care, there is no reason to discontinue the National Formulary. Concerns exist in a number of areas, such as the addition of drugs, the nonformulary process, therapeutic interchange, and patient and physician acceptance. The absence of good data on quality effects is a particular concern, as is the need for better data to enable prudent management of the National Formulary. The VA should focus its health services research capacity on National Formulary and drug treatment issues and should improve operational data. It is the responsibility of an important national program to illuminate these issues, which have implications beyond the boundaries of the VHA.

COMPARISONS

Almost all managed care organizations offer pharmacy benefits and have formularies. PBMs frequently either manage these benefits, pay claims, or both. Most of the formularies are closed or partially closed, although it is not clear precisely what is meant by this, since formulary systems are extremely varied in managed care plans and PBMs. Copayments are a common practice in managed care, often amounting to the entire cost of a brand drug if generics are available. Other formulary management strategies in managed care include generic substitution, therapeutic interchange, DUR, exclusion of certain specific drugs or drug classes, and prior approval. The committee reviewed a number of publicly available managed care or PBM formularies and described some classes that are closed in these formularies and also in the VA National Formulary. The numbers and varieties of drugs or drug classes that are excluded or subject to prior approval in some managed care formularies were listed. New information of this kind was collected by the Academy of Managed Care Pharmacy and is discussed in Chapter 2.

In general, managed care formularies employ exclusions, prior approvals, and copayments, which are not features of the VA National Formulary. Some of these—for example, prescription copayments—are insensitive to medical need. Reacting to data such as these and to public concerns, legislatures in many states have enacted legislation requiring public disclosure of formulary and nonformulary processes. Some states have imposed requirements on the nonformulary process, mandating that it be expeditious or that requests be approved within 24 hours and that a 72-hour supply of the drug be provided. Other states have set criteria for the approval of nonformulary requests. Many states have laws that set limits on therapeutic interchange, prohibit increased cost sharing or copayments, or prohibit eliminating or decreasing coverage during a contract year. These state requirements for managed care generally are not relevant to the National Formulary, which is already characterized by disclosure on the Internet (although the nonformulary process is in practice not transparent), low or no copayments, and relatively stable drug coverage.

Because the VA is a government health care program, the committee decided to review two public-sector programs with formularies and formulary systems. The Medicaid program has the largest government pharmacy benefit and has been functioning with formularies for several decades. The committee also decided to review the DOD formulary and formulary system. The DOD health system and pharmacy benefit are roughly the same size as those of the VA. Unlike Medicaid recipients who are primarily poor women and children, the DOD population consists of military personnel (that is, persons who are or will be veterans and dependents of veterans) with many similarities to the VHA population.

The Medicaid fee-for-service program provides coverage for prescription drugs in every state under Title XIX of the Social Security Act and applicable state law. In addition to Title XIX, the current Medicaid benefit is governed by provisions enacted in the Omnibus Budget Reconciliation Act (OBRA) of 1990 and 1993. Prior to OBRA 1990, states faced fewer limits on drug management strategies, such as formularies, prescription limits, generic substitution, prior approval systems, refill limits, and copayments. In OBRA 1990, Congress prohibited restrictive state Medicaid formularies, allowed prior approval under certain conditions, required Medicaid programs to reimburse all new drugs for at least 6 months after FDA approval, and required that manufacturers rebate to Medicaid the lesser of an approximately 15% discount below average wholesale price or the best price offered to other purchasers.

OBRA 1993 softened the prohibition on restrictive formularies. Currently manufacturers are required to sign rebate agreements to qualify their products for Medicaid reimbursement. Medicaid may exclude only a list of drugs or drug classes specified in the legislation. Prior approval is allowed as long as the approval system provides a response within 24 hours and a 72-hour emergency supply of the drug under review. The limits on exclusions and the requirements for listing all drugs under rebate agreements have left prior approval as one of the last flexible drug management strategies available to state Medicaid programs. States may adopt their own clinical or nonclinical criteria for approving a prior approval request. States may restrict a particular drug to patients of a certain age, those with a specific diagnosis, or those who have been treated with another drug first. States also can impose small copayments ($0.50 to $3.00) on certain categories of recipients, and many states impose prescription limits.

The different formulary system controls and the types of formularies, open or closed, in each state are listed in Table 5.1. Most states use some combination of prior approval, exclusions, prescription limits, and copayments. The effects of these controls are not clear. They depend on the design and rigor of implementation. Since the states are so different, comparisons with the VA National Formulary are uncertain. The VA provides a standardized national entitlement through the National Formulary, but this uniformity is diluted by the variability among VISNs in their formularies and formulary system policies and procedures. The VA nonformulary system is perhaps more variable than Medicaid's, although data are limited for both systems. Exclusion of OBRA classes and some kinds of limits on the amount and frequency of dispensing by Medicaid are more restrictive than VA controls. The National Formulary provides fewer choices in some drug classes, particularly closed classes, although Medicaid prior approval in some of these classes may limit access.

The committee reviewed 15 studies of formulary system controls in Medicaid fee-for-service programs. Many of these studies had significant deficiencies, including short follow-up periods and a lack of control groups, which limited any conclusions that could be drawn from them. In spite of this, the committee suggested certain inferences. Programs to decrease utilization or costs through a particular control sometimes result in offsetting utilization or costs in another part of the pharmacy or other benefits of the health care system. Controls that do not allow for medical need-based exceptions sometimes cause undesirable changes in utilization, costs, or quality of care. Most of the restrictions or characteristics of Medicaid formularies and formulary systems studied in the 15 reports that the committee reviewed are not features of the VA National Formulary, however. Therefore, these reports are of limited usefulness in evaluating the restrictiveness or effects on cost and quality of the VA formulary system.

Medicaid managed care has expanded dramatically in the past 10 years. Currently, more than half of Medicaid recipients are enrolled in almost 600 different plans. Two states, Tennessee and Arizona, administer their entire program through managed care plans. Only two states do not use managed care (Alaska and Wyoming). Most plans are authorized through federal approval of waivers of Title XIX requirements—Section 1915b or Section 1115 waivers. The Balanced Budget Act of 1997 made it easier for states to enroll recipients in managed care. Most plans have enrolled women and children, not the more vulnerable and costly aged and disabled population which is more like the VHA population. The pharmacy benefit in Medicaid managed care varies with the plan, but is based on the contract between the state and the plan, the provisions of the waivers, and an underlying requirement that it should not be more restrictive than the fee-for-service benefit. At present, 13 states have carved out their pharmacy benefit from managed care and administer it separately. Insufficient information was available to the committee to make detailed comparisons between Medicaid managed care and the VA National Formulary. It is likely that findings would be similar to those for Medicaid fee-for-service programs.

The committee briefly reviewed the Department of Defense pharmacy benefit, which has a somewhat lesser cost than the VA benefit. The DOD formularies and formulary systems are variable across a number of facilities. The benefit varies because it is in part available at more than 500 military treatment facilities worldwide and in part available through contract mail order or thousands of retail pharmacies. Substantial deductibles and copayments are a part of the system for some non-active duty personnel. The DOD Basic Core Formulary, which is a national requirement at all military treatment facilities, is a very limited formulary with 159 listings.

The DOD benefit, formularies, and formulary systems are in transition under provisions of the National Defense Authorization Act for FY 2000 (P.L. 106-65, Section 701), which requires a new Uniform Formulary, data systems, and advisory committees, among others. The committee observed that the present DOD Basic Core Formulary, mail order formulary, and multiple treatment facility formularies are not comparable counterparts to the VA National Formulary and formulary system. They are in earlier stages of development. How they will compare after full implementation of the National Defense Authorization Act is unknown and presumably will depend on the details of changes.

In examining public and private-sector formularies in comparison to the VA, the committee concluded that some are more open. Medicaid programs are required to offer all drugs on the Federal Supply Schedule that manufacturers list for rebates. Some are more restricted. They require prior approvals and exclude some drugs. All are variable, some probably more so than the VA's (for example, DOD's). Some controls that are not part of the VA system, such as relatively costly deductibles and copayments, may present real barriers to needed drugs, especially for low-income patients. These controls are part of DOD requirements for some eligibles or employed by some managed care plans.

Other controls, such as generic substitution and therapeutic interchange, are in common use in many systems. The important element for quality and restrictiveness is timely availability of a safe and effective, medically necessary drug, if not listed, through an exceptions process. A good formulary supports this element and, through its capacity to make quality choices, enhances price negotiations and prudent purchasing.

References

Academy of Managed Care Pharmacy (AMCP). *Where We Stand*. Alexandria, VA: AMCP; 1997.

Academy of Managed Care Pharmacy. Common practices in formulary management system. *Acad. Managed Care Pharm. Newsl*. In press.

Achusim LE. Therapeutic interchange as a cost-containment measure. *Pharmaco-Economics*. 1992; 2(5):347–351.

Aetna US Health Care. Members and Consumers. *2000 Precertification List* [on line]. Available at: http://www.aetnaushc.com/products/rx/precert_00.html.

American Association of Health Plans (AAHP). *Formularies*. Washington, DC: AAHP; 1998.

American College of Clinical Pharmacy (ACCP). ACCP position statement guidelines for therapeutic interchange. *Pharmacotherapy*. 1993; 13(3):252–256.

American College of Physicians (ACP). Therapeutic substitution and formulary systems. *Ann. Intern. Med.* 1990; 113(2):160–163.

American Hospital Association (AHA). *Statement of Guiding Principles on the Operation of the Hospital Formulary System*. Chicago: AHA; 1974.

American Hospital Association. *Operation of the Hospital Formulary System*. Chicago: AHA; 1975.

American Hospital Association. American Hospital Association Statement on National Patient Safety Partnership Press Conference Attribute to Jack Lord, M.D., Chief Operating Officer, AHA. Chicago: AHA; 1999.

American Medical Association (AMA). AMA policy on drug formularies and therapeutic interchange in inpatient and ambulatory patient care settings. *Am. J. Hosp. Pharm.* 1994; 51:1808–1810.

American Medical Association. *Pharmaceutical Benefits Management Companies , Report of the Board of Trustees* . Chicago: AMA; 1997.
American Society of Health-System Pharmacists (ASHP). *Best Practices for Health-System Pharmacy* . Bethesda, MD: ASHP; 1998.
American Society of Hospital Pharmacists. ASHP guidelines for the scientific and therapeutic evaluation of drugs for hospital formularies. *Am. J. Hosp. Pharm.* 1981; 38:1043–1044.
American Society of Hospital Pharmacists. *Therapeutic Interchange* . Bethesda, MD: ASHP; 1982.
American Society of Hospital Pharmacists. ASHP statement on the formulary system. *Am. J. Hosp. Pharm.* 1983; 40:1384–1385.
American Society of Hospital Pharmacists. ASHP technical assistance bulletin on the evaluation of drugs for formularies. *Am. J. Hosp. Pharm.* 1988; 45:386–387.
American Society of Hospital Pharmacists. *Am J. Hosp. Pharm.* 1991.
American Society of Hospital Pharmacists. ASHP statement on the pharmacy and therapeutics committee. *Am. J. Hosp. Pharm.* 1992; 49:2008–2009.
American Society of Hospital Pharmacists. 1996
American Society of Hospital Pharmacists, APA, AHA, AMA. Statement of guiding principles on the operation of the hospital formulary system. *Am. J. Hosp. Pharm.* 1964; 21:40–41.
Anonymous. An interview with John Ogden. *Am. Pharm.* 1988; NS28:8:22–23.
Ascione FJ, Bagozzi RP, Mannebach MA, et al.. *Analysis of the Internal and External Factors Related to Performance of Pharmacy and Therapeutic Committees* . Ann Arbor: University of Michigan; 1998.
Avorn J, Chen M, Hartley R. Scientific versus commercial sources of influence on the prescribing behavior of physicians. *Am. J. Med.* 1982; 73:4–8.
Avorn J, Soumerai SB. Improving drug-therapy decisions through educational out-reach—A randomized controlled trial of academically based "detailing." *N. Engl. J. Med.* 1983; 308 (24):1457–1463.
Baciewicz AM, Cowan RI, Michaels PE, Kyllonen KS. Quality and productivity assessment of clinical pharmacy interventions. *Hosp. Formul* 1994; 29:773–779.
Bajpai SK, Pathak DS. Predicting formulary decisions in health maintenance organizations involving nonsteroidal anti-inflammatory drugs. *J. Res. Pharmaceut. Econ.* 1998; 9(1):57–70.
Bakke OM. How many drugs do we need? *World Health Forum* . 1986; 7:252–255.
Barents Group LLC. *Analysis of Benefits Offered by Medicare HMOs, 1999: Complexities and Implications* . Menlo Park, CA: The Henry J. Kaiser Family Foundation; 1999a.
Barents Group LLC. *Factors Affecting the Growth of Prescription Drug Expenditures* . Washington, DC: National Institute for Health Care Management Research and Educational Foundation; 1999b.
Barksdale Air Force Base. Dihydropyridine switch program deemed not cost effective. *Formulary* . 1998; 33:12.
Bartlett S, Marshall JA, Prochazka A, et al. *A Study of the Short-Term Clinical and Economic Outcomes of Converting Hypertensive Patients from Long-Acting Nifedipine to Short-Acting Nifedipine* . Denver: Department of Veterans Affairs Medical Center (unpublished) ; 1996.

REFERENCES

Basskin L. Pharmacoeconomics and the formulary decision-making process. *Formulary* . 1998; 33:460.
Baugh D, Pine P, Blackwell S. Trends in prescription drug utilization and payments. *Health Care Financing Rev.* 1999; 20:3 :79–105.
Berkowitz HS. Formulary designation of cimetidine as the primary intravenous histamine H_2-receptor antagonist. *Am. J. Hosp. Pharm.* 1992; 49:134–135.
Black J, Griffin TN, Beisel WBMD. Implementation of an outpatient prescription drug formulary in a managed-care system. *Am. J. Hosp. Pharm.* 1988; 45:561–565.
Bloom BS, Jacobs J. Cost effects of restricting cost-effective therapy. *Med. Care* . 1985; 23(7):872–880.
Bodenbender, R. Henry. PVA, personal communication , 1999.
Bootman JL, Milne RJ. Costs, innovation and efficacy in anti-infective therapy. *PharmacoEconomics* . 1996; 9(Suppl. 1):31–39.
Boston D, Collins C. Safety, efficacy, and lipid profile of doxazosin at a VA medical center. *Hosp. Formul.* 1995; 30:233–236.
Briscoe TA, Dearing CJ. Clinical and economic effects of replacing enalapril with benazepril in hypertensive Patients. *Am. J. Health-Syst. Pharm.* 1996; 53:2191–2193 .
Brook RH et al.. Does free care improve adults' health? Results from a randomized trial. *N. Engl. J. Med.* 1983; 309(23) :1426–1434 .
Brown GR, Clarke AM. Therapeutic interchange of cefazolin with metronidazole for cefoxitin. *Am. J. Hosp. Pharm.* 1992; 49:1946–1950 .
Brown JS. Review of State Medicaid Formularies. Unpublished manuscript ; 1999.
Brown JS, Bienz-Tadnor B, Lasagna L. Availability of anticancer drugs in the United States, Europe, and Japan from 1960 through 1991. *Clin. Pharmacol. Therapeut.* 1995; 58: (3):243–256.
Brunsting J, Johnson M. Paper presented at the Western States Residents Conference , Pacific Grove, CA ; .
Buchanan R, Smith S. Medicaid policies for HIV-related prescription drugs. *Health Care Financing Rev.* 1994; 15:(3):43–61.
Bull S, Shoheiber O, Bailey M, et al. Utilization of pharmacy claims data to evaluate therapeutic interchange programs. *J. Managed Care Pharm.* 1999 : 331–334.
Calvo MV, Fruns I, Domínguez-Gil A. Decision analysis applied to selection of histamine H_2-receptor antagonists for the formulary. *Am. J. Hosp. Pharm.* 1990; 47:2002–2006 .
Cantrell W, Kimber G, Morrill G. Evaluation of blood pressure and adverse effects in patients converted from lisinopril to benazepril. *J. Managed Care Phar.* 1999; 5:52–54.
Carroll NV. Formularies and therapeutic interchange: The health care setting makes a difference. *Am. J. Health-System Pharm.* 1999; 56:467–471 .
Cascio M, Williams J. Impact of non-formulary drug notification form. *Am. J. Hosp. Pharm.* 1982; 39:1039–1041 .
Centeon. Reimbursement alert. The debate over drug formularies. October December 1999 [on line]. Available at: www.adventisbehring.com/na/med/reimbursementrc/x_8med_99_4.asp.
Center for Drug Evaluation and Research (CDER). 1998. CDER 1998 Report to the Nation: Improving Public Health Through Human Drugs [on line]. Available at: http://www.fda.gov/cder/reports/rptntn98.pdf.

Center for Health Policy Research. *Negotiating the New Health System: A Nationwide Study of Medicaid Managed Care Contracts*. Washington, DC: George Washington University; 1998.
Chassin M.R., Galvin RW. The urgent need to improve health care quality. *J. Am. Med. Assoc.* 1998; 280(11):1000–1005.
Chinburapa V, Larson LN. The availability of new drugs in health maintenance organizations. *J. Res. Pharmaceut. Econ.* 1991; 3(1):91–110.
Chon HS, Suzuki NT. Evaluation of omeprazole to lansoprazole conversion in a VA medical center. *ASGO Midyear Clin. Meet*. 1998; P-122E.
Chren M-M, Landefield S. In reply letter. *J. Am. Med. Assoc.* 1994; 272:(5):355.
Congressional Budget Office (CBO). *How the Medicaid Rebate on Prescription Drugs Affects Pricing to the Pharmaceutical Industry*. Washington, DC: CBO; 1996.
Congressional Budget Office. *How Increased Competition from Generic Drugs Has Affected Prices and Returns in the Pharmaceutical Industry*. Washington, DC: CBO; 1998.
Cook A, Kornfield T, Gold M. *The Role of PBMs in Managing Drug Costs: Implications for a Medicare Drug Benefit*. Washington, DC: Mathematica Policy Research, Inc.; 2000.
Covington TR, Thornton JL. *The Formulary System: A Cornerstone of Drug Benefit Management*. Alexandria, VA: Foundation for Managed Care Pharmacy; 1995.
Crawford SY, Santell JP. ASHP national survey of pharmaceutical services in federal hospitals—1993. *Am. J. Hosp. Pharm.* 1994; 51:2377–2393.
Cromwell DM, Bass EB, Steinberg EP, et al. Can restrictions on reimbursement for anti-ulcer drugs decrease Medicaid pharmacy costs without increasing hospitalizations? *Health Serviees Res.* 1999; 33(6):1593–1610.
Department of Veterans Affairs, Veterans Health Administration. *Pharmacy Benefits Management: A Valuable Product Line*. Washington, DC: Department of Veterans Affairs; 1989.
Department of Veterans Affairs, Veterans Health Administration. *ADE Report*. Washington, DC: Department of Veterans Affairs; 1999a.
Department of Veterans Affairs, Pharmacy Benefits Management Strategic Health Group. Criteria for Use of Selected Drugs [on line]. Available at: http://www.dppm.med.va.gov/newsite/criteriadrop.html.
Department of Veterans Affairs, Pharmacy Benefits Management Strategic Health Group. Drug Class Reviews [on line]. Available at: http://www.dppm.med.va.gov/newsite/reviews.html.
Department of Veterans Affairs, Pharmacy Benefits Management Strategic Health Group. Treatment Guidelines [on line]. Available at: http://www.dppm.med.va.gov/newsite/treatment1.htm.
Department of Veterans Affairs, Pharmacy Benefits Management Strategic Health Group. Pharmacologic Management of Congestive Heart Failure [on line]. Available at: http://www.dppm.med.va.gov/newsite/DSMCHF.htm
Department of Veterans Affairs, Pharmacy Benefits Management Strategic Health Group [on line]. Available at: http://www.dppm.med.va.gov.
Desai N, Vigil JM, Wood MJ. Effects on lipids and liver function tests when patients are converted from lovastatin to fluvastatin. Paper presented at the Western States Residency Conference, Monterey, CA; 1997.

DeTorres OH, White RE. Effect of aminoglycoside-use restrictions on drug cost. *Am. J. Hosp. Pharm.* 1984; 41:1137–1139.

Dillon M. Drug Formulary Management. In: Navarro RP, ed. *Managed Care Pharmacy Practice*. Gaithersburg, MD: Aspen Publishers, Inc.; 1999.

DiMasi JA, Brown JS, Lasagna L. An analysis of regulatory review times of supplemental indications for already-approved drugs: 1989–1994. *Drug Inform. J.* 1966; 30:(2):315–337.

Doering PL, Russell WL, McCormick WC, Klapp DL. Therapeutic substitution in the health maintenance organization outpatient environment. *Drug Intell. Clin. Pharm.* 1988; 22 (2):125–130.

Donabedian A. *Explorations in Quality Assessment and Monitoring, Vol 1: The Definition of Quality and Approaches to Its Assessment*. Ann Arbor, MI: Health Administration Press; 1980.

Dranove D. Medicaid drug formulary restrictions. *J. Law Econ.* 1989; 32(1):143–162.

Dunagan WC, Medoff G. Formulary control of antimicrobial usage: What price freedom? *Diag. Microbiol. Infect. Dis.* 1993; 16:265–274.

Dzierba S, Reilly RT, Caselnova DAI. Cost savings achieved through cephalosporin use review and restriction. *Am. J. Hosp. Pharm.* 1986; 43:2194–2197.

Edwards DE, Triplett JW, Izquierdo-San Juan AB. Conversion from pravastatin or fluvastatin to simvastatin through a protocol: Outcome study. *ASHP Midyear Clin Meet*. 1998; P-9R.

Edwards JG, Anderson I. Systematic review and guide to selection of selective serotonin reuptake inhibitors. *Drugs*. 1999; 57(4):507–533.

Farrow, H.M. ; Personal communication, VISN 16. 1999.

Fink JL, Vivian JC, Reid KK, et al. *Facts and Comparisons*. St Louis, MO: Wolters Kluwer Co.; 1998.

Fonseca ML, Smith ME, Klein RE, Sheldon G. The Department of Veterans Affairs medical care system and the people it serves. *Med. Care*. 1996; 34(3 Suppl.):MS9–MS20.

Food and Drug Administration (FDA). FDA seeks help in evaluating consequences of therapeutic interchange. *Am. J. Health-System Pharm.* 1997; 54:(10):1149.

Food and Drug Administration. *Letter to Health Practitioners on Therapeutic Equivalence of Generic Drugs*. Washington, DC: FDA; 1998a.

Food and Drug Administration. *TalkPaper*. Washington, DC: FDA; 1998b.

Food and Drug Administration. *Electronic Orange Book: Approved Drug Products with Therapeutic Equivalence Evaluations*. Washington, DC: Department of Health and Human Services, Public Health Service; 1999a.

Food and Drug Administration. *TalkPaper*. Washington, DC: FDA; 1999b.

Food and Drug Administration. Manual of Policies and Procedures [on line]. Available at: www.fda.gov/MAPP.

Frank, G., et al. Prescription Drug Policy Issues in California, 1999.

Francke DE. The formulary system: Product of the teaching hospital. *J. Am. Hosp. Assoc.* 1967; 41:110–116.

Friedmann YM, Hanchak NA. Pharmacy Program Performance Measurement. In: Navarro RP, ed. *Managed Care Pharmacy Practice*. Gaithersburg, MD : Aspen Publishers, Inc.; 1999.

Fudge KA, Moore KA, Schneider DN, et al. Change in prescribing patterns of intravenous histamine2-receptor antagonists results in significant cost savings without adversely affecting patient care. *Ann. Pharmacother*. 1993; 27:232–237.

Furberg CD, Herrington DM, Psaty BM. Are drugs within a class interchangeable? *Lancet*. 1999; 354:1202–1204.

Ganz MB, Saksa B. Switching long-acting nifedipine. The large elderly population of a VAMC made an ideal setting to study the effects of changing antihypertensive therapy. *Fed Practioner*. 1997 : 71 , 72 , 75.

General Accounting Office (GAO). *Prescription Drugs in the Elderly: Many Still Receive Potentially Harmful Drugs Despite Recent Improvements*. Washington, DC: GAO; 1995.

General Accounting Office. *VA's Management of Drugs on Its National Formulary*. Washington, DC: GAO; 1999.

Gerbrandt KR, Yedinak KC. Formulary management of ACE inhibitors. *Pharmaco-Economics*. 1996; 10(6):594–613.

Gibaldi M. Vertical Integration: The drug industry and prescription benefits managers. *Pharmacotherapy*. 1995; 15:265–271.

Glassman PA, Good CB, Kelley M, et.al. Physician perceptions of a national formulary. *J. Int. Med*. [submitted] . 1999.

Glennie JL, Woloschuk DMM, Hall KW. High-technology drugs for cancer: The decision process for adding to a formulary. *PharmacoEconomics*. 1993; 4(6):405–413.

Gold M, Joffe M, Kennedy TL, et al. Pharmacy benefits in health maintenance organizations. *Health Affairs*. 1989 : 182–190.

Goldberg RA. Managing the pharmacy benefit: The formulary system. *J. Managed Care Pharmacy*. 1997; 3(5):565–573.

Grabowski H. Medicaid patients' access to new drugs. *Health Affairs*. 1988; 7(5):103–114.

Grabowski H, Mullins CD. Pharmacy benefit management, cost-effectiveness analysis and drug formulary decisions. *Soc. Sci. Med*. 1997; 45(4):535–544.

Grabowski HG, Schweitzer SO, Shiota SR. The effect of Medicaid formularies on the availability of new drugs. *PharmacoEconomics*. 1992; 1(Suppl. 1):32–40.

Gray DR. Documentation and assessment of pharmacist-initiated drug therapy intervention. *Topics Hosp. Pharm. Management*. 1992; 11:69–79.

Gray DR. Evaluation of a Formulary Switch from Alodipine to Felodipine in a Veterans Affairs Medical Center [unpublished manuscript]. Long Beach, CA, VA Long Beach Healthcare System; 1999.

Green ER, Chrymko MM, Rozek SL, et al. Clinical consideration and costs associated with formulary conversion from tobramycin to gentamicin. *Am. J. Hosp. Pharm*. 1989; 46:714–719.

Green M. *Pharmaceutical Payola: How Secret Commercial Deals Are Dictating Your Next Prescription and Harming Your Health*. New York: New York City Public Advocate; 1997.

Gross JD. Prescription drug formularies in managed care: Concerns for the elderly population. *Clin. Therapeutics*. 1998; 20(6):1277–1291.

Guastella C. Cost savings realized from interchanging ceftizoxime for cefoxitin. *Am. J. Hosp. Pharm*. 1988; 45:2376–2377.

REFERENCES

Gustin G, White WB, Taylor S. Clinical outcome of a mandatory formulary switch for dihydropyridine calcium channel blocker therapy at a Veterans Administration medical center. *Am. J. Hypertens*. 1996; 9(4 Pt 1):312–316.

Guze BH. Selective serotonin reuptake inhibitors: Assessment for formulary inclusion. *PharmacoEconomics*. 1996; 9(5):430–442.

Haig GM, Kiser LA. Effect of pharmacist participation on a medical team on costs, charges, and length of stay. *Am. J. Hosp. Pharm.* 1991; 48:1457–1462.

Hanson C, Shepherd M, Pleil A. How P&T committee members in HMOs make formulary decisions. *P&T.* 1992 : 247–254.

Hatcher RA, Stainsby WJ. The hospital formulary. *J. Am. Med. Assoc.* 1933; 101:1802–1807.

Hatoum HT, Freeman RA. The use of pharmacoeconomic data in formulary selection. *Topics Hosp. Pharm Manage*. 1994; 13(4):47–53.

Hazlet TK, Hu T-W. Association between formulary strategies and hospital drug expenditures. *Am. J. Hosp. Pharm.* 1992; 49:2207–2210.

Health Care Financing Administration (HCFA). Medicare and Medicaid statistical supplement. *Health Care Financing Rev.* 1966.

Health Care Financing Administration. Medicaid Program Statistics (HCFA-2082 Report) [on line]. Available at: http://www.hcfa.gov/medicaid/mstats.htm.

Health Care Financing Administration. Drug Policy. Medicaid Coverage of Viagra [on line]. Available at: http://www.hcfa.gov/medicaid/drpolicy.htm.

Health Care Financing Administration. Medicaid Managed Care Enrollment Report [on line]. Available at: http://www.hcfa.gov/medicaid/omc1998.htm.

Health Care Financing Administration. Medicaid Program Statistics (HCFA-2082 Report) [on line]. Available at: http://www.hcfa.gov/medicaid/mstats.htm.

Herstek J. *Managed Care Drug Formularies*. Washington, DC: National Conference of State Legislatures; 1999.

Hilleman DE, Mohiuddin SM, Wurdeman RL, Wadibia EC. Outcomes and cost savings of an ACE inhibitor therapeutic interchange. *J. Managed Care Pharm.* 1997; 3(2):219–223.

Hisnanick JJ, Gujral SS. Veterans' health insurance status and their use of VA medical facilities: A joint-choice analysis. *Soc. Sci. Q.* 1996; 77(2):393–407.

Hoechst Marion Roussel. *Managed Care Digest Series 1998, HMO-PPO/Medicare/ Medicaid Digest*. Hoechst Marion Roussel; 1998.

Hoffmann RP. Perspectives on the hospital formulary. *Hosp. Pharm.* 1984; 19(5):359–361 , 364.

Holdford D, Smith S. Improving the quality of outcomes research involving pharmaceutical services. *Am. J. Health-System Pharm.* 1997; 54(12):1434–1442.

Horn S, Sharkey P, Gassaway J. Managed care outcomes project: Study design, baseline patient characteristics, and outcome measures. *Am. J. Managed Care*. 1996; 2:237–247.

Hudson T. State Medicaid officials battle drug firms in war to cut costs. *Hospitals*. 1990; 64(7):30–34.

Iglehart JK. The American health care system: Expenditures. *N. Engl. J. Med.* 1999; 340(1):70–76.

IMS Health. Direct-to-Consumer Prescription Drug Advertising in U.S. Reaches $1.5 Billion for Twelve Months Through March; TV Ad Expenditures Reach $825 Mil lion, Up 24 Percent. [on line] Available at: http://www.imshealth.com/html/news_arc/06_07_1999_211.htm.

Institute of Medicine. *Clinical Practice Guidelines . Directions for a New Program* . Washington, DC: National Academy Press; 1990a.

Institute of Medicine. *Medicare: A Strategy for Quality Assurance* . Washington, DC: National Academy Press; 1990b.

Institute of Medicine. *To Err Is Human: Building a Safer Health System* . Washington, DC: National Academy Press; 1999.

Ito MK, Stolley SN, Morreale AP, et al. Rationale, design, and baseline results of the Pravastatin-to-Simvastatin Conversion Lipid Optimization Program (PSCOP). *Am. J. Health-Syst Pharm.* 1999; 56:1107–1113.

Jackson R. Practice guidelines, physician groups, and drug formularies. *J. Managed Care Pharm.* 1997; 3:489–492.

Jang R. Medicaid formularies: A critical review of the literature. *J. Pharmaceut. Market. Manage* . 1988; 2(3):39–61.

Jay GT, Quercia RA, Gousse G et al. Procedure for evaluating nonformulary drug orders. *Am. J. Hosp. Pharm.* 1993; 50:2554–2556.

Johnson RE, Goodman MJ, Hornbrook MC, et al. The impact of increasing patient prescription drug cost sharing on therapeutic classes of drugs received and on the health status of elderly HMO members. *Health Services Res.* 1997; 32(1):103–122.

Joint National Committee on the Prevention, Detection, and Treatment of High Blood Pressure. The Sixth Report of the Joint National Committee on Prevention, Detection, Evaluation, and Treatment of High Blood Pressure. *Arch. Int. Med.* 1997; 157:2413–2446.

Jones WN. *Statin Conversion Study, Memo to Coussens* , IOM . 1999.

Kazis LE, Miller DR, Clark J, et al. Health-related quality of life in patients served by the Department of Veterans Affairs. *Arch. Intern. Med.* 1998; 158:626–632.

Kellick KA, Burns K, McAndrew E, et al. Outcome monitoring of fluvastatin in a Department of Veterans Affairs lipid clinic. *Am. J. Cardiol.* 1995; 76:(2):62A–64A.

King N. Pharmacopoeias and Formularies. In: King N , ed. *A Selection of Primary Source for the History of Pharmacy in the United States: Books and Trade Catalogs from the Colonial Period to 1940* . Madison: American Institute of the History of Pharmacy, University of Wisconsin-Madison ; 1987; 8–25.

Kinnon A, Bourne J, Blizzard S, et al. Outcome analysis of a formulary transition from nifedipine to felodipine at a Veterans Affairs medical center. *J. Managed Care Pharm.* 1999; 5(5):425–428.

Kittel JF, Swatzell RH, Williams MP, Forrester CW, Bancroft WH. Development of a flexible formulary for a Veterans Administration hospital. *Hosp. Formul.* 1978; 13(1):46–48.

Kizer KW. Transforming the veterans health care system— The "new VA." *J. Am. Med. Assoc.* 1996; 275(14):1069.

Kizer KW. The "new VA": A national laboratory for health care quality management. *Am. J. Med. Qual.* 1999; 14(1):3–20.

Kotzan JA, McMillan JA, Jankel CA, Foster AL. Initial impact of a Medicaid prior authorization program for NSAID prescriptions. *J. Res. Pharmaceut. Econ.* 1993; 5(1):25–41.

Kozma C.M., Reeder CE, Lingle EW. Expanding Medicaid drug formulary coverage: Effects on Utilization of related services *Med. Care* . 1990; 28(10):963–977.

Kozma CM, Reeder CE, Schultz RM. Economic, clinical and humanistic outcomes: A planning model for pharmacoeconomic research. *Clin. Ther.* 1993; 15:1121–1132.

Kreling DH, Mucha RE. Drug product management in health maintenance organizations. *Am. J. Hosp. Pharm.* 1992; 49:374–381

Kreling DH, Collins T, Lipton HL, et al. *Assessment of the Impact of Pharmacy Benefit Managers* . Washington, DC: Health Care Financing Administration; 1996a.

Kreling DH, Knocke DJ, Hammel RW. Changes in market share for internal analgesic products after a Medicaid formulary restriction. *J. Pharmaceut. Market. Manage* . 1989a; 3(2):65–76.

Kreling DH, Knocke DJ, Hammel RW. The effects of an internal analgesic formulary restriction on Medicaid drug expenditures in Wisconsin. *Medical Care* . 1989b; 27(1):34–44.

Kreling DH, Lipton HL, Collings T, Hertz KC. *Assessment of the Impact of Pharmacy Benefit Managers* . Springfield, VA: U.S. Department of Commerce, National Technical Information Service; 1996b.

Kresel J, Hutchings C, MacKay D, et al. Application of decision analysis to drug selection for formulary addition. *Hospital Formul.* 1987; 22:658–676.

Laetz T, Silberman G. Reimbursement policies constrain the practice of oncology (erratum, *J. Am. Med. Assoc.* 1992; 267[24]:3287) . *J. Am. Med. Assoc.* 1991; 266(21):2996–3000 .

Langley PC. *Guidelines for Formulary Submissions for Pharmaceutical Product Evaluation* . Denver: Blue Cross Blue Shield of Colorado, Blue Cross Blue Shield of Nevada; 1998.

Langley PC, Sullivan SD. Pharmacoeconomic evaluations: Guidelines for drug purchasers. *J. Managed Care Pharm.* 1996; 2:(6):671–677.

Leape LL, Bates DW, Cullen DJ, et al. Systems analysis of adverse drug events. *J. Am. Med. Assoc.* 1995; 274(1):35–43.

Leape LL, Brennan T, Laird N, et al. The nature of adverse events in hospitalized patients. *N. Engl. J. Med.* 1991; 324:377–384.

Leape LL, Cullen DJ, Clapp MD, et al. Pharmacist participation on physician rounds and adverse drug events in the intensive care unit. *J. Am. Med. Assoc.* 1999; 282(3):267–270 .

Lederle FA, Rogers EM. Lowering the cost of lowering the cholesterol: A formulary policy for lovastatin. *J. Gen. Int. Med.* 1990; 5:459–463.

Lehmann DF, Frey HS, Smalley WE, Griffin MR, Ray WA. Effect of a prior-authorization requirement on the use of non-steroid antiinflammatory drugs. *N. Engl. J. Med.* 1995; 333 (19):1289–1290.

Leibowitz A, Manning WG, Newhouse JP. The demand for prescription drugs as a function of cost-sharing. *Soc. Sci. Med.* 1985; 21(10):1063–1069.

Levit K, Cowan C, Braden B, et al. National health expenditures in 1997: More slow growth. *Health Affairs* . 17,(6) :99–119.

Levy RA, Cocks D. Component Management Fails to Save Health Care System Costs: The Case of Restrictive Formularies (2nd Ed.). Reston, VA: National Pharmaceutical Council; 1999.

Liang FA, Greenberg RB, Hogan GF. Legal issues associated with formulary product-selection when there are two or more recognized drug therapies. *Am. J. Hosp. Pharm.* 1988; 45:2372–2375.

Liang FZ, Greenberg RB, Hogan GF. New Medicare conditions of participation for hospitals. *Am. J. Hosp. Pharm.* 1987; 44:1119–1122.

Lin JC, Ito MK, Stolley SN, Morreale AP, Marcus DB. The effect of converting from pravastatin to simvastatin on the pharmacodynamics of warfarin. *J. Clin. Pharmacol.* 1999; 39:86–90.

Lindgren-Furmaga E, Schuna A, Wolff N, Goodfriend T. Cost of switching hypertensive patients from enalapril maleate to lisinopril. *Am. J. Hosp. Pharm.* 1991; 48:276–279.

Lipsy RJ. Institutional formularies: The relevance of pharmacoeconomic analysis to formulary decisions. *PharmacoEconomics*. 1992; 1(4):265–281.

Lipton HL, Kreling DH, Collins T et al. Pharmacy benefit management companies: Dimensions of performance. *Annu. Rev. Public Health*. 1999; 20:361–401

Lowe JC, Trilli LE. Development of a multifacility core formulary. *ASHP Midyear Clin. . Meeting*. 1995; 30:P-485(D).

Luce BR, Lyles CA, Rentz AM. The view from managed care pharmac*y*. *Health Affairs*. 1996; 15 (4):168–176.

Lyles A, Luce B, Rentz A. Managed care pharmacy, socioeconomic assessments, and drug adoption decisions. *Soc. Sci. Med.* 1997; 45:511–521.

MacPherson P. The FDA just says yes. *Hosp. Health Network*. 1996; 70(10):34–36, 38.

Majercik PL, May JR, Longe RL, et al. Evaluation of pharmacy and therapeutics committee drug evaluation reports. *Am. J. Hosp. Pharm.* 1985; 42:1073–1076.

Mannebach MA, Ascione FJ, Gaither CA, et al. Activities, functions, and structure of pharmacy and therapeutics committees in large teaching hospitals. *Am. J. Health-Syst. Pharm.* 1999; 56 (7):622–628.

Martin BC, McMillan JA.. *Med. Care.* 1996; 34(7):686–701.

Massachusetts Out Patient Formulary Guide. 1999. Mather DB, Sullivan SD, Augenstein D, Fullerton PDS, Atherly D. Incorporating Clinical Outcomes and Economic Consequences into Drug Formulary Decisions: A Practical Approach. *The American Journal of Managed Care*. 1999; 5(3):277–285.

McAllister FA, Laupacis A, Wells GA, et al. Users' guides to the medical literature XIX. Applying clinical trial results. B. Guidelines for determining whether a drug is exerting (more than) a class effect. *J. Am. Med. Assoc.* 1999; 282(14):1371–1377.

McDonough KP, Weaver RH, Viall GD. Enalapril to lisinopril: Economic impact of a voluntary angiotensin-converting enzyme-inhibitor substitution program in a staff-model health maintenance organization. *Ann. Pharmacother*. 1992; 26:399–404.

McMillan K. Considerations in the formulary selection of hydroxymethlglutaryl-coenzyme A reductase inhibitors. *Am J. Health-SystPharm.* 1996; 53(18):2206–2214.

Mehl B, Santell JP. Projecting future drug expenditures—1998. *Am J Health-Syst Pharm.* 1998; 55:127–136.

Mehl B, Santell JP. Projecting future drug expenditures—1999. *Am J Health-Syst Pharm.* 1999; 56 (1):31–39.

Meier JL, Swislocki ALM, Lopez JF. Implementation of VA guidelines for Self-Monitoring of Blood Glucose (SMBG): Effect on Glucose Control and Pharmacy Costs. *Medicaid Managed Care Program*. 1998; Summary.

Meyer MC, Bates H Jr, Swift RG. The role of state formularies. *J. Am. Pharmaceut. Assoc.* 1974; NS14(12):663–666.

Minnilch BN, Swanson KM, Dutro MP. *Conversion from Amlodipine to Felodipine in VISN 18*. Monterrey, CA.: Western States Conference for Pharmacy Residents; 1997.

Mitchell J, Greenberg J, Finch K, et al. Effectiveness and economic impact and antidepressant medications: A review. *Am. J. Managed Care*. 1997; 3(2):323–330.

Moisan J, Vaillancourt R, Gregoire J-P, Gaudet M, Cote I, Leach A. Preferred hydroxymentyglutaryl-coenzyme A reductase inhibitors: treatment-modification program and outcomes. *Am. J. Health-Syst. Pharm.* 1999; 56:1437–1441.

Moore W, Newman R. Drug formulary restrictions as a cost-containment policy in medicaid programs. *J. Law Econ.* 1993; 36:71–97.

Nash DB, Catalano ML, Wordell CJ. The formulary decision-making process in a U.S. academic medical centre. *PharmacoEconomics*. 1993; 3(1):22–35.

Nash DB, Shulkin DJ, Owerbach J., et al. Physician attitudes toward managed care formularies: An initial survey. *J. Res. Pharmaceut. Economy*. 1992; 4(2):31–41.

National Academy for State Health Policy. *Medicaid Managed Care: A Guide for States*. Portland, ME: National Academy for State Health Policy; 1999.

National Committee to Review Current Procedures for Approval of New Drugs for Cancer and AIDS. *Final Report of the National Committee to Review Current Procedures for Approval of New Drugs for Cancer and AIDS*. Washington, DC: National Cancer Institute; 1990.

National Pharmaceutical Council. *Pharmaceutical Benefits Under State Medical Assistance Programs*. Washington, DC: National Pharmaceutical Council; 1973.

National Pharmaceutical Council. *Pharmaceutical Benefits Under State Medical Assistance Programs*. Washington, DC: National Pharmaceutical Council; 1989.

National Pharmaceutical Council. 1998.

Navarro RP, Cahill JA. The U.S. Health Care System and the Development of Managed Care. In : Navarro RP , ed. *Managed Care Pharmacy Practice*. Gaithersburg, MD: Aspen Publishers, Inc.; 1999.

New York Office of Mental Health . *Guidelines for Monitoring Committee Approval Process for Clozapine Treatment*. Albany, NY: Office of Mental Health; 1991.

Nightingale CH, Gousse GC, On A, et al. Antibiotic use and formulary considerations. *J. Pharmacy Pract.* 1991; 4(3):153–157.

Nightingale SL. Therapeutic Equivalence of Generic Drugs: Letter to Health Practitioners [on line]. Available at: http://www.fda.gov/cder/news/nightgenlett.htm. Food and Drug Administration; 1998.

Nightingale SL, Morrison JC. Generic drugs and the prescribing physician. *J. Am. Med. Assoc.* 1987; 258(9):1200–1204.

Novartis. *Pharmacy Benefit Report: Trends and Forecasts*. East Hanover, NJ: Novartis Pharmaceuticals Corp.; 1999.

Novartis. *Pharmacy Benefit Report*. East Hanover, NJ: Novartis Pharmaceuticals Corp.; 1998.

Omnibus Budget Reconciliation Acts 1990, 1993.

Ogden JE, Muniz A, Patterson AA, Ramirez DJ, Kizer KW. Phamaceutical services in the Department of Veterans Affairs. *Am J Health–Sys Pharm.* 1997; 54(7):761–765.

Oh T, Franko TG. Implementing therapeutic interchange of intravenous famotidine for cimetidine and rantidine. *Am. J. Hosp. Pharm.* 1990; 47:1547–1551.

Owens MK. Medicaid Pharmacy Benefit Management. In : Navarro RP , ed. *Managed Care Pharmacy Practice*. Gaithersburg, MD: Aspen Publishers, Inc.; 1999.

Packer LA, Mahoney CD, Rich DS, et al. Effect of pharmacists' clinical interventions on nonformulary drug use. *Am. J. Hosp. Pharm.* 1986; 43:1461–1466.

Patterson AA, Pierce RAI, Powell AP. Prime vendor purchasing of pharmaceuticals in the Veterans Affairs health care system. *Am. J. Health-Syst. Pharm.* 1995; 52(17):1886–1889.

Pear R. *Drug Industry Gathers a Mix of Voices to Bolster Its Case* . New York: New York Times; 1993.

Pennstate Geisinger Health Plan, Formulary 1999.

Petitta A, Ward RE, Anandan JV, et al. The cost-effectiveness impact of a preferred agent HMG-CoA reductase inhibitor policy in managed care population *J. Managed Care. Pharm.* 1997; 3(5):548–553.

Pharmaceutical Manufacturers Association. *Waxman Airs Plan to End OBRA 90's Medicaid Formularies Ban* . Washington, DC: Pharmaceutical Manufacturers Association; 1993.

Pharmaceutical Manufacturers Association (PMA). *Towns Urge Black Caucus Oppose Planned Medicaid Restrictive Formulary* . Washington, DC: Pharmaceutical Manufacturers Association; 1993.

Pharmacy Benefits Management in a Valuable Product Line. 1995.

Phillips CR, Larson LN. Evaluating the operational performance and financial effects of a drug prior authorization program. *J. Managed Care Pharm.* 1997; 3(6):699–706.

Pollard M, Coster J. Savings for Medicaid drug spending. *Health Affairs* . 1991; Summer:196–206.

Portner TS, Srnka QM, Gourley DR, et al. Comparison of Department of Veteran Affairs pharmacy services in 1992 and 1994 with strategic-planning goals. *Am J. Health-Syst. Pharm.* 1996; 53(9):1032–1040.

Premier. Summary of Premier's Products and Services . 1998.

Quigley MA, Brown WM. A survey of selective administration procedures in formulary maintenance. *Hosp. Pharm.* 1981; 16:371–380.

Raiford D, Shulman S, Lasagna L. Determining appropriate reimbursement for prescritionn drugs: off-label uses and investigational therapies. *Food Drug Law J.* 1994; 49(1):37–76.

Rascati KL. Survey of formulary system policies and procedures. *Am. J. Hosp. Pharm.* 1992; 49:100–103.

Reeder CE. Overview of pharmacoeconomics and pharmaceutical outcomes evaluations. *Am. J. Health-Syst Pharm.* 1995; 52(Suppl. 4):S5–S8.

Reeder CE, Dickson M, Kozma CM, et al. ASHP national survey of pharmacy practice in acute care setting—1996. *Am. J. Health-Syst. Pharm.* 1997; 54:653–669.

Rich DS. Experience with a two-tiered therapeutic interchange policy. *Am. J. Hosp. Pharm.* 1989; 46:1792–1798.

Richton-Hewett S, Foster E, Apstein CS. Medical and economic consequences of a blinded oral anticoagulant brand change at a municipal hospital. *Arch. Intern. Med.* 1988; 148:806–808.

Rindone JP, Arriola G. Conversion from fluvastatin to simvastatin therapy at a dose ratio of 8 to 1: Effect on serum lipid levels and cost. *Clinical Therapeutics*. 1998; 20(2):340–346.

Roberts MJ, Summerfield MR. Formulary management to reduce costs: P&T committee strategies. *Hosp Formul.* 1986; 21:481–490.

Rucker TD. Formularies: conceptual and experimental factors related to product selection. *Drug Inform. J.* 1982a; 16(3):115–121.

Rucker TD. Formularies: principles, problems, and prognosis. *Hosp. Pharm.* 1982b; 17(9):460–461.

Rucker TD. A public policy strategy for drug formularies: preparation or procrastination necessity for implementing an effective national formulary. 1999.

Rucker TD. Quality control of hospital formularies. *Pharmaceutisch Weekblad Scient. Ed.* 1988; 10:145–150.

Rucker TD. Restricted formulary drugs: An exploratory study. *Hosp. Pharm.* 1982c; 17:246–253.

Rucker TD. Superior hospital formularies: A critical analysis. *Hosp. Pharm.* 1982d; 17(9):465–471, 474–475, 477–479.

Rucker TD, Schiff G. Drug formularies: Myths-in-formation. *Med. Care*. 1990; 28(10):928–939.

Rucker TD, Visconti JA. Hospital formularies: Organizational aspects and supplementary components. *Am. J. Hosp. Pharm.* 1976; 33:912–917.

Rucker TD, Visconti JA. How Effective Are Drug Formularies? A Descriptive and Normative Study. *USDA*. 1978.

Sax M, Emigh R. Managed care formularies in the United States. *J. Managed Care Pharm.* 1999; 5 (4):289–295.

Schulman KA, Rubenstein LE, Abernathy DR, Seils DM, Sulmasy DP. The effect of pharmaceutical benefits managers: Is it being evaluated? *Ann. Int. Med.* 1996 ; 124 (10):906–913.

Schwartz RK, Soumerai SB, Avorn J. Physician motivations for nonscientific drug prescribing. *Soc. Sci. Med.* 1989; 28(6):577–582.

Schweitzer, SO, Shiota S. Access and cost implications of state limitations on Medicaid reimbursement for pharmaceuticals. *Annu. Rev. Public Health*. 1992; 13:399–410.

Segal R, Pathak DS. Formulary decision making: identifying factors that influence P&T committee drug evaluations. *Hosp. Formul.* 1988 ; 23:174–178.

Shea BF, Churchill WW, Powell SH, Cooley TW, Maguire JH. P&T committee over-view: Bringham and Women's Hospital. *Pharm. Pract. Manage. Q.* 1998; 17(4):76–83.

Shepherd MD, Salzman RD. The formulary decision-making process in a health maintenance organization setting. *PharmacoEconomics*. 1994; 5(1):29–38.

Shulman SR, Brown JS. The Food and Drug Administration's early access and fast-track approval initiatives: How have they worked? *Food Drug Law J.* 1995; 50(4):503–531.

Siegal D, Lopez J. Trends in antihypertensive drug use in the United States. *J. Am. Med. Assoc.* 1997; 278(21):1745–1748.

Siegel D, Meier JL, Lopez JR. Academic Detailing to Promote Hyperension (HTN) clinical Practice Guidelines. *Am. J. Hypertension.* 1999; 12(4):2 (37A).

Sloan FA. Drug Formularies, Prior Authorization, and Medicaid Cost Containment: Is There a Relationship. Unpublished manuscript ; 1989.

Sloan FA, Whetten-Goldstein K, Wilson A. Hospital pharmacy decisions, cost containment, and the use of cost-effectiveness analysis. *Soc. Sci. Med.* 1997; 45(4):523–533.

Smalley WE, Griffin M, Fought RL, et al. Effect of a prior authorization requirement on the use of nonsteroidal antiinflammatory drugs by medicaid patients. *N. Engl. J. Med.* 1995; 332 (24):1612–1617.

Smith DM, McKercher PL. The elimination of selected drug products from the Michigan Medicaid formulary: a case study. *Hosp. Formul* 1984; 19(5):366–372.

Smith DG. The effects of copayments and generic subsitution on the use and costs of prescription drugs. *Inquiry* . 1993; 30:189–198.

Smith KS, Briceland LL, Nightengale CH, Quintiliani R. Formulary conversion of cefoxitin usage to cefotetan: experience at a large yeaching hospital. *DICP Ann. Pharmacother.* 1989; 23:1024–1030.

Sonnedecker G. Earliest formulary for a civilian hospital, U.S.A. *Drug Intell. Clin. Pharm.* 1972; 6:425–434.

Sonnedecker G. *Kremers and Urdang's History of Pharmacy.* Philadelphia: J.B. Lippincott Co.; 1976.

Soumerai SB, Avorn J, Ross-Degnan D, Gortmaker S. Payment restrictions for presecription drugs under Medicaid: Effects on therapy, cost, and equity. *N. Engl. J. Med.* 1987; 317(9):550–556.

Soumerai SB, Lipton HJL. Computer based drug utilization review–Risk, boondoggle? *N. Engl. J. Med.* 1995; 332(24):1641–1645.

Soumerai SB, McLaughlin TJ, Ross-Degnan D, Casteris CS, Bollini P. Effects of limiting Medicaid drug-reimbursement benefits on the use of psychotropic agents and acute mental health services by patients with schizophrenia. *N. Engl. J. Med.* 1994; 331(10):650–655.

Soumerai SB, Ross-Degnan D. Experience of state drug benefit programs. *Health Affairs.* 1990; 9 (3):36–54.

Soumerai SB, Ross-Degnan D, Avorn J et al. Effects of Medicaid drug-payment limits on admission to hospitals and nursing homes. *N. Eng. J. Med.* 1991; 325(15):1072–1077.

Soumerai SB, Ross-Degnan D, Fortess EE et al. Examining product risk in context: market withdrawal of Zomepirac as a case study. *J. Amer. Med. Assoc.* 1993; 270(16):1937–1942.

Soumerai SB, Ross-Degnan D, Fortess EE, Abelson J. A critical analysis of studies of state drug reimbursement policies: research in need of discipline. *Milbank Q.* 1993a; 71(2): 217–252.

Spencer NA, Crouse MT. Drug Policy and Regulation in Managed Care. In : Navarro RP , ed. *Managed Care Pharmacy Practice* . Gaithersburg, MD: Aspen Publishers, Inc.; 1999.

Sprague MS, Gray DR. Impact of a formulary switch from amlodipine to felodipine. *ASHP Midyear Clin. Meet* . 1998; P-424E.

Stanaszek MB, Foss, ND. Lansoprazole-associated diarrhea: Case report and experience at a Veterans Affairs medical center.

Stock AJ, Kofoed L. Therapeutic interchange of fluoxetine and sertraline: Experience in the clinical setting. *Am. J. Hosp. Pharm.* 1994; 51:2279–2281.

Streja DA, Hui RL, Streja E, McCombs JS. Selective contracting and patient outcomes: A case study of formulary restrictions for selective serotonin reuptake inhibitor anti-depressants. *Am. J. Managed Care*. 1999; 5(9):1133–1142.

Strom BL. Generic drug substitution revisited. *N. Engl. J. Med.* 1987; 316(23):1456–1462.

Summers KH, Szeinbach SL. Formualries: The role of pharmacy-and-therapeutics (P&T) committees. *Clin. Ther.* 1993; 15(2):433–441.

Taniguchi R. Pharmacy benefit management companies. *Am. J. Health-System Pharm.* 1995; 52:1915–1917.

The Office of the Medical Inspector, Veterans Health Administration. *Special Report: VA Patient Safety Event Registry: First Nineteen Months of Reported Cases Summary and Analysis*. Washington, DC: Department of Veterans Affairs, 1999.

The Pink Sheet. Florida Medicaid prior authorization for four drug categories. *Pink Sheet*. 1993.

Tufts Health Plan. Prescription Alternative Program: Non-Covered Drugs [on line]. Available at: http://www.tuftshealthplan.com/members/pharmacy-index.html.

United Health Care. Preferred Drug List [on line]. Available at: http://www.unitedhealthcare.com/pharmacy/pdl00/pdl00.html

Vivian E, Morreale A, Boyce E, Lowry K, Ereso O, Hlavin P. Efficacy and cost effectiveness of lansoprazole versus omeprazole in maintenance treatment of symptomatic gastroesophageal reflux disease. *Am. J. Managed Care*. 1999; 5(7):881–886.

Wall DS, Abel SR. Therapeutic interchange algorithm for multiple drug classes. *Am. J. Health-Syst. Pharm.* 1996; 53(11):1295–1296.

Walser B, Ross-Degnan D, Soumerai SB. Do open formularies increase access to clinically useful drugs? *Health Affairs*. 1996; 15(3):95–107.

Weintraub M. *The United States: Hospital Formularies in Controlling the Use of Therapeutic Drugs: An International Comparison*. Washington, DC: American Enterprise Institute for Public Policy Research; 1978.

Weintraub M, Singh S, Byrne L, et al. Consequences of the 1989 New York State triplicate benzodiazepine prescription regulations. *J. Am. Med. Assoc.* 1991; 266(17):2392–2397.

Wilson J, Burke S. Member Satisfaction Strategies. In : Navarro RP , ed. *Managed Care Pharmacy Practice*. Gaithersburg, MD: Aspen Publishers, Inc.; 1999.

Wilson NJ, Kizer KW. The VA health care system: An unrecognized national safety net. *Health Affairs*. 1997; 16(4):200–204.

Wyeth Ayerst Laboratories. *The Wyeth Ayerst Prescription Drug Benefit Cost and Plan Design Survey Report*. Albuquerque, NM: Wellman Publishing, Inc. 1998.

Yankelovich Partners. *VA Physicians Study*. Washington, DC, unpublished report ; 1999.

Zellmer WA. Medication error versus medication misadventure—What's in a name? *Am. J. Hosp. Pharm.* 1993; 50:315–318.

Zhanel GG, Gin AS, Przybylo A, Louie TJ, Otten NH. Effect of interventions on prescribing of antimicrobials for prophylaxis in obstetric and gynecologic surgery. *Am. J. Hosp. Pharm.* 1989; 46:2493–2496.

Zimmerman DL, Daley J. *Using Outcomes to Improve Health Care Decision Making*. Boston: Department of Veterans Affairs, Office of Research and Development; 1997.
Zoeller J. Does therapeutic interchange hurt patients? *Am. Druggist.* 1991; 66–79.

Acronyms

AAHP	American Association of Health Plans
ACCP	American College of Clinical Pharmacy
ACEI	angiotensin-converting enzyme inhibitor
ACP	American College of Physicians
ADE	adverse drug event
ADR	adverse drug reaction
AFDC	Aid to Families with Dependent Children
AMA	American Medical Association
AHA	American Hospital Association
AMCP	Academy of Managed Care Pharmacy
AMP	average manufacturer price
APhA	American Pharmaceutical Association
ASHP	American Society of Health-System Pharmacists
AWP	average wholesale price
BCF	Basic Core Formulary
BPA	blanket purchase agreement
CCB	calcium channel blocker
CHAMPUS	Civilian Health and Medical Programs of the Uniformed Services
CMOP	consolidated mail outpatient pharmacy
COPD	chronic obstructive pulmonary disease
COX-2	cyclooxygenase-2

ACRONYMS

DAV	Disabled American Veterans
DESI	drug efficacy study implementation
DOD	Department of Defense
DUR	drug utilization review
FDA	Food and Drug Administration
FSS	Federal Supply Schedule
GAO	General Accounting Office
H_2R	histamine$_2$ receptor
5-HT$_3$	5-hydroxytryptamine
HCFA	Health Care Financing Administration
HCTZ	hydrochlorothiazide
HMG-CoA RI	hydroxymethylglutaryl-coenzyme A reductase inhibitor
HMO	health maintenance organization
ICD-9	*International Classification of Diseases,* Ninth Edition
IOM	Institute of Medicine
IPA	Independent practice association
IV	intravenous
JCAH, JCAHO	Joint Commission on Accreditation of Hospitals, now Joint Commission on Accreditation of Healthcare Organizations
MAP	Medical Advisory Panel
MCO	managed care organization
MTF	military treatment facility
NAC	National Acquisition Center
NCQA	National Committee for Quality Assurance
NDAA	National Defense Authorization Act
NPC	National Pharmaceutical Council
NRC	National Research Council
NSAID	nonsteroidal anti-inflammatory drug
OBRA	Omnibus Budget Reconciliation Act
OTC	over the counter
1P	FDA priority (drug)
P&T	pharmacy and therapeutics
PBM	pharmacy benefits management organization
PVA	Paralyzed Veterans of America
RFP	request for proposal

SSA	Social Security Administration
SSI	Supplemental Security Income
SSRI	selective serotonin reuptake inhibitor
TANF	Temporary Assistance for Needy Families
UM	utilization management
USP	U.S. Pharmacopoeia
VA	Department of Veterans Affairs
VFW	Veterans of Foreign Wars
VHA	Veterans Health Administration
VISN	Veterans Integrated Service Network
VSO	veterans service organization

ACRONYMS

APPENDIX A

Interim Report of the Committee on VA Pharmacy Formulary Analysis to the Department of Veterans Affairs and the Congress of the United States

JANUARY 28, 2000

This is the interim report specified in VA contract No V101(93)P-1637, Task 10, on the VA pharmacy formulary analysis between the Department of Veterans Affairs (the VA) and the Institute of Medicine (IOM) of the National Academy of Sciences (NAS), effective April 12, 1999. That contract scheduled this report 6 months after the beginning of the project. The report was to be in a form determined by the IOM committee on the VA pharmacy formulary analysis. The IOM committee, meeting in Washington, D.C., on September 30–October 1, 1999, and December 13–14, 1999, decided that the interim report should consist of this short document describing the implementation of the study, progress to date, and the anticipated schedule to completion, supplemented by a briefing by the IOM committee chairman, Dr. David Blumenthal, to the VA and to interested parties and committees of jurisdiction in the Congress. These latter include the House Committee on Appropriations (Congressman Freylinghuysen) and the Senate and House Committees on Veterans Affairs. The IOM committee discussed and approved this interim report, subject to revisions, at its December meeting.

The VA contract for this study requires the IOM to analyze and report on four major congressional concerns. House Report 105-610, which accompanied legislation providing an appropriation for the VA for fiscal year 1999, directed the VA to enter into the contract with the IOM and expressed the four concerns of the Committee on Appropriations. These were also concerns of the Senate and House Committees on Veterans Affairs, and they formed the basis of an audit of the VA National Formulary requested in October 1998 of the General Accounting Office (GAO) by Senator Rockefeller, ranking minority member of the Senate Committee on Veterans Affairs. These concerns or questions included whether the VA National Formulary is overly restrictive, what effect it has on the cost of drugs and related products to the Veterans Health Administration (VHA), what effect it has on quality of care delivered by the VHA to veterans, and how it compares with other formularies in the public and private sector. The IOM study will address and analyze these four issues.

At the outset, the IOM reviewed a number of candidates for director of this project, and decided against recruiting new staff from outside the Institute. Instead, Roger Herdman, M.D., Senior Scholar at IOM, was asked to assume the position of responsible study officer. Dr. Herdman was completing a study, the Safety of Silicone Breast Implants, for the House Committee on Appropriations and the Department of Health and Human Services, which was delivered June 14, 1999. This caused some delay in the initial phases of this work. Early contacts were made and discussions held with staff of Congressman Freylinghuysen of the House Appropriations Committee and both majority and minority sides of the Senate and House Committee on Veterans Affairs, however. Follow-up contacts have provided congressional staff with additional information on the project and the study committee. Representatives from the Pharmacy Benefits Management Group of the VA, Mr. Ogden and Mr. Muniz, visited the IOM, briefed IOM staff, and provided helpful information on the National Formulary. Staff began to gather literature on the VA pharmacy benefit and formulary system and formulary systems in general. A list of literature accumulated and reviewed to date is appended to this report.

In late spring and early summer of 1999, IOM staff solicited recommendations of candidates for the IOM committee on the VA pharmacy formulary analysis. Recommendations were received from the Pharmaceutical Research and Manufacturers of America, the National Pharmaceutical Council, the American Association of Health Plans, the Academy of Managed Care Pharmacy, members of the academic pharmacy community, a Washington, D.C. consultant on veterans affairs, IOM members, the President of the IOM, and, after his selection and preliminary approval, the committee chairman, Dr. Blumenthal, among others. Responding in part to these recommendations and to independent evaluations, 14 committee appointments were approved in the summer of 1999 by the President of the IOM and the President of the NAS. They represented experience and expertise in veterans affairs, veterans health care and veterans service organizations, clinical medicine and geriatrics, clinical epidemiology, pharmacy and therapeutics committees, managed care and managed care pharmacy, pharmacy benefits management, Medicaid drug benefits, drug utilization review, pharmaceutical standards, clinical pharmacology, the science and practice of pharmacy, nursing, health services research and health care policy, health care management and health economics, pharmacy law, and public health, among others.

Committee members came from two veterans service organizations, U.S. medical schools and academic health centers, managed care organizations, schools of pharmacy and nursing, pharmacy benefit management companies, the United States Pharmacopoeia, academic departments of health care policy, law and economics, and major health care systems and clinics. They were from all sections of the United States, for example, the District of Columbia and the states of Arizona, California, Maryland, Massachusetts, Minnesota, New Jersey, New York, North Carolina, Pennsylvania, and Utah. The Presidents of the IOM and NAS appointed an experienced internist actively seeing patients as chairman of the committee. This appointment and the presence of five physicians on the committee were intended to ensure that this study would focus on quality health care to veterans. The committee roster is attached to this report.

During the summer of 1999, IOM staff met with staff of the General Accounting Office (GAO) responsible for the audit of the VA National Formulary to coordinate the IOM and GAO projects and avoid duplication of effort. Coordination meetings with GAO have continued periodically during the course of the IOM study. By August, the IOM recruited and retained the staff for this project, Christine Coussens, Ph.D., Research Associate, and Rita Gaskins, Project Assistant. Also during the summer of 1999, the IOM identified consultants for the VA pharmacy formulary analysis project as specified in the VA contract. After discussion with advisors and potential consultant organizations, the IOM determined that the Harvard Department of Health Care Policy met the requirements for performing the cost analysis of the National Formulary in terms of professional qualifications and experience and could carry out the necessary analyses within the amount budgeted for this subcontract. Staff assigned to this project at Harvard included Richard Frank, Ph.D., Haiden Huskamp, Ph.D., health economists, Arnold Epstein, M.D., medical consultant, and other supporting professionals. These named individuals were made official consultants to the IOM to allow full participation in this work and in meetings of the committee as economic and medical advisors as well as staff responsible for the cost assessment portion of the VA contract. The report of this group, which will comprise the chapter on costs in the final IOM report, was scheduled for completion and delivery to IOM on April 1, 2000. To prepare the separate VA contractual commissioned paper on Medicaid formularies, the IOM selected Jeffrey Brown, a Ph.D. student at Brandeis who was also made an official IOM consultant. He was identified by, and worked under the supervision of, Stephen Soumerai, Sc.D., Professor of Ambulatory Care and Prevention and Director, Drug Policy Research Group, Harvard Medical School. This paper was scheduled for delivery to IOM on February 1, 2000, and has been delivered.

On August 18, 19, and 20, 1999, IOM staff, Dr. Haiden Huskamp from the Harvard group performing the cost analysis of the VA formulary, and a member of the IOM committee visited the VA Pharmacy Benefits Management Strategic Healthcare Group and the National Acquisition Center in Chicago to collect information on the management of the National Formulary and formulary system and on price negotiations, contracting and availability of price and other cost data. During this visit, staff and a committee member attended the August 19 and 20 meeting of the VA Medical Advisory Panel to observe the functioning of this VA analogue of a conventional pharmacy and therapeutics committee. During this meeting, presentations and discussions on adding drugs to the formulary, drug class reviews, policies on pill splitting, pharmacogenomics, therapeutic guidelines for COX-2 inhibitors, a second RAND survey of VA physician attitudes and experience with the National Formulary, and dosing schedules, among others, were held. Staff also visited the Lakeside VA hospital in Chicago and discussed formulary matters with medical and pharmacy representatives of that hospital's staff.

In September 1999, IOM staff prepared for the first meeting of the IOM committee on VA pharmacy formulary analysis. This meeting took place in the Foundry Building in Georgetown, on September 30 and October 1, 1999, with 100% of the committee in attendance for all or part of the sessions. After a "bias discussion" among committee members to identify and discuss potential biases and conflicts of interest, the meeting was open to the public from 2:30 PM to 5:30 PM on September 30th. During that time the committee heard from Ms. Kim Lipsky, staff to Senator Rockefeller of the Senate Committee on Veterans Affairs. Staff from all the known interested congressional committees had been invited to speak, but except for Ms. Lipsky, were unable to attend due to the press of congressional business. Ms. Lipsky's remarks were followed by a presentation from the VA Pharmacy Benefits Group central and Chicago offices and representatives of the VA Medical Advisory Panel. They provided the committee with information on the formulary and an opportunity to ask questions of responsible VA pharmacy benefit leaders. Thereafter, GAO staff addressed the committee, describing their study of National Formulary operations and responded to committee questions. The committee met in closed session on October 1, 1999, and discussed information on VA formulary policies and procedures, the various tasks or components of the IOM study, the plans of the Harvard Department of Health Care Policy to implement the formulary cost analysis, an outline of the Medicaid commissioned paper, and plans for the committee's continued work. The next meeting of the committee was scheduled for December 13 and 14, 1999.

In the interval before the next committee meeting, staff continued to gather data from the literature and from the VA. Repeated contacts for information on policies, procedures, results, and outcomes were made to the VA central office, the Chicago office, each of the 22 regional offices (veterans integrated service networks or VISNs), and many medical centers. In these interactions IOM found VA personnel responsive to requests for data and examples of forms and policies, although IOM staff, the Harvard group, and the committee noted that some VA data that would have informed in a useful way analyses responding to the four major tasks and congressional concerns of the study were not generated by the VA system and therefore not available. VA cost data that were essential to the cost analysis of the National Formulary were not always available in a timely way or contained errors and gaps.

Before the December meeting of the committee, draft material relating to several of the study tasks and supporting sections of the report were prepared, including various tables and graphs displaying data obtained from the VA. The second meeting of the committee was held in closed sessions on December 13 and 14 in the Foundry Building. All committee members attended the sessions at least in part. At this meeting the prepared drafts were reviewed and suggestions, made. The Harvard group reported on progress to date and entertained suggestions and comments. A draft of the commissioned paper on Medicaid formularies was available and was reviewed and subject to critique by the committee. Again, the various major components of the study were extensively discussed in light of accumulating data on VA policies and procedures and available draft documents. The committee reviewed data collected from the VA pharmacy benefits managers and VISNs. Data and a survey provided by Pfizer, Inc., were also reviewed and discussed. The committee considered possible conclusions and recommendations for the final report. The draft of this interim report was approved subject to suggested revisions. The third meeting of the committee was scheduled for March 8 and 9, 2000.

In January 2000, the IOM and the Harvard group notified the VA that price data that had been requested for relevant years and drugs were not on hand for some of those years and drugs. The Harvard group cautioned that if these data were not available to them by early February 2000, the descriptions and analyses of cost effects of the National Formulary that had been agreed upon with the committee could not be completed in time to meet the congressionally imposed report delivery schedule. After a telephone conference mutually clarifying the needs of the IOM and Harvard and the capacity of the VA, the requisite data began to be rapidly delivered. By the day of this report, the remaining data that the VA system can generate and that the IOM and Harvard need were committed to delivery by no later than the end of January. This would allow performance of the cost subcontract in time for the final IOM report.

By the time of this interim report, the committee had reviewed and amended the introduction and chapters on restrictiveness, quality, and comparisons with other formularies (which incorporated the consultant report on Medicaid). Extensive data on elements of restrictiveness current in PBMs and MCOs covering about 200 million lives were being collected nationally. Additional graphs and tables were constructed. At the third meeting of the committee, given timely delivery of the VA data as committed, the committee will discuss the preliminary findings from the Harvard Department of Health Care Policy, and comments and suggestions can then be incorporated into the Harvard preparation and delivery of the cost chapter of the final report by April 1st. At this third meeting, the committee plans to review a final draft of the report (except for the pending cost chapter), and make comments, corrections, and suggestions which will be incorporated into a draft report suitable for review by the National Academy of Sciences' report review process. Reviewers for this final report should be selected by April 1, 2000, and it is anticipated that review comments will be returned by mid-May. It is hoped that reviewer comments can be incorporated and the report approved by the IOM and the NAS sometime in June 2000, preparatory to delivering a prepublication copy of the final report to the sponsor and the Congress, with release to the public to follow. The contractual deadline for completion of the final, full report specified in the VA contract is the 15th month of the project. Subsequent to the contract terms, the Congress in House Report 106-379 specified July 11, 2000, as the delivery date for the final report. The IOM and the committee on VA pharmacy formulary analysis have planned, scheduled, and intend to meet this delivery deadline.

APPENDIX B

Academy of Managed Care Pharmacy's Managed Care Formulary and Pharmacy Benefit Design Survey

AMCP MANAGED CARE FORMULARY AND PHARMACY BENEFIT DESIGN SURVEY (JANUARY 2000)

Plan/Company name: ___ (for in-house use only)
Please list the total number of covered/managed lives serviced. ___

The P&T Committee

What is the composition (number of members) of your P&T committee:

A. Pharmacists ___
B. Physicians ___
C. Other Healthcare Professionals ___

Exclusion of Coverage

Regardless of the existence of a formulary or a system of nonformulary prior authorizations for exceptions, how many covered lives are enrolled in plans that exclude the following drug classes for reimbursement as a benefit design restriction:

DESI drugs? ___

Experimental drugs ___

Off-label use? ___

OTC? ___

Cosmetic drugs or life-style drugs? ___

Survey sent by the Academy of Managed Care Pharmacists to eight members covering 200 million lives in the United States.

Other? (please specify the drug class) ___

How many covered lives are in plans with:

A. 1–2 excluded classes? ___
B. 3–5 excluded classes? ___
C. >5 excluded classes? ___

Closed Formularies

How many covered lives are in plans that have a pharmacy benefit with a closed or partially closed formulary; that is, a formulary that limits and requires justification for use of drugs not listed on the formulary independent of those drugs excluded through benefit design? ___

How many covered lives are in plans with: (See top of page 2 for definition)

1–2 closed classes? ___
3–5 closed classes? ___
>5 closed classes? ___

(That is, classes in which some drugs are not listed on the formulary, are not covered or reimbursed, and can be obtained only through a nonformulary exceptions process.)

How many covered lives are in plans with closed classes that contain only one drug? ___

What are the closed classes in your plans? ___ ___ ___

Which processes are in place in closed formulary environments to allow for access to nonformulary drugs? (check all that apply)

None, all nonformulary drugs are not covered. ___

Nonformulary drugs may be covered through an informal exceptions process. ___

Nonformulary drugs may be covered through a formal prior authorization process. ___

Other, describe. ___

Open–Preferred Formularies

How many covered lives are in plans that have nonclosed formularies but have preferred classes, that is, classes in which there are drugs whose use is encouraged by incentives (lower copay, academic detailing, DUR, soft edits), or usage criteria, or in which prescribing of nonpreferred drugs is discouraged. ___

How many covered lives are in plans with:
1–2 preferred classes? ___
3–5 preferred classes? ___
>5 preferred classes? ___
What are the preferred classes in your plans? ___

Open–Passive Formularies

How many covered lives are in plans where an open formulary is used but the items listed are only passively promoted (use of educational materials, few soft edits)? ___

Other Types of Formularies

How many covered lives are in plans:

that have no formulary, but selected drugs are labeled as "Require Prior Authorization?" ___

that have no formulary or prior authorization process, but pharmacists perform DUR and physicians are notified when inappropriate use is identified? ___

that have no formulary, no controls, or no checks on physician practice patterns. All drugs go through as covered and access is open? ___

Drug Restrictions

How many covered lives are in plans that restrict coverage or reimbursement of specific drugs or classes of drugs to specific prescribers, settings, or disease conditions? ___

Generic Drugs

How many covered lives are in plans that require generic substitution? ___

Access to Nonformulary Drugs

How many covered lives fall under formulary systems which:
Have a nonformulary exceptions process for coverage? ___
Use copay design controls to influence use of nonformulary drugs? ___

Cost-Containment Measures

How many covered lives fall under plans whose system edits include:
Limits on numbers of prescriptions per patient at any time or per unit time?

Limits on refills of prescriptions (number of drugs with such limits)? ___
Limits on duration of use of some drugs (number of drugs with such limits)? ___
Limits on the supply of drugs per prescription or on hand? ___
Presence of a prior approval process for some drugs (number of drugs requiring prior approval)? ___

Addition of New FDA-Approved Drugs

How many covered lives are in plans that limit formulary addition of new FDA-approved drugs by requiring waiting periods? ___

How many covered lives are in plans that require waiting periods of more than 6 months? ___

Do any enrollees participate in plans that have policies in place to actively review or monitor activities at the FDA such that reviews of new drugs are done concurrently (proactively) with FDA approval?
Yes ___ No ___

If yes, the number of covered lives in plans that proactively review/monitor for new AIDS/cancer medications. ___

If yes, the number of covered lives in plans that proactively review/monitor for new FDA "1P" drugs. ___

If yes, the number of covered lives in plans that proactively review/monitor for new FDA "standard" designation drugs. ___

Appeals Process

How many covered lives are in plans that:
have an internal appeals process for denials of drug coverage or reimbursement for excluded drugs? ___
have an internal appeals process for denials of nonformulary drug requests? ___
have an appeals process subject to independent external review? ___

Continuation of Care

1. How many covered lives are in plans that provide continuation of coverage after removal of a drug from the formulary? (Choose which one applies)
   Policy applies to a few specific drugs. ___
   How many covered lives? ___
   Policy applies to all drugs. ___
   How many covered lives? ___
2. Are there financial penalties incurred by patients? (Please describe)
   ___
   ___

APPENDIX C
Additional Cost Information

This appendix contains additional graphs that are relevant to the analysis of the potential cost effects associated with the National Formulary (see chapter 3 for discussion).

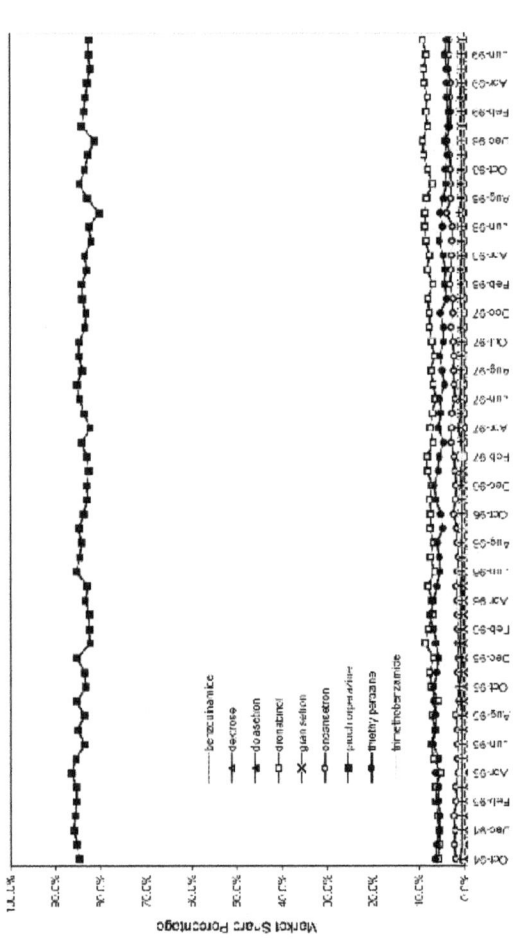

FIGURE C.1 National formulary policy has no effect on market share distribution of antiemetics (open class).

APPENDIX C

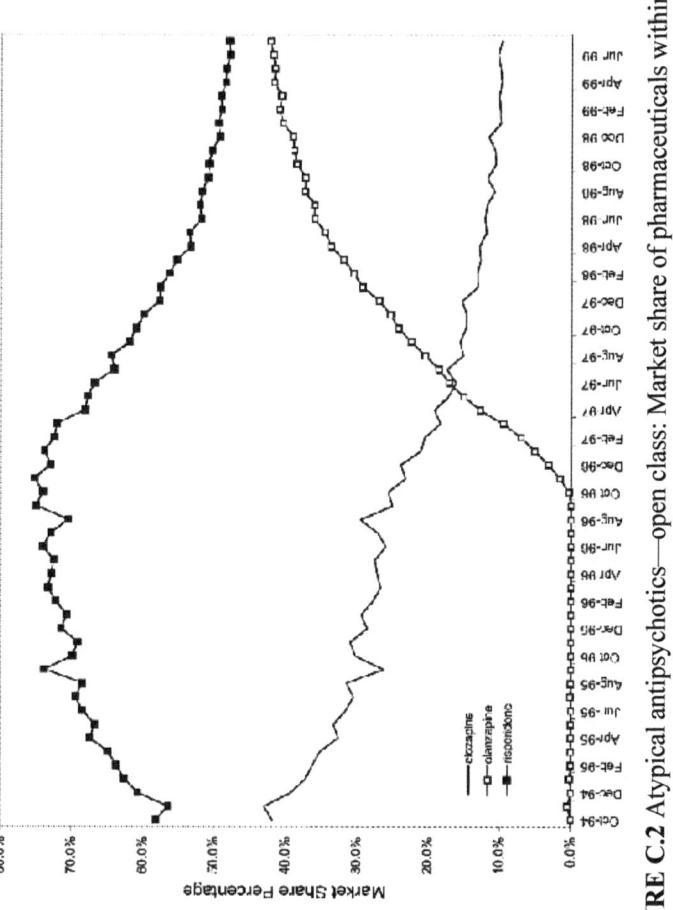

FIGURE C.2 Atypical antipsychotics—open class: Market share of pharmaceuticals within the class.

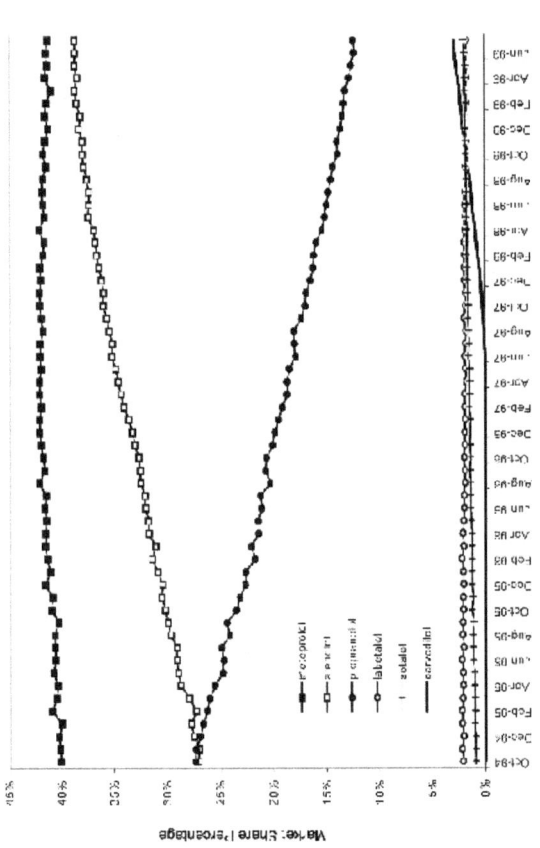

FIGURE C.3 Beta-blockers—open class: Market share of pharmaceuticals within the class. NOTE: Some drug products (timolol, pindolol, nadolol, bisoprol, betaxolol, and acebutolol) had negligible market share and were removed for clarity.

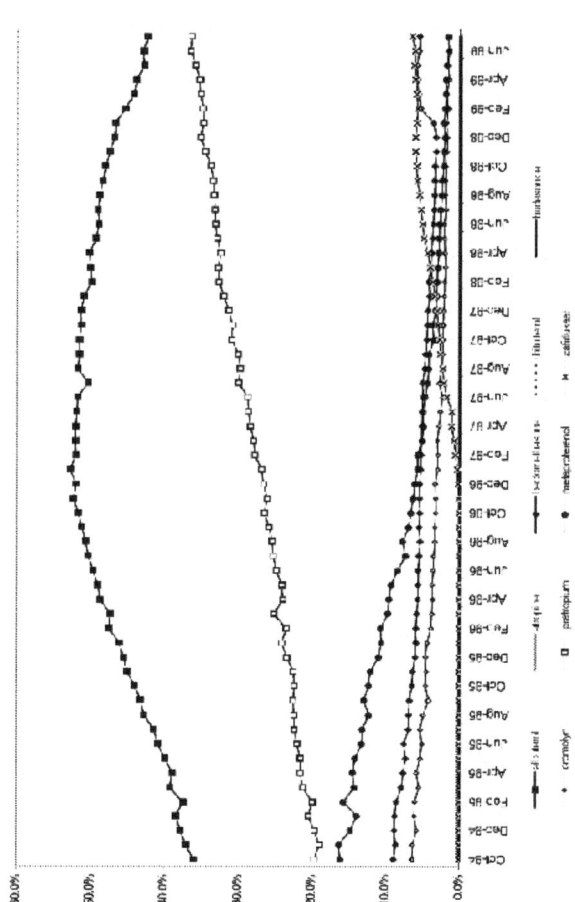

FIGURE C.4 Inhaled antiasthma agents—open class: Market share of pharmaceuticals within the class. NOTE: Some drug products (triamcinolone, salmeterol, pirbuterol, nedocromil, montelukast, fluticasone, mometasone, levalbuterol, isoetharine, flunisolide, and epinephrine) had negligible market share and were removed for clarity.

APPENDIX C   236

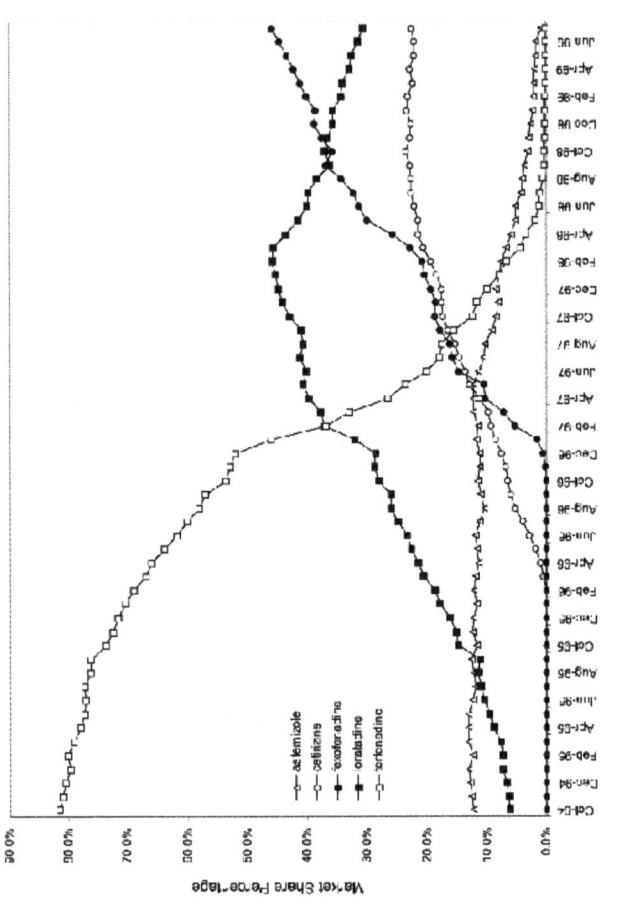

FIGURE C.5 Nonsedating antihistamines—open class: Market share of pharmaceuticals within the class.

APPENDIX C 237

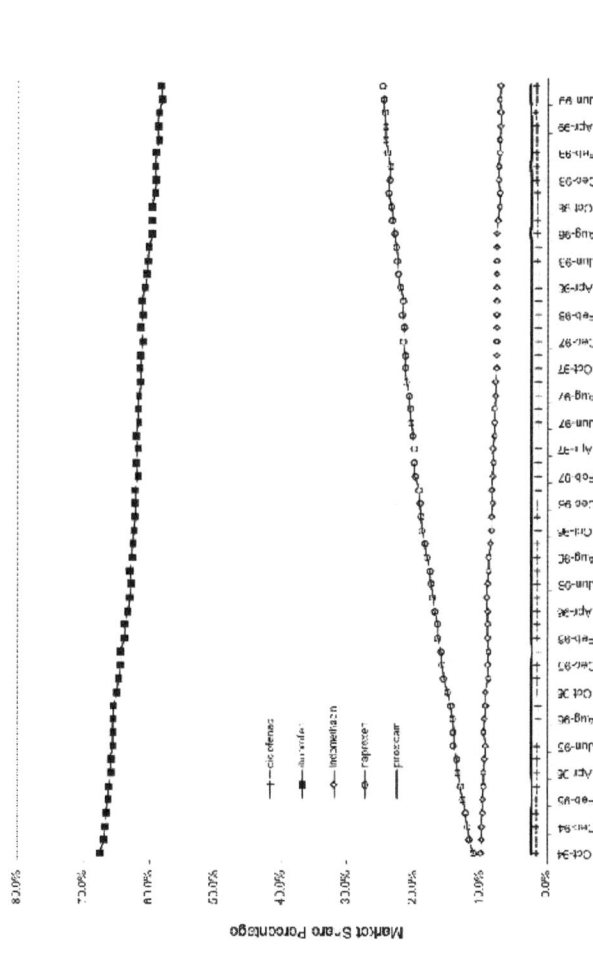

FIGURE C.6 Nonsteroidal anti-inflammatory drugs—open class: Market share of pharmaceuticals within the class. NOTE: Some drug products (tolmetin, phenylbutazone, meclofen, ketoprofen, flurbiprofen, fenoprofen, diflunisal, sulindac, and nabumetone) had negligible market share and were removed for clarity.

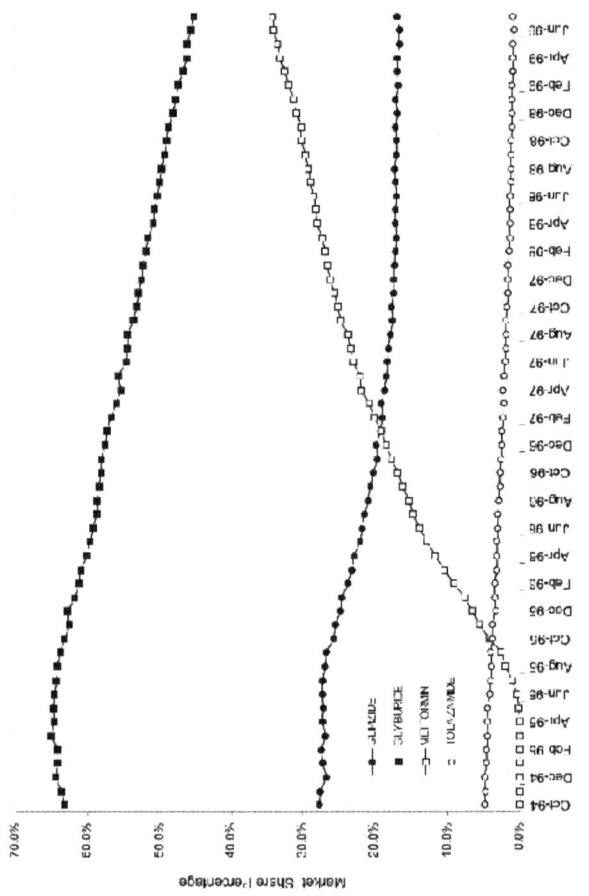

FIGURE C.7 Oral diabetic—open class: Market share of pharmaceuticals within the class. NOTE: Some drug products (dextrose, diazoxide, tolbutamide, acarbose, troglitazone, rosiglitazone, repaglinide, miglitol, chlorpropamide, glucose, glucagon, acetohexamide, and glimepiride) had negligible market share and were removed for clarity.

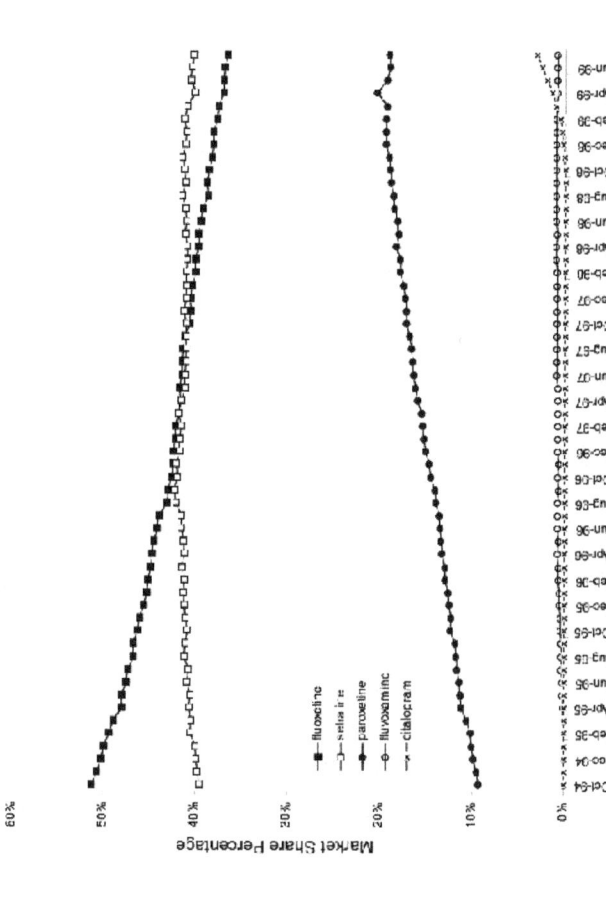

FIGURE C.8 Selective serotonin-reuptake inhibitors—open class: Market share of pharmaceuticals within class.

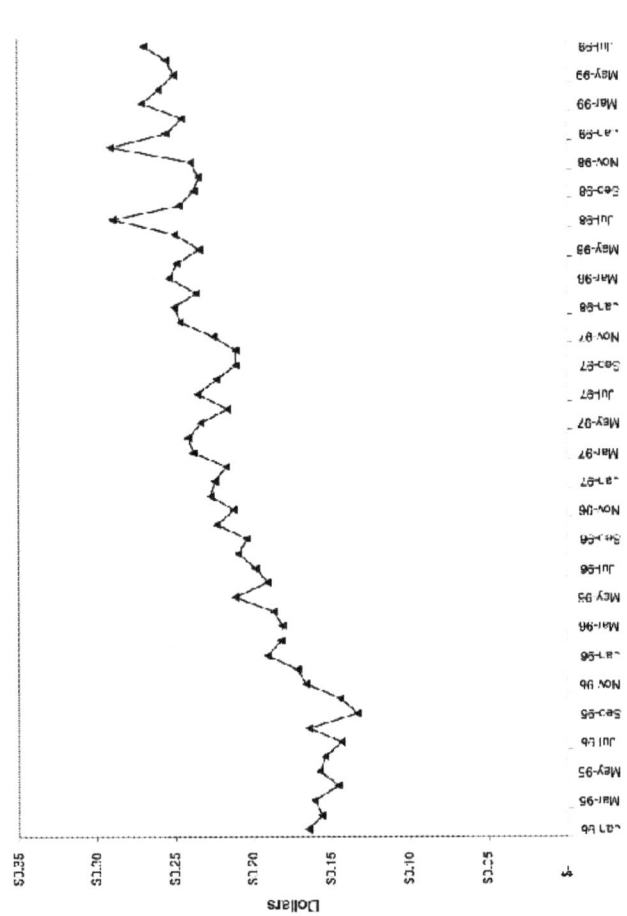

FIGURE C.9 Average outpatient pharmacy spending per outpatient user by month on antiemetics

APPENDIX C 241

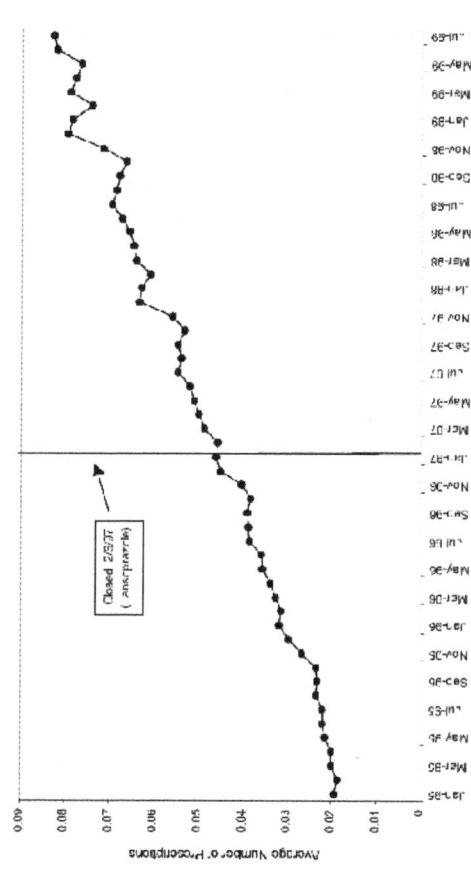

FIGURE C.10 Average number of prescriptions per outpatient user by month for proton pump inhibitors.

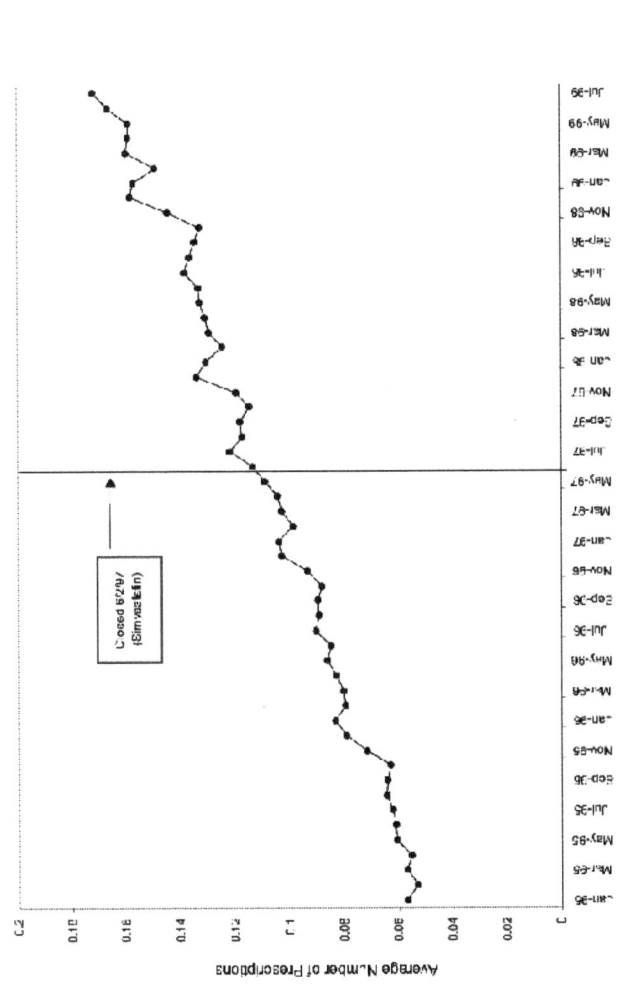

FIGURE C.11 Average number of prescriptions per outpatient user by month for hydroxymethylglutaryl coenzyme A reductase inhibitors.

APPENDIX C

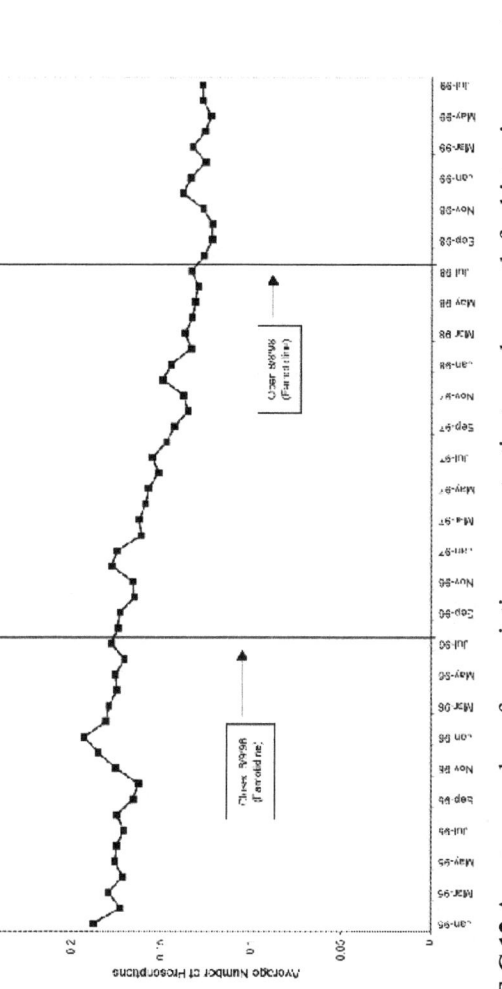

FIGURE C.12 Average number of prescriptions per outpatient user by month for histamine$_2$ receptor blockers.

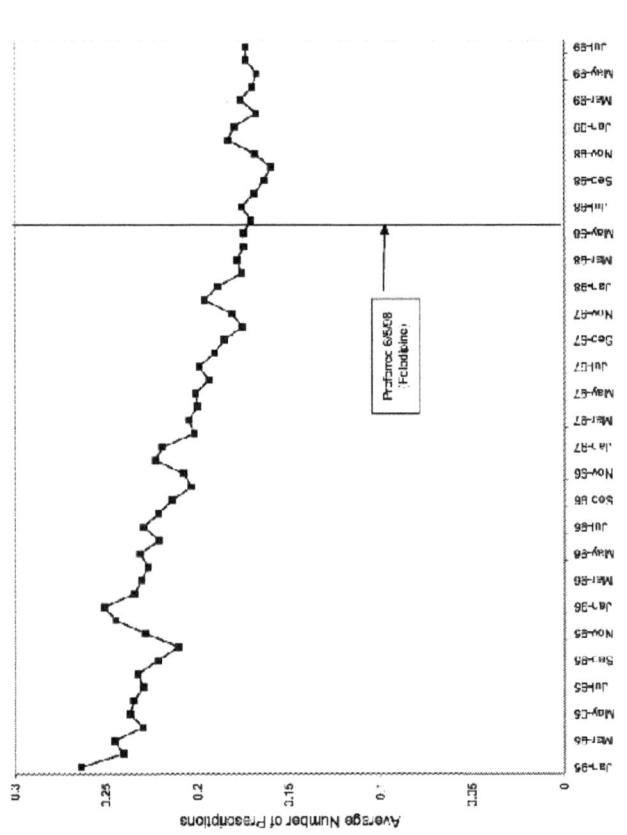

FIGURE C.13 Average number of prescriptions per outpatient user by month for calcium channel blockers (CCBs).

APPENDIX C 245

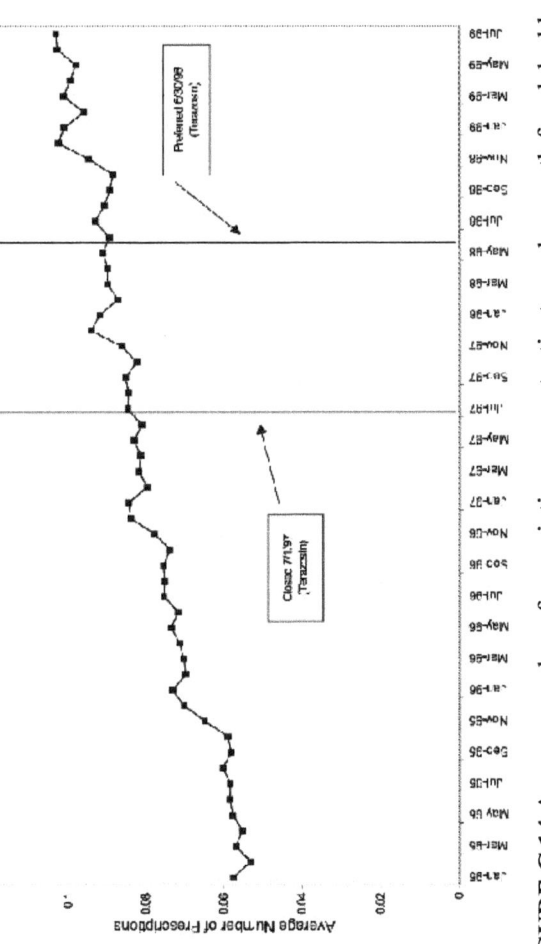

FIGURE C.14 Average number of prescriptions per outpatient user by month for alpha blockers.

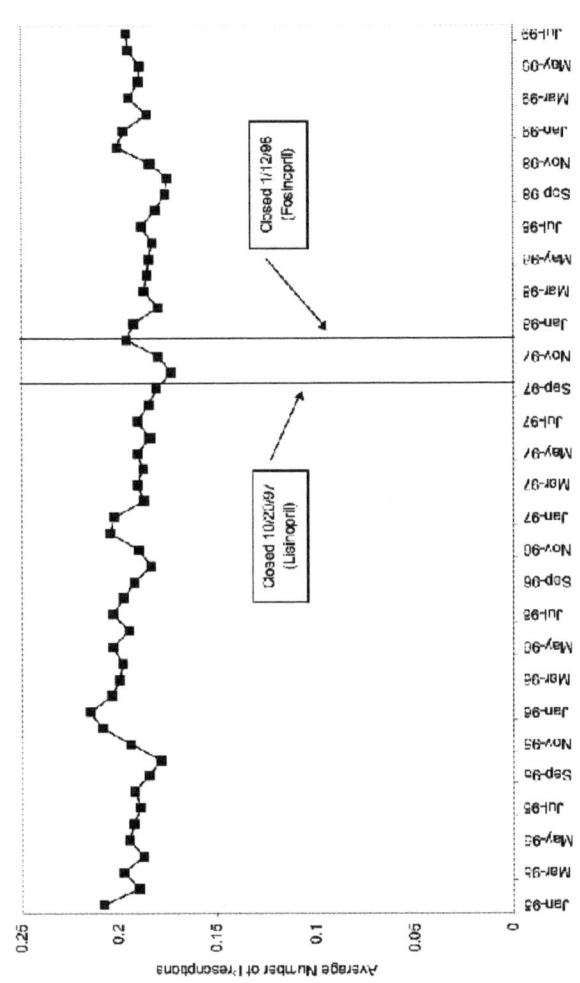

FIGURE C.15 Average number of prescriptions per outpatient user by month for angiotensin converting enzyme inhibitors (ACEI).

APPENDIX C   247

TABLE C.1 Implementation Date of VHA National Contracts Across the VISNs

	HMG CoA RIs lovastatin/simvastatin	LHRHs goserelin	PPIs lansoprazole	ACE inhibitors		H₂R blocker[a] famotidine	Alpha blockers[b] terazosin
				lisinopril	fosinopril		
National	06/02/1997	01/13/1997	02/06/1997	10/20/1997	01/02/1998	8/9/1996–8/8/1998	7/1/1997–6/30/1998
VISN 1	06/02/1997	01/13/1997	02/06/1997	10/20/1997	01/02/1998	8/9/1996–8/8/1998	07/01/1997
VISN 2	06/02/1997	01/13/1997	02/06/1997	10/20/1997	01/02/1998	8/9/1996–8/8/1998	07/01/1997
VISN 3	06/02/1997	01/13/1997	02/06/1997	10/20/1997	01/02/1998	8/9/1996–8/8/1998	07/01/1997
VISN 4	06/02/1997	01/13/1997	02/06/1997	10/20/1997	01/02/1998	8/9/1996–8/8/1998	07/01/1997
VISN 5	06/02/1997	01/13/1997	02/06/1997	10/20/1997	01/02/1998	8/9/1996–8/8/1998	07/01/1997
VISN 6	06/22/1997	01/13/1997	02/06/1997	10/20/1997	01/02/1998	8/9/1996–8/8/1998	07/01/1997
VISN 7	06/02/1997	01/13/1997	02/06/1997	10/20/1997	01/02/1998	8/9/1996–8/8/1998	07/01/1997
VISN 8	07/02/1997	02/13/1997	03/06/1997	11/20/1997	02/02/1998	9/9/1996–9/8/1998	08/01/1997
VISN 9	06/02/1997	01/13/1997	02/06/1997	10/20/1997	01/02/1998	8/9/1996–8/8/1998	07/01/1997
VISN 10	06/02/1997	01/13/1997	02/06/1997	10/20/1997	01/02/1998	08/09/1996	07/01/1997
VISN 11	06/02/1997	01/13/1997	02/06/1997	10/20/1997	01/02/1998	8/9/1996–8/8/1998	07/01/1997
VISN 12	06/02/1997	01/13/1997	02/06/1997	10/20/1997	01/02/1998	8/9/1996–8/8/1998	07/01/1997
VISN 13	06/02/1997	01/13/1997	02/06/1997	10/20/1997	01/02/1998	8/9/1996–8/8/1998	07/01/1997
VISN 14	06/02/1997	01/13/1997	02/06/1997	10/20/1997	01/02/1998	8/9/1996–8/8/1998	07/01/1997
VISN 15	08/28/1997	06/11/1996	06/11/1996	10/20/1997	06/01/1996	01/02/1997	07/11/1997
VISN 16	06/02/1997	01/13/1997	02/06/1997	10/20/1997	01/02/1998	8/9/1996–8/8/1998	07/01/1997
VISN 17	06/02/1997	01/01/1997	01/01/1997	10/01/1997	12/01/1998	08/09/1996	07/01/1997
VISN 18	06/02/1997	01/13/1997	02/06/1997	10/20/1997	01/02/1998	8/9/1996–8/8/1998	07/01/1997
VISN 19	7/1/1997–9/1/1997	3/1/1997–7/1/1997	3/1/1997–4/1/1997	2/1/1997–12/1/1997	2/1/1997–12/1/1997	9/1/1996–12/1/1996	7/1/1997–10/1/1997
VISN 20	06/01/1997	12/01/1996	05/01/1997	10/20/1997	01/02/1998	8/9/1996–8/8/1998	7/1/1997–6/30/1998
VISN 21	06/02/1997	12/23/1996	01/24/1997	09/19/1997	09/19/1997	07/26/1996	08/15/1998
VISN 22	07/02/1997	02/13/1997	03/06/1997	11/20/1997	05/02/1998	9/9/1996–9/8/1998	08/01/1997

[a] H₂R blockers were closed (8/9/1996) and reclassified as open (8/8/1998).
[b] Alpha blockers were closed (7/1/1997) and reclassified as preferred (6/30/1998).

TABLE C.2 Regression Results on Natural Logarithm of Spending per Veteran Outpatient User

Variable	ACEI	Alpha	HMG	PPI	CCB	H_2R
Closed	−0.185 (8.60)	−0.193 (9.10)	−0.085 (5.92)	−0.076 (5.45)		−0.529 (11.26)
Subsequent change in formulary status*	−0.089 (3.93)	−0.195 (4.91)				−0.0605 (7.73)
preferred					0.076 (1.83)	
% Male	−0.007 (1.99)	0.013 (2.69)	0.017 (4.87)	0.041 (12.03)	0.010 (2.20)	0.005 (0.46)
%<45 years	0.0001 (0.06)	0.011 (3.33)	−0.002 (0.85)	0.003 (1.11)	0.004 (1.32)	0.022 (3.13)
% 45–65	0.019 (2.96)	−0.001 (0.14)	−0.005 (0.79)	−0.050 (7.99)	−0.020 (2.38)	0.011 (0.63)
Time	−0.019 (15.27)	−0.046 (24.45)	0.036 (29.43)	0.054 (43.48)	0.010 (6.06)	0.014 (3.15)
$Time^2$	0.0002 (8.55)	−0.0004 (10.86)	−0.0002 (10.56)	−0.003 (21.11)	−0.0002 (8.57)	−0.0004 (5.74)
Constant	1.203 (3.01)	−1.819 (3.39)	−0.642 (1.66)	−1.941 (5.16)	1.362 (2.71)	−0.388 (0.35)
VISN fixed-effects included						
R^2	0.83	0.83	0.92	0.96	0.66	0.66
F	198.43	201.2	507.5	944.3	85.86	80.12

NOTE: ACEI= angiotensin converting enzyme inhibitor; alpha= alpha blocer; CCB= calcium channel blocker; HMG= hydroxymethylglutaryl coenzyme A reductase inhibitor; PPI= proton pump inhibitor; VISN= veteran integrated service network; t statistics in parentheses.

* For ACEIs, this variable represents the addition of a second closed drug, fosinopril, to the National Formulary. For alpha blockers, this variable represents the change in formulary status from closed to preferred. For H2R blockers, this variable represents the reopening of the class.

TABLE C.3 Regression Results on Natural Logarithm of Inpatient Discharge Rates*

Variable	ACEI-Related Discharges	PPI-Related Discharges
Closed	−0.014 (0.89)	−0.051 (1.54)
% Male	0001 (0.26)	0.009 (1.13)
%<45 years	−0.021 (7.76)	−0.125 (2.34)
% 45–65 years	0.011 (1.58)	0.006 (0.44)
Time	−0.081 (10.17)	−0.019 (6.15)
Time^2	−0.00001 (0.85)	0.00004 (0.93)
Constant	−5.74 (13.53)	−6.602 (7.66)
VISN fixed-effects included		
R^2	0.81	0.64
F	183.54	79.00

NOTE: ACEI = angiotensin converting enzyme inhibitor; PPI = proton pump inhibitor, VISN = veteran integrated service network.

* The discharge rate is the number of discharges for the selected diagnoses divided by the number of veteran outpatient users. The unit of observation is a VISN-month.

APPENDIX D

Glossary

Adverse Drug Event (ADE)— An injury caused by medical management rather than by the underlying disease or condition of the patient.

Adverse Drug Reaction (ADR)— Unwanted or unintended effects of a medicine that occur during its proper use.

Average Wholesale Price (AWP)— The standard charge for a pharmacy item, derived by a pricing service from the average charge of a large representation of wholesale suppliers. Actual wholesale prices may differ; discounts are common.

Bioavailability— The extent to which the active ingredient or active moiety is available from a drug product.

Bioequivalent Drug Products— Chemically equivalent drug products that display comparable bioavailability when studied under similar experimental conditions.

Blanket Purchase Agreement— A VISN (or local) agreement with manufacturers on terms of drug purchasing.

Clinical Guidelines or Drug Treatment Guidelines— Systematically developed statements to assist practitioner and patient decisions about appropriate health care for specific clinical circumstances.

Closed Class— A drug class in which the number of members listed on the formulary is limited.

Drug Class—The grouping of drug products based on various criteria, which may include similarity of chemical structure, clinical indications, pharmacology, and therapeutic activity.

Drug Efficacy Study Implementation (DESI) Drugs—A group of drugs of insufficient efficacy based on decisions resulting from a review by the National Academy of Sciences and the Food and Drug Administration (FDA) pursuant to federal law. These drugs are not reimbursable by U.S. government programs.

Drug Utilization Review (DUR; also called drug use evaluation, or medication use evaluation)—A formal performance improvement program for assessing data on drug use against explicit, prospective standards (criteria) and, as necessary, introducing remedial strategies to achieve some desired end.

Federal Supply Schedule (FSS)—A manufacturer-level price catalog with about 23,000 drug products (includes the same drugs in different dosage and package sizes) administered by the National Acquisition Center (NAC) for drug (and other) purchases by federal agencies. The Veterans Health Care Act of 1992 requires "covered" drugs (innovator single- and multiple-source drugs, insulin, and biological products) to be sold through the FSS to the four largest federal agencies (the VA, DOD, PHS, and Coast Guard) with a statutorily required discount amounting to no more than 76% of the nonfederal average manufacturer price. Manufacturers must also list their brand name drugs on the FSS to be eligible for Medicaid coverage. The VA accounts for about 70% of FSS pharmaceutical purchases annually.

Formulary—A continuously revised list of pharmaceuticals that meet pharmacopoeial standards. A list of preferred drugs that are considered by physicians and other professional staff of a health care organization to be the most useful in caring for the patients served by the organization.

- **Open or Unrestricted Formulary**—An open formulary is a very comprehensive listing of medications typically offering almost every commercially available product in each therapeutic category. Physicians who prescribe from an open formulary are not restricted and may prescribe virtually any drug. Payers, including employers, health plans, and third-party administrators, provide coverage for all medications since there are no restrictions.
- **Closed Formulary**—Closed formularies are exclusive lists of specific drugs that often limit prescribers to only some of the commercially available products in each therapeutic class. Drugs that do not appear on the list of approved products (nonformulary drugs) are not covered by the health plan, PBM, or employer, and patients must pay additional out-of-pocket expenses to obtain nonformulary prescriptions (or use a prior approval or nonformulary exceptions process).
- **Partially/Selectively Closed Formulary**—These are formulary hybrids that limit prescribing choices within certain therapeutic classes and offering unlimited choice within other drug classes. Such formularies direct prescribers to preferred agents within therapeutic classes, which may be included

in a treatment protocol or clinical guideline. In some cases, entire categories, such as drugs used solely for cosmetic purposes, may be closed to prevent payment for those drugs that are excluded from coverage. In the VA system, drugs not listed may be available through the nonformulary process, and only very rarely is a drug excluded (that is, not available through the system under any circumstances).

Formulary System— A method whereby the medical staff of an organization, working through a P&T committee or an equivalent group of physician and pharmacy experts, objectively evaluates, appraises, and selects from among numerous available drug entities and drug products those that are considered most useful in patient care—the management of a formulary.

Generic Drug— A nonproprietary drug approved by the FDA that is tested against a standard of bioavailability and bioequivalence.

Generic Substitution— The substitution of drug products that contain the same active, chemically identical ingredient(s) and are identical in strength, concentration, dosage form, and route of administration to the drug product prescribed.

Medical Advisory Panel (MAP)— A committee that is part of the management and medical decision-making structure of the VA PBM. The committee consists of 11 physicians in practice at VA medical centers and 1 DOD physician.

Medicare— A federal program of health insurance for the elderly enacted in 1965 as Title XVIII of the Social Security Act. **Part A** is primarily a hospital benefit to which beneficiaries are automatically entitled. **Part B** is primarily a physician benefit, which requires beneficiaries to enroll and pay a monthly premium.

National Acquisition Center (NAC)— A combined contracting activity within the VA responsible for purchasing drugs and medical supplies for the VA as well as other government agencies and administering the Federal Supply Schedule, National Contract, and Prime Vendor Distribution Programs.

Nonformulary Request— The process by which a drug product not on the formulary is approved for dispensing.

OBRA (Omnibus Budget Reconciliation Act, 1990) Drugs These are drugs that may be excluded from Medicaid formularies: for example, drugs for anorexia; weight loss or gain; fertility; cosmetic purposes or hair growth; symptomatic relief of cough and colds; smoking cessation; prescription vitamins and minerals (except prenatal); nonprescription drugs; covered outpatient drugs that require associated tests purchased from the manufacturer; barbiturates; and benzodiazepines.

Off-Label Prescribing The prescribing of medications for conditions not approved by the FDA.

Open Class	A drug class that contains numerous drug products, all of which are covered.
Over-the-Counter (OTC) Drugs—	Drugs that are available from retail stores without a prescription.
Pharmaceutical and Therapeutics (P&T) Committee	An advisory committee of the medical staff that represents the official, organizational line of communication and liaison between the medical staff and the pharmacy department; its recommendations are subject to medical staff approval.
Pharmacopoeia—	A compendium of drug standards for purity and strength.
Preferred Class—	A drug class listed in a formulary in which specific drugs are named as the "preferred agent" for use.
Prescription Drugs—	Any drugs or biologics that by federal or state law, rule, or regulation require a written prescription to dispense and that are listed as Federal Legend Drugs, State Restricted Drugs, or compendial medications.
Prior Approval or Authorization—	A cost-containment procedure that requires a prescriber to obtain permission to use medications prior to prescribing.
Step Protocol—	A treatment protocol that recommends beginning a trial of drug therapy for a medical condition with one drug or class of drugs (often of lower cost or risk) before proceeding to other drugs or drug classes.
Therapeutic Alternates—	Drug products differing in composition or in their basic drug entity, but of the same pharmacological and/or therapeutic class, that are considered to have very similar pharmacological and therapeutic activities and adverse reaction profiles when administered to patients in therapeutically equivalent doses.
Therapeutic Equivalence—	Similar pharmacological and therapeutic activity of drugs.
Therapeutic Interchange—	Authorized exchange of various therapeutic alternates by pharmacists under arrangement between pharmacists and authorized prescribers who have previously established written guidelines or protocols within a formulary system and jointly agreed on conditions for interchange or who give permission individually at the time of exchange.
Veterans Integrated Service Network (VISN)—	One of 22 regional health systems created under the VA reorganization of 1994–1995. This reflected a shift of funding from facilities to population and a shift of emphasis from hospital to ambulatory and community-based settings. Over time, these VISNs have evolved to become analogous to a managed care organization.

APPENDIX E
Drug Classes and Drug Index

There are several hundred classifications of drugs using various systems such as the American Hospital Formulary System. Although, many drugs fit into more than one category, they are commonly classified by therapeutic indication (for example, cardiovascular drugs for use in treating conditions such as hypertension, congestive heart failure, and cardiac arrhythmias). Classification of drugs and drug classes is a complicated subjected. The interested reader is referred to *The Physicians' Desk Reference, Drug Facts and Comparisons, American Hospital Formulary System,* or *Drug Information for the Health Care Professional.* Information can also be found on-line at www.ditonline.com, and www.intelihealth.com. For brevity and clarity, the committee has included in this index only the listing and definitions of drug classes and class members cited in this report.

DRUG CLASSES

Angiotensin-Converting Enzyme Inhibitors (ACEI)—Drugs for the treatment of high blood pressure that inhibit an enzyme, angiotensin-converting enzyme, which produces a blood-pressure-elevating substance.

- Captopril, a generic ACE inhibitor
- Enalapril, brand name Vasotec (Merck)
- Fosinopril, brand name Monopril (Bristol Myers Squibb)
- Lisinopril, brand name Prinivil (Merck) and Zestril (Zeneca)
- Quinapril, brand name Accupril (Parke-Davis)

- Ramipril, brand name Altace (Hoechst Marion Roussel)
- Trandolapril, brand name Mavik (Knoll Pharmaceuticals)

Alpha Blockers—Drugs that block receptors in arteries and smooth muscle. This action relaxes the blood vessels and leads to an increase in blood flow and a lower pressure for the control of hypertension. The action in the urinary tract enhances urinary flow in prostatic hypertrophy.

- Doxazosin, brand name Cardura (Pfizer)
- Prazosin, brand name Minipress (Pfizer)
- Terazosin, brand name Hytrin (Abbott)

Analgesic Drug—A drug for the control of pain.

Angiotensin II Receptor Blockers— Drugs for the treatment of high blood pressure that act to block the receptor for Angiotensin II, a blood-pressure-elevating substance.

- Losartan, brand names Hyzaar (Merck) and Cozaar (Merck)
- Irbesartan, brand name Avapro (Bristol Myers Squibb and Sanofi)

Antipyretic Drug—A drug for the control of fever.

Calcium Channel Blockers (CCBs)— Drugs that inhibit the movement of calcium through cellular membranes and cause blood vessels to relax thereby increasing flow and lowering blood pressure.

- Amlodipine, brand names Lotrel (Novartis) and Norvasc (Pfizer)
- Diltiazem, a generic CCB
- Felodipine, brand names Lexxel and Plendil, extended release (Astra)

Cyclooxygenase-2 (COX-2) Inhibitors—Drugs for the treatment of pain, arthritis, and primary dysmenorrhea that inhibit prostaglandin synthesis by inhibiting the enzyme cyclooxygenase-2.

- Celecoxib, brand name Celebrex (Pfizer)
- Refecoxib, brand name Vioxx (Merck)

Histamine $_2$ Receptor ($H_2 R$) Blockers— Drugs for ulcers and acid reflux that diminish acid by blocking a receptor in the acid-producing system in the stomach.

- Cimetidine, brand name Tagamet (SmithKline Beecham), also OTC
- Famotidine, brand name Pepcid (Merck), also OTC
- Nizatidine, brand name Axid (Eli Lilly)
- Ranitidine, brand name Zantac (Glaxo Wellcome), also OTC

Hydroxymethylglutaryl Coenzyme A Reductase Inhibitors (HMG CoA RIs) —Drugs that inhibit a liver enzyme involved in the synthesis of cholesterol, thus reducing cholesterol levels and the risk of cardiovascular disease.

- Atorvastatin, brand name Lipitor (Parke-Davis, Pfizer)
- Cerivastatin, brand name Baycol (Bayer)
- Fluvastatin, brand name Lescol (Novartis)
- Lovastatin, brand name Mevacor (Merck)
- Pravastatin, brand name Pravachol (Bristol Myers Squibb)
- Simvastatin, brand name Zocor (Merck)

Luteinizing Hormone-Releasing Hormone (LHRH) Analogues—Drugs that suppress endogenous sex hormone production and are used to treat prostate cancer.

- Leuprolide, brand name Lupron (TAP)
- Goserelin, brand name Zoladex (Zeneca)

Nonsteroidal Anti-Inflammatory Drug (NSAID)—An analgesic and anti-inflammatory drug that is not a corticosteroid analogue.

- Diflunisal, brand name Dolobid (Merck)
- Ketorolac tromethamine, brand name Toradol (Roche Laboratories)

Prokinetic Agents—Drugs used in the treatment of gastroesophageal reflux and delayed gastric emptying.

Proton Pump Inhibitors (PPIs)—Drugs for the treatment of ulcers and acid reflux disease that inhibit the enzyme system that produces stomach acid.

- Lansoprazole, brand name Prevacid (TAP)
- Omeprazole, brand name Prilosec (Astra)

Selective Serotonin Reuptake Inhibitors (SSRIs)—Drugs that selectively block the uptake of the neurotransmitter serotonin and are used in the treatment of depression and certain other mental health disorders.

- Citalopram, brand name Celexa (Forest Pharmaceuticals)
- Fluoxetine, brand name Prozac (Dista)
- Fluvoxamine, brand name Luvox (Solvay)
- Paroxetine, brand name Paxil (SmithKline Beecham)
- Sertraline, brand name Zoloft (Pfizer)

OTHER DRUGS

Aldesleukin Interleukin-2—Drug for the treatment of adults with metastatic renal cell carcinoma, brand name Proleukin (Chiron Corp).

Alendronate Sodium—Drug used for the prevention and treatment of osteoporosis in postmenopausal women, brand name Fosamax (Merck).

Alglucerase—Modified form of the enzyme Beta-glucocerebrosidase used in the treatment of patients with type I Gaucher's disease, brand name Ceredase (Genzyme).

Alprostadil— A drug that has vasodilatory effects and is used in the treatment of erectile dysfunction, brand name Caverject (Pharmacia and Upjohn).

Bupropion—A member of the drug class aminoketones used for the treatment of depression. The mechanism of action is unknown but may be related to preventing the reuptake of neurotransmitters, brand name Welbutrin (Glaxo Wellcome).

Clopidogrel— A drug that, like aspirin, inhibits cells involved in blood clotting and decreases heart attacks and strokes, brand name Plavix (Bristol Meyers Squib, Sanofi).

Clozapine— An atypical antipsychotic used for the treatment of schizophrenia, brand name Clozaril (Novartis).

Donepezil Hydrochloride—A drug that inhibits acetylcholinesterase and is used for the treatment of Alzheimer's disease, brand name Aricept (Eisai).

Epoetin Alpha—A drug that stimulates red blood cell production and is used in the treatment of patients with chronic renal failure, brand names Epogen (Amgen) and Procrit (Ortho Biotech).

Etanercept— A drug that blocks tumor necrosis factor from binding to its receptor, thus preventing normal inflammatory and immune responses. It is currently used in the treatment of rheumatoid arthritis, brand name Enbrel (Immunex).

Filgrastim Granulocyte Colony Stimulating Factor (G-CSF)— A drug used to stimulate blood production of white cells and decrease the incidence of infection in cancer patients, brand name Neupogen (Amgen).

Finasteride— A drug used in the treatment of symptomatic benign prostatic hyperplasia in men with an enlarged prostate, brand name Proscar (Merck).

Fluconazole—drug for the treatment of fungal infections, brand name Diflucan (Pfizer).

Fluticasone Propionate—A synthetic corticosteroid for the treatment of allergic rhinitis, brand name Flonase (Glaxo Wellcome).

Imiglucerase—A recombinant DNA form of the enzyme beta-glucocerebrosidase (alglucerase) used in the treatment of patients with type I Gaucher's disease, brand name Cerezyme (Genzyme).

Interferon Beta-1—Drug used in the treatment of ambulatory patients with multiple sclerosis to reduce the frequency of clinical exacerbations, brand name Betaseron (Berlex).

Isotretinoin—A drug that inhibits sebaceous gland function and is used in the treatment of severe acne, brand name Accutane (Roche Laboratories).

Itraconazole—A drug used in the treatment of fungal infections, brand name Sporanox (Janssen).

APPENDIX E

Rizatriptan Benzoate—A selective serotonin agonist used in the treatment of migraines, brand name Maxalt (Merck).

Sumatriptan—A selective serotonin agonist used in the treatment of migraines, brand name Imitrex (Glaxo Wellcome).

Tacrine Hydrochloride—A drug that is a reversible inhibitor of cholinesterase and is used in the treatment of Alzheimer's disease, brand name Cognex (Parke-Davis).

Terbinafine—A drug for the treatment of fungal infections, brand name Lamisil (Novartis).

Troglitazone—A drug that lowers blood glucose by improving target cell response to insulin and was used (recalled by FDA) in the treatment of type II diabetes, brand name Rezulin (Parke-Davis).

Zolmitriptan— A selective serotonin agonist used in the treatment of migraines, brand name Zomig (Zeneca).

Committee Biographies

DAVID BLUMENTHAL, M.D., M.P.P., is director of the Institute for Health Policy and a physician at the Massachusetts General Hospital/Partners Health Care System in Boston. He is also professor of medicine and professor of health care policy at Harvard Medical School. He is a member of the Institute of Medicine and serves on several journal editorial boards. He is currently executive director for the Commonwealth Fund Task Force on the Future of Academic Health Centers and chairman of the Board of the Massachusetts Peer Review Organization.

R. HENRY BODENBENDER, M.D., is the director of medical services for the Paralyzed Veterans of America. He previously served as acting deputy commander for personnel management at the Naval Medical Command in Washington, D.C., until his retirement from active duty as a captain in the Navy Medical Corps in 1988. He is a board-certified pediatrician. His military awards include the Meritorious Service Medal with Gold Star and the Legion of Merit.

J. LYLE BOOTMAN, Ph.D., is dean and professor of the University of Arizona College of Pharmacy. He is the founding and executive director of the University of Arizona Center for Health Outcomes and PharmacoEconomic (HOPE) Research. Dr. Bootman has authored over 200 research articles and monographs and has been an invited speaker at more than 300 professional healthcare meetings and symposia throughout the world. He is a member of the

Institute of Medicine and currently serves as president of the American Pharmaceutical Association.

JOHN P. BURKE, M.D., is director of the Department of Clinical Epidemiology, LDS Hospital/Intermountain Health Care and professor of medicine at the University of Utah, where he holds the Ann G. and Jack Mark Presidential Endowed Chair in Medicine. Dr. Burke's primary research interests are in the epidemiology and prevention of adverse clinical outcomes using computer-assisted decision support systems. He is an elected member of the American Epidemiological Society and a Fellow of both the American College of Physicians and the Infectious Diseases Society of America.

ELIZABETH DICHTER, M.P.H., is head of strategic marketing at PCS, where she is responsible for creating market opportunities. During her 9 years at PCS, the organization became the leader in managed pharmaceuticals and grew from 15 million to 55 million members. Ms. Dichter spent over 15 years in health policy at both the federal and state levels at the Department of Health and Human Services in Washington, D.C., and in the states of Colorado and Ohio. She has served as advisor to health information and research organizations such as Health Data Institute, Codman Research Group, Knowledge Data Systems, and the Association for Health Services Research.

THOMAS R. FULDA, M.A., is program director for Drug Utilization Review at the U.S. Pharmacopoeia, Division of Drug Information Development. He is responsible for the Pharmacopoeia's development of pharmaceutical therapy choice criteria and evidence-based drug-specific criteria for use in prospective DUR, disease management environments. He is also responsible for the development of a disease-specific, annotated, and evaluated bibliography of outcomes and pharmacoeconomic literature. Before joining US Pharmacopoeia, Mr. Fulda was employed by the Health Care Financing Administration, where he received the Department of Health and Human Services Secretary's Special Achievement Award

MARTHA N. HILL, R.N., Ph.D., is a professor and director of the Center for Nursing Research at the Johns Hopkins University School of Nursing. She holds joint appointments in the School of Hygiene and Public Health and the School of Medicine at Johns Hopkins. Dr. Hill was the 1997–1998 president of the American Heart Association; she also serves on numerous review panels, editorial boards, and advisory committees including the Coordinating Committee of the National High Blood Pressure Education Program, the board of directors of the International Society of Hypertension in Blacks, and the American Society of Hypertension.

JOHN D. JONES, J.D., is director of Pharmacy Networks, Public, and Legal Affairs at Prescription Solutions, a pharmacy benefit management company owned by PacifiCare Health Systems. He has been involved in managed care pharmacy practice for 9 years and has been a pharmacist for 24 years. He is also licensed as an attorney in California, where he has applied his legal knowledge in the fields of managed healthcare regulation, pharmacy health insurance, health care contracting and interstate regulatory compliance. Mr. Jones is president for the Academy of Managed Care Pharmacy. He currently sits on the California State Board of Pharmacy.

JAMES J. LIPSKY, M.D., is director of clinical pharmacology and professor of medicine and pharmacology at the Mayo Clinic in Rochester, Minnesota. His research involves many aspects of clinical pharmacology, including studies of the mechanism of drug action and toxicity, phamacokinetics, and clinical trials. He serves on the American Board of Clinical Pharmacology and is also a member of the Board of Directors of the American Society for Clinical Pharmacology and Therapeutics. He is a board-certified internist and is a Fellow of the American College of Physicians. He serves on the Minnesota Drug Utilization Review Board and on the Antiviral Drugs Advisory Committee of the Food and Drug Administration

ALBERT L. SIU, M.D., is the Clifford L. Spingarn, M.D., Professor of Medicine at the Mount Sinai School of Medicine. He is currently chief of the Division of General Internal Medicine in the Samuel Bronfman Department of Medicine and director of Adult Primary Care (with responsibilities for coordinating the activities of Mount Sinai's Internal Medicine Associates, Coffey Geriatrics Associates, and the Medicine/Pediatrics Associates). He is also a senior associate editor of *Health Services Research,* a trustee of the Nathan Cummings Foundation, and a member of National Committee for Quality Assurance's Measurement Advisory Panel on geriatrics.

FRANK A. SLOAN, Ph.D., has been the J. Alexander McMahon Professor of Health Policy and Management and professor of Economics at Duke University since 1993. He is also director of the Center for Health Policy, Law, and Management at Duke, which was founded in 1998. Previously, he was chair of the Department of Economics at Vanderbilt from 1986 to 1989. His current research interests include alcohol use prevention, long-term care, medical malpractice, and cost-effectiveness analyses of medical technologies. Dr. Sloan also has a long-standing interest in hospitals, health care financing, and health manpower. He is a member of the Institute of Medicine and was recently a member of the Physician Payment Review Commission.

RICHARD A. WANNEMACHER, JR., a combat-disabled Vietnam veteran, is the associate national legislative director of the Disabled American Veterans (DAV). As a member of the DAV's legislative team, he works to promote reasonable and responsible legislation to assist disabled veterans and their families, as well as guarding current veteran's benefits and services from legislative erosion. Mr. Wannemacher earned an associate's degree in business administration from Erie Community College and a bachelor's degree in environmental studies from Buffalo State College. He has been with the DAV in various capacities since 1978.

OTTO F. WOLKE is currently president and chief executive officer of Schellen and Partners, USA, Inc., a healthcare consulting company. He was formerly vice president of pharmacy for Penn State Geisinger Health Plan, in Danville, Pennsylvania. In this capacity, he served on the Penn State Geisinger System therapeutics team and provided managed care insights, including on formulary selection, contracting, and utilization management. He currently serves on the Commonwealth of Pennsylvania Medicaid Drug Utilization Review Board, the Technical Advisory Committee for the State of Pennsylvania Pharmaceutical Assistance to the Elderly (PACE) program, and several pharmaceutical company advisory boards.

ALLAN ZIMMERMAN is currently senior executive vice president and general manager of National Prescription Administrators, Inc. (NPA), a privately held, independent pharmacy benefit management company serving over 7 million members nationally. He directs the marketing, industry relations, professional services, professional relations, vision service, information systems and data administration departments at NPA. He has written numerous articles on managed care pharmacy. He served as president of both the Academy of Managed Care Pharmacy and the Foundation for Managed Care Pharmacy.